Amalgam Illness
diagnosis and treatment

Copyright © 1999 Andrew Hall Cutler
(425) 557-8299 voice (425) 557-2104 fax
3006 230th Lane SE #X103
Sammamish, WA 98075-8230
AndyCutler@aol.com

First edition, ISBN 0-9676168-0-8

Available from the author for $35 in US funds payable by a US
bank or otherwise readily negotiable in the US.
Customary distributor terms available to retailers.

Disclaimer:

I have written this book to provide information on a controversial subject - chronic mercury poisoning from dental amalgam and other sources.

The purpose of this book is to educate any interested reader. This book as complete and as accurate as I could make it. The author assumes no liability for errors or omissions. Much of this book is a statement of opinion in areas where the facts are controversial or do not exist.

I do not advocate the use of any particular form of health care. I am not offering a diagnosis or suggesting treatment for any specific individual. This book is not a substitute for medical counseling and is not intended as such. Each person's own particular situation is unique.

The author assumes no liability or responsibility for any loss, damage, or injury caused or alleged to be caused directly or indirectly by the information contained in this book or information omitted from it. This book is sold with the understanding that the author is not liable for misunderstanding, misinterpretation, misuse or misapplication of the information in it. There is always some risk involved in health care. Please do not use this book unless you are willing to assume that risk.

Acknowledgements

The extensive comments and contributions of Amy L. Riskedahl, OD, have been invaluable in bringing this book to its present form. Idelle Port's also provided a helpful review. Extensive technical discussions with Alise Dobrot and Patti Belsky were very helpful, informative and motivating. Some exceptionally helpful people will be acknowledged in spirit only as they want it that way.

Preface

Both traditional and alternative physicians wait for something to go so wrong it overwhelms you. The doctor then listens to your worst symptom or two, maybe pokes a few places to see how high you jump, and sends you for a lab test to confirm that he did indeed guess right about what you have. Then he looks in his "cookbook" for the "recipe" to "fix" you. Mainstream doctors prescribe surgery or drugs, alternative doctors prescribe vitamins or herbs. But the basic philosophy is the same - use a repair manual to fix things that went wrong. Don't try to understand what is going on. Don't consider the underlying biochemistry. Don't try to catch things before they break. Don't try anything that isn't in the repair manual. This is today's medical paradigm.

This paradigm led to the current mercury catastrophe. Any analytical thinker would have read the mercury literature and realized that millions of people are being poisoned by mercury compounds the medical profession is exposing them to. But this isn't in most repair manuals, so health care providers think of it as controversial. Their repair manuals tell them to avoid controversy, so they won't explore the issue - even going so far as to insist sick people in front of them are well rather than disobey their repair manual and consider a controversial diagnosis like mercury poisoning from amalgam.

The mercury catastrophe shows that is time for a paradigm shift away from thoughtless adherence to the "repair manual" approach. It is time to include an understanding of basic biochemistry and scientific problem solving in the practice of medicine.

With a doctorate in chemistry[1], a bachelor's in physics[2], experience in both basic research and practical problem solving in chemistry and engineering[3], and extensive self study in biochemistry and medicine I hope I can follow the new paradigm. This new paradigm consists of viewing the human body as a system where biochemistry leads to metabolism which in turn becomes physiology. The new paradigm is to see disease as a slow progression from health to death rather than the sudden onset of a "disease" once a certain number of symptoms occur. The new paradigm doesn't seek to replace either mainstream or alternative medicine, but simply to enhance and extent them in areas where the cookbook doesn't contain the right recipes yet. Chronic mercury poisoning is such an area.

---

[1] Princeton, 1985.
[2] University of California, 1978.
[3] Registered professional engineer, California and Colorado, 1995.

Contents

List of figures

List of tables

Introduction

Where to start if you think you have amalgam illness

You will have to:

1) Start taking appropriate nutritional supplements and medication (which is likely to help regardless of what you have)
2) Decide how to tell if you have amalgam illness
3) Find a dentist who will safely replace your fillings
4) Find some doctors who will help you
5) Get ready for a year or so of getting well
6) Avoid getting hurt by bad choices early on

All of these are covered in this book.

1) Read the first subsection on what to do right now in the treatment section, and read item number two in the protocol.

2) Read the symptom description. Did that convince you? If not, read the practical procedure for diagnosis. Do the checklists. Read the history and physical examination part. Did that convince you? If not, find a doctor who is open minded and will help both of you decide. Don't find one who has already decided you don't have it. Use whatever kind of doctor you are comfortable with - it doesn't have to be a regular allopathic MD type if you don't want.

3) Start asking around to find a mercury free dentist. Call DAMS and ask for a local chapter leader (800-311-6265 or NatlDAMS@aol.com). Talk to doctors, chiropractors, acupuncturists etc. who deal with this kind of thing. Then talk to the dentists as described later or in other books on the subject. Decide who makes sense to you.

4) Ask around among friends, family, DAMS members, mercury free dentists, etc. to find some doctors who might help you. Call them and talk to them. They should be willing to do this for free, or to let you fax or mail a brief note over to which they respond. Ask them what they think of amalgam illness and whether they want to help you with it. See what they say. Go to see them if you are comfortable with their answer. The basic thing you will want out of them if you get your fillings replaced is prescriptions for chelating agents plus testing and assistance to keep you reasonably well while you go through detoxification and get rid of your mercury. If you are not yet sure you have amalgam illness, you may want them to start by helping you decide.

5) It takes a while to get better. Even if you do everything perfectly. Be realistic. Prepare yourself, your plans, your job and your finances for a rough year or two. Tell your friends and family it is going to be a rough time and you will need their help. Count on the ones who indicate they understand and act like they want to help. Don't fool yourself into depending on people because they are "supposed" to help. Depend on the ones who are WILLING to help, regardless of who is supposed to.

6) There are some people in the medical profession who wrongly believe they know how to treat amalgam illness. They can hurt you very badly, or kill you, by doing the wrong thing. Some "trendy" treatments have gotten talked up and a lot of physicians hear about them, try them, and don't realize they are dangerous until someone gets hurt. Don't let it be you. Dangerous things you should never do: a "DMPS challenge test." A "DMSA challenge test" other than under strict safety guidelines such as those described later. Therapy using DMPS injections except under the extremely limited circumstances described later in the few days after fillings are out. Therapy using DMSA capsules administered every other day, or every

1

week, or on some schedule where you don't take small amounts frequently. A therapeutic dietary or supplement program where you take a lot of cysteine, or glutathione, or eat large amounts of foods like onions and broccoli and garlic. Physicians who insist on doing this kind of thing can't help you - you will have to go elsewhere. Physicians who have administered such therapy but are open minded enough to learn more appropriate therapeutic approaches may be quite helpful.

How to use this book

If you are a patient, this book presents a wealth of information on mercury poisoning, how to tell if you have it, what to do about it, how to get help, and how to deal with physicians. Much of this information is covered several times at different levels of technical depth so that you can find the one that best suits your knowledge and needs. The book is quite straightforward and factual. It is not an attempt to convince you this disease exists, or to convince you that you indeed have it. I present the information and let you make the decision. The book is simply a tool for you to use in trying to sort out an intractable health problem you or someone close to you may have. It covers amalgam illness and related topics. Since it addresses symptoms and their causes it may be useful even if mercury poisoning isn't the root of your problem - but in that case you are well advised not to stop seeking knowledgeable medical help just because you have brought your symptoms under control for a while.

The parts that sound like they are addressed to doctors are for patients too. If the doctor isn't doing what those parts say, you need to find a real doctor who wants to make you well, not somebody who goes through the motions in order to collect a hefty fee for not solving hard problems.

If you are a physician, this book contains the information you need to relate to the mercury toxic patient, confirm or exclude the diagnosis, understand the physiological effects of this toxin on your patient, and

select a suitable therapeutic approach that will cure him in a reasonable period of time without excessive side effects or undue risk. Much information is also presented on how to control symptoms since even a 'rapid' cure may take 6 months to a year. Much of the book is written in layman's language. Detailed technical information such as that found in textbooks of internal medicine or endocrinology is omitted if it would not be useful and clear to at least some nonphysician readers.

The chapters are intended to stand alone. This book need not be read cover to cover or in any particular order. Figures and tables have been included to rapidly convey how the different symptoms are interrelated through the disease process, and how different medicines and nutritional supplements can be used therapeutically.

I list a lot of medicines, nutritional supplements, and other measures. This is NOT meant to imply the patient should try them all or the physician should prescribe them all! This book has somewhat the nature of a laundry list - everything is here. Thus there will be SOMETHING that each individual patient's metabolism tolerates, and SOMETHING that each physician is familiar and comfortable with on the list. Start with the familiar, comfortable stuff. When you find something that works, stick with it.

There are many potential sources of mercury poisoning, and there are many similar conditions (like lead or arsenic poisoning). I have mentioned these at appropriate points throughout the text. Much of the material on how to determine the physiological basis of symptoms and how to ameliorate them doesn't really depend on what is causing them. It can be used regardless of whether mercury is the culprit. Much of the detoxification chemistry works for other heavy metals, and this is discussed in adequate detail to permit therapy to be adapted to other related toxins. If mercury from some source other than amalgam is the problem, it can be detoxed pretty much the same way amalgam is detoxed. In that case I would strongly recommend removing any amalgams because they will contribute in an unknown and uncontrollable manner to re-poisoning someone already sensitized to the effects of mercury.

This book discusses methods to diagnose and treat some of the physiological and metabolic dysfunctions which are a part of chronic fatigue, fibromyalgia, and environmental illness arising from other sources, or of unclear origin. Thus some of the information herein will be helpful to people who got these diseases from some cause other than mercury.

What is in this book

This book discusses the reasons to believe chronic mercury poisoning is common, and its physiology, effects, diagnosis, and treatment. The most common cause of chronic mercury poisoning today is dental amalgam. Mercury poisoning is an unrecognized root cause of chronic fatigue, environmental illness, multiple chemical sensitivities, intractable allergies, developmental disabilities, mental illness and many other conditions. Some of the information in this book may also be helpful in diagnosing or treating these conditions if there is some other root cause.

Since amalgam illness and other mercury poisoning syndromes are so politicized, there is little good research on them and decreasing ability to get it done today. I have had to rely on the best information available. Some of this information is not very good. Some is highly reliable. It is not all that clear which is which. Thus I have given you my best opinion of what is true.

Much of the information in this book could have been written in either layman's terms or medical jargon. I have tried to use everyday terms when possible. Thus "low thyroid" instead of "hypothyroid," "poisoned" instead of "intoxicated," etc. The more technical sections use more fancy medical words. Sometimes a medical word has to be used, and I have explained it where that is important.

I have included an appendix of a few books I found particularly helpful and clear, as well as providing information on other literature I cite. I have used the convention of giving the author's name in the text, and having the papers alphabetized by author's last name in the references. Paper titles are also included so you can use the references cited section as a bibliography if you wish. Most of the journal articles will only be available in major academic libraries. Some of the popular books are more likely to be found in public libraries.

I am a chemist and chemical engineer who has done lots of research and written chemistry journal articles. This has had quite an influence on how I think about things. This book is the kind of book you'd expect a chemist to write - one that is mechanistic, interrelated, and views the body as a complex chemical factory to be measured and controlled by adding a bit of the right reagent over here, taking something out over there, and sprinkling on "magic pixie dust" where needed. This isn't necessarily the best way to understand the body or explain what I have to say. It is just the way I knew how to say it.

My omission of certain treatments or treatment modalities is not intended to disparage them. I have written the book that my knowledge and experience leads me to write. Thus it is pretty "allopathic" and mechanistic in approach. Much of the omission is of chiropractic, oriental medicine, homeopathy and acupuncture. My best understanding is that these are effective in ameliorating the symptoms of mercury intoxication, but not so effective for detox. As with standard allopathic medicine, some practitioners of any technique are very talented and knowledgeable and can quickly help people, while others may take more time and generate more expense to do so.

There are a couple of places to look for some quick information on those areas I don't understand but which help a lot of people. Van Benschoten has described the use of chinese herbal medicines and acupuncture diagnosis to treat amalgam illness. Ellen Cutler has described the alternative allergy control technique NAET which many have found useful during treatment of amalgam illness.

This book is NOT the last word. There are few certainties. Among those certainties are:

• many people have unrecognized chronic mercury poisoning at the root of their (physical or mental) health problems;

• these health problems can be cured by treating the mercury toxicity;

• most physicians will never accept this;

• DMPS injections once a month and DMSA pills every other day, or every week, do not help patients and do have the risk of adverse reactions;

• effective treatments do exist (some are spelled out in this book);

• amalgam and other exposure sources must be completely removed to effect a cure;

• chelation is essential to heal the brain;

• not everyone who thinks he has mercury poisoning really does - some actually do have some other medical problem.

The uncertain, imperfect information that I have today is here. It covers:

• how to find and work with good doctors;

• the effects of chronic mercury poisoning, and how mercury causes these effects;

• how to diagnose chronic mercury poisoning;

• how to treat chronic mercury poisoning;

• why you should believe a lot of people are mercury poisoned.

Using other books

Anyone with a technical background is encouraged to find the nearest library with medical textbooks, the physician's desk reference, etc. These are surprisingly clear and well written compared to what you will experience in all too many doctor's offices. They certainly aren't light reading, but physics, chemistry, math, and all engineering books are much more difficult to read at the upper division level. Most places that have these books also have a medical dictionary, so the vocabulary can eventually be mastered.

I don't mean to imply that you need a college education to get anything out of these books either! Many people are able to puzzle out the important parts when their health or that of a loved one is at stake. In fact, supposedly "unsophisticated" people sometimes see important things long before the "properly educated professionals" who have been taught not to look for them!

There is one other important reason to read up on things. If it makes your physician insecure, or if s/he tries to demonstrate you don't know what you are talking about instead of explaining things so you do, then you know you need to find a real doctor instead. Getting over amalgam illness takes time and can be complicated. You need to be involved in your own therapy and understand what is going on. Your doctor has to be secure enough in his or her knowledge to help you learn.

The main advantage of popular books other than this one is to convince you, your physician, and your friends and family that you do have amalgam illness and will get well if you treat it. They do not otherwise offer useful advice.

Using the internet

The internet is a place to find a few tidbits of valuable information you won't find anywhere else among an enormous mountain of incorrect, misleading, prejudicial or

Introduction

dogmatic material. Unfortunately most of it is not appropriately identified.

If you really aren't finding anything relevant in the printed literature the internet is a good place to go. Search around. Look at lots of websites. Try lots of listservers or newsgroups. Find the ones that have information that is relevant to you, makes sense, and that you can try out. Find people who are willing to explain things to you as best they can and who will share information and experiences. Newsgroups and listservers are a lot easier to use and enjoy if you learn whose messages are always wild, raving, inflammatory and seldom useful, and delete them unread.

Traditional media (e. g. medical books and journals) have a good editorial process in place that ensures that what is in them is accurate as far as it goes. This process works about 90% of the time. The major problem is that the process is somewhat political, so controversial things - as all new discoveries are - do not show up here for some time. When you need controversial information, go to the internet. Find some leading information. Then do as much of the learning as you can out of more traditional media - the information you find in the library will be a lot more accurate and easy to digest.

One of the most interesting and useful things on the internet is the medline database. There are also other databases like toxline that are relevant. These can be accessed a number of ways. Medline can easily be found by searching for "pubmed." Medline presents the titles (and sometimes abstracts) of journal articles that the National Library of Medicine receives. Being original research literature, this material is NOT presented in a clear, comprehensible and organized fashion like the material in a medical textbook. However, you can find lots of interesting and useful things that haven't made it into medical textbooks yet. You can also find the most up to date research results relevant to something you are interested in (e. g. something discussed in this book). Do remember that medicine is highly political and what is said in the abstract does not always follow from the material in the paper, or agree with the conclusions drawn. Medline only shows you the abstract, not the entire text.

If you find something in a traditional peer reviewed medical journal, you know that it passed some level of quality control. You also know that it has been accepted at some level of political correctness. There is a good chance it contains some truth, but there is no chance it contains much that is controversial. If you find something on the internet it is very likely to be controversial, but you have no idea at all how much truth it contains. Try as they might, nobody has managed to make editing completely neutral or free speech completely dispassionate yet. The internet is where you find those elements of truth that are passionately politically incorrect mixed in with highly opinionated screeches of intellectual pain.

The biggest reason to use the internet? It is easy. You will actually do it. It is always better to do something instead of feeling guilty about not reading that medical textbook you are worried might not understand even if you could find it at the library.

Medicine, controversy, and mercury

The mercury controversy and me

There is a debate in the medical community regarding the prevalence of iatrogenic (doctor caused) chronic mercury poisoning from dental amalgam (silver fillings) and assorted health care products. Understandably this is a very heated and dogmatic debate since it implies that a major health care problem in America today may be damage done by doctors and dentists while they were supposed to be helping us, and that products the regulators and professional associations certified as safe were in fact far more dangerous than most things they criticized or banned.

If people are getting mercury poisoned by their dental amalgams, contact lens cleaning solutions, contraceptives, antiseptics, over the counter salves and lotions, etc., then a large number of people are actually mercury poisoned, but are not diagnosed that way. They are instead diagnosed with chronic and generally incurable conditions. These conditions have substantial morbidity, mortality, and cause tremendous suffering - in plain english the victims hurt a real whole lot, then die young. If these problems are indeed due to mercury intoxication they are unlikely to be cured by treatments which do not reduce the body burden of mercury. If even a few of these people actually have mercury poisoning it is a terrible tragedy since mercury poisoning can be cured.

Typical conditions that might be caused by chronic mercury exposure through health care or other routes are: allergies, asthma, autoimmune diseases, ALS, myasthenia gravis, Parkinson's, Alzheimers', schizophrenia spectrum disorders, borderline personality disorder, anxiety, panic attacks, atheroschlerosis, attention deficit hyperactivity disorder, learning disabilities, endocrine dysfunction, depression, obsessive-compulsive disorder, manic depressive disorder, rheumatoid arthritis, juvenile arthritis, lupus erythromatosus, multiple chemical sensitivity, environmental illness, chronic fatigue, fibromyalgia, sciatica, gastritits, irritable bowel syndrome, colitis, Crohn's disease, sleep disorders, anorexia nervosa, bulimia, yeast syndrome, etc.

Personally, I believe many people with these and other conditions are actually mercury poisoned. I am sure I will be subjected to extremely harsh and severe criticism for this belief. Other people who bothered to investigate the issue also came to the conclusions I have and were subjected to extreme criticism and harassment by authorities who made no effort to investigate their claims and took no responsibility to check facts widely available in the medical literature. The powers that be will assure you that people like Andy Cutler or Hal Huggins or Michael Ziff simply do not know what they are talking about and must be hallucinating the cures they observed (Huggins, also Ziff) or personally experienced (myself, or Pleva, or Stock[1], who verified their cures as due to properly treated mercury intoxication by using their well developed skills at scientific research). People with chronic debilitating conditions may wish to draw their own conclusions regarding the likelihood that they are mercury poisoned, since mercury poisoning can be cured in a year or two, and much can be done to ameliorate symptoms in the meantime.

Regardless of how glib the criticism levelled at me is, I will remain convinced amalgam illness is a real condition since I had it. I became quite seriously ill while most doctors told me there was nothing wrong. After an "environmental medicine" doctor

---

[1] as described in english rather than german by Hanson and Pleva.

Medicine, controversy, and mercury

suggested I had amalgam illness I had to read lots of medical literature to figure out what was going on and what to do about it, and got well after having my fillings replaced and taking appropriate chelating agents. I also know a lot of other people to whom this happened.

I was very lucky when I got sick. Not lucky to get sick! That was a terrible experience! But I was lucky to have received exactly the right education before I needed it - a PhD in chemistry (Princeton, 1985) - close enough to medicine to be able to read physician's textbooks, but not close enough to share all the myths and be sure of the things "everyone knows." I was lucky to have had some business experience so I viewed physicians as professional service providers and knew how to get the services I needed from them. This made me comfortable enough to browbeat, wheedle, sweet talk, and cajole physicians into helping[2]. I had the right political experience to realize I could get lots of valuable information by just talking to enough people - and I learned lots from fellow patients. I also learned how much people suffer from this terrible condition. I learned how poor the understanding is of how to diagnose and treat chronic mercury poisoning. I wanted to write this book so that other people don't have to do all their own detective work when they get sick. So that people could start with the best information I could find. So that future victims of mercury poisoning won't have to suffer unnecessarily because nobody really knows what to do.

Many people have similar experiences to mine - having lots of problems their physicians were unable to help with which disappear in the months following amalgam

---

[2] Most physicians really do want to help sick people, but they are very strongly trained not to do that in medical school. State licensing boards also take a dim view of it. Physicians are under a tremendous amount of pressure to follow a cookbook and not be at all creative about it. If they don't find the right recipe for you they need a lot of courage and self confidence to try to come up with something new.

removal. Indeed, there are many case reports of this in the mainstream medical literature. I also personally know people who have gone through it. While not uncommon, physicians routinely disbelieve it even when they have observed one of their own patients get well following amalgam removal.

This is not the first time in the history of modern medicine that a very obvious disease was belittled and ignored for political reasons. Until recently it was believed that ulcers were entirely psychosomatic. Ulcer sufferers underwent prolonged treatment, were seldom cured, and often ended up under the surgeon's knife. After years of intense criticism and ridicule - about 20 years after the research was published - it has finally been accepted that most ulcers are due to helicobacter pylorii infection which can be easily cured with appropriate antibiotic therapy. At least by the medical schools and licensing boards. Yet it is still common to find physicians who still treat ulcers by prescribing acid suppressors - as if they resulted from too much stomach acid.

Cholesterol was held out as the root cause of atherosclerosis and coronary artery disease for about 30 years during which the correct evidence that elevated homocysteine played a major role was ridiculed and ignored.

Older physicians still remember when "there was no such thing as Epstein Barr Virus (mononucleosis)."

And who can forget Lyme disease? A housewife fell ill. Her arthritis and other symptoms were diagnosed as psychosomatic. When her husband and children came down with similar symptoms, this was regarded as some kind of projection of her psychosomatic complaint. She was eventually able to convince physicians that the only crazy thing was assuming that something psychosomatic could be contagious!

Chronic Fatigue Immune Deficiency Syndrome is still routinely considered a psychiatric disorder despite the repeated publication of physical and laboratory abnormalities always found in victims of it. When it can no longer be ignored, it is dismissed with a bit of namecalling - "Yuppie flu."

And in less recent times, another form of mercury poisoning - acrodynia - was endemic for 150 years until physicians recognized mercury as the causal agent. The disease was promptly eliminated by changing the formulation of certain infant care products.

I saw a large number of physicians during my illness. Most of them simply ignore anything not in their textbooks. In fact, few of them even remember all the textbook stuff! Some physicians understand that patients come to them because there is something wrong and try to help even if it isn't a textbook case. These physicians were always able to do something helpful, but never able to do all that was necessary. A few physicians reject the idea that the textbooks are filled with useful knowledge, diagnose and treat all kinds of politically incorrect conditions, but routinely make serious errors in treatment and case management by not remembering the useful and correct stuff that IS in their medical school texts. Between the open minded mainstream physicians and the alternative ones I was able to muddle through to the point where I could read up on stuff in the textbooks and medical journals so I could figure out what the best choices were for me.

The root of this problem appears to be toxicologists' unwarranted belief, generally propagated in medical texts, that blood and urine levels of mercury are an accurate measure of toxicity. Yet to quote the Handbook on the Toxicology of Metals, volume 2, pg 402, "At present, there is no suitable biological index of the mercury concentration in critical organs such as the brain..." Thus diagnosis must depend on tests other than those standard medical textbooks instruct physicians to use. It is not surprising that mercury poisoning is incorrectly excluded by most physicians even in obvious cases of mercurialism.

I have written this book to share what I know about mercury poisoning and related subjects so that people with apparently intractable health problems can see whether they actually have one - mercury poisoning - that is readily curable, and, if so, treat it effectively.

Scientific or dogmatic medicine?

Science is the system of thought where observers collect data which is taken to be true if it is reproducible, then construct theories which are the simplest explanation of all data known at the time. Any observer may make a new observation that present theories can't explain. In fact, one of the less well known requirements of a scientific theory is that there must be some hypothetical future observations which would prove it false. If these observations are made, the theorists should go back to the drawing board and science should advance. Theories consistent with all possible observations (e. .g any symptoms not corresponding to a disease in my medical school textbooks are psychosomatic) do not qualify as science - they are more akin to religion.

Progress is difficult due to people's natural tendency to hold on to the old theories they learned in school which are their preconceived notions. Thus experiments are designed to disprove theories rather than prove them (to falsify the hypothesis in techncial terms) to account for the natural human tendency to become attached to their theories and their experiments.

The morality of science is that observation is truth. Theories are just clever poetry written to describe observations. Observers perform the most fundamental task of science, and there is never a growing burden of proof for an observer - each observation is as true as any other.

Thus in medical SCIENCE, the ordinary physician in his clinic is a key figure. He observes truth. Real data. Real patients with real symptoms. Any clinician may stumble upon new data that proves existing theory inadequate and forces the medical school professors to come up with new theories and write new textbooks.

Since each physician has observed different patients and knows different things, each will have a different set of facts to base his theories on. Thus in scientific medicine there is disagreement between different physicians in the details of how they understand and explain a patient's clinical condition and each physician may have a slightly different approach to helping any given patient.

To be scientific, a hypothesis must meet three criteria. It must be consistent with other reproducible observations. It must be simple. There must be an obvious and objective test to prove whether it is right or wrong.

Dogmatic thinking consists of defining a body of theory as true, igoring observations that are not consistent with the dogma, and inventing some catch all explanation for the observations that can't be ignored. Medicine is taught as dogma today, and psychiatric or behavioral explanations like somatization disorder as used in practice are the dogmatic catch all explanations that lack the scientific requirement of falsifiability to be a valid theory. In dogmatic medicine, symptoms are either in the textbook or in the patient's head. In real science, there is always the choice that the theory (the textbook) is wrong - or perhaps just incomplete. New diseases like amalgam illness can be discovered scientifically, but not dogmatically.

In the dogmatic system some authority figures are considered purveyors of TRUTH and everyone else is a thoughtless receiver of it who has nothing to contribute. Thus, dogma demotes the clinician to the bottom of the intellectual totem pole and raises the theorizer with minimal clinical experience to the level of exhalted expert. One can certainly see why dogma is popular with professors and researchers!

There is no requirement in scientific medicine for placebo controlled trials, etc. before something is 'scientifically proven.' This is a dogmatic requirement. Controlled trials, when properly designed, are just a sophisticated way of testing a scientific theory. There are many other ways to test theories, and until tested and found wanting the simplest theory that fits known observations is the scientific truth.

Mainstream and alternative medicine

These are more properly characterized as two different segments of the medical community, one of which currently happens to control AMA leadership and the state licensing boards.

It is common for two conflicting but legitimate segments of the medical community to be at oods as to the methods for diagnosing and treating certain conditions. Where there is more than one recommended method of diagnosis or therapy and none of them are used exclusively and uniformly by all physicians, a physician is acting ethically and in accordance with the law if he uses one of these approved methods, even if it later turns out to be the wrong one.

Thus, in controversial areas, the burden really is on the patient to decide whether to accept the physician's diagnosis and proposed treatment plan, or to seek another. This is why patients' rights exist and are strongly protected by law. So if you are getting diagnoses like "there is nothing wrong," or "it's all in your head" and proposed treatment plans like "try ignoring it and seeing if it goes away," you have no obligation to accept these. If you want another diagnosis or treatment plan, you have to find another physician who follows different methods of diagnosis and treatment for this kind of condition.

This all sounds nicely dispassionate until you run across the adversarial nature and lack of objectivity which characterizes the current debate within the medical community. This great polarization leads to most physicians on both sides of the divide having an inappropriately emotional rejection of discussions based on the other paradigm. Certain elements of the "mainstream" community - e. g. Quackwatch - make dramatic pronouncements and proclamations which do not foster much interest in discussion.

This book is an attempt to learn from a constructive combination of mainstream and alternative concepts. I have tried to leave out the religious fervor of protectionism that makes it so difficult for caring physicians to find the information they need to help sick people.

In real science - the kind I tried unsuccessfully to teach premeds a few times - we can precisely determine and predict a great deal once we know all the variables in a closed system. In medicine, we don't even know what all the variables are, and the system is open! Some creativity is needed to imagine what might be going on since we don't even know what to measure. That is why medicine is an art, not a science. As with any art, the physician who has a wider variety of techniques in his repertoire will do better work. I think the physician who is well versed in both mainstream and alternative techniques has be best hope of curing you, or me, of our ailments. It is a shame that the social strictures medicine imposes on itself make it so hard to find such physicians when we need them.

Physical versus mental illness

The symptoms of mercury poisoning could be misdiagnosed as various psychiatric conditions depending on exactly how mercury affects the patient. This is very unfortunate since psychiatry is unable to cure most conditions and in only a few is able to prescribe medications - which generally have serious side effects - that control the problem somewhat. However, if the problem is really mercury it can be cured easily.

A quick perusal of assorted medical textbooks (e. g. the porphyria section in *Harrison's Principles of Internal Medicine*) or some creative searching on medline will show that many physical diseases have primarily psychiatric symptoms. These diseases are often misdiagnosed as psychiatric diseases and the patients treated ineffectively - often for years while under confinement at a mental hospital - before someone has the sense to run a few simple laboratory tests, get a correct diagnosis, and cure them.

Under the circumstances it is unlikely that many people who appear to have psychiatric illnesses will be tested for chronic mercury intoxication, or treated for it.

Psychiatric illness has a great stigma both inside and outside the medical community. If you have been diagnosed with psychiatric problems, or believe you have them, you will have to conduct a vigorous search to find a physician who is willing to help you by seeking a physical cause for your problem.

Given the protracted course, great suffering, and poor prognosis of most psychiatric conditions when subjected to standard psychiatric treatment, it is very wise to seek all possible physical causes before relying solely on mentally directed drug and talk therapy. Anyone with an apparent psychiatric problem would be wise to explore the issue of mercury intoxication thoroughly.

How can a doctor help you?

A physician can do a lot more for you than just sign test orders and write prescriptions. Even physicians who are not so open minded will often have something useful to say that you can benefit from. An open minded physician can give you more perspective on your case than you are ever going to get out of a book even if she is not familiar with amalgam illness and isn't sure she believes it exists.

Medicine, controversy, and mercury

You need to find a physician who has the self confidence to trust his clinical observations instead of med school dogma and the humility to understand that finding the simplest explanation for what he is seeing in front of him can be surprisingly difficult. This physician is practicing medicine scientifically. This physician can help you.

Your doctor can give you expert help in identifying what you really NEED when you ask for a specific drug or test if they will talk to you about what you are trying to figure out or do. After all, doctors spend years and years studying what all the tests mean and what all the drugs do, and they have a lot of experience seeing what the drugs actually do to people. Talk to them about what you are trying to accomplish. Insist they do something reasonable, but don't be inflexible if they get interested in what you are saying and discuss alternatives that might work better.

Note that there are many different specialties in medicine, and while in theory the people in each one should actually help you with problems in their field of expertise, it seldom works out this way. Don't worry about having your endocrine problems handled by an endocrinologist, etc. Worry about finding a doctor who will help you figure out what to do, and will help you do it. All specialization means is that a particular doctor has memorized some of the "cookbook" recipes by heart. Since you aren't a cookbook case a doctor who specializes in one specific sort of recipe isn't more likely to help you than any other doctor.

Why doctors should read this book

Based on the discussion given later, statistical estimates of how many people's health is adversely affected by mercury exposure can be made. While these are not highly accurate estimates they are adequate for motivational purposes. At least 1% and possibly as much as 5% of the population is definitely experiencing serious and life limiting adverse health effects due to their body burden of mercury. These health problems can be cured by therapy that removes the mercury. Other therapies cannot cure these problems.

One to five percent of the population is a HUGE number of people. Being able to recognize and treat or refer them appropriately is very important in providing quality health care.

Proper treatment for mercury toxicity is relatively inexpensive and has a low complication rate. Many of the current treatments are quite expensive and also have a high complication rate - leading to even greater expense. Suggesting the treatments described in this book and warning patients away from those known to have a high rate of adverse reactions - regardless of whether you believe a particular patient is mercury toxic or even believe that mercury intoxication is a real public health problem - is appropriate to reduce unnecessary suffering and control health care costs.

I addition, many people believe they are mercury toxic and that physicians are unknowledgeable about the diagnosis and treatment of this condition. At least some of these people actually are not mercury toxic[3]. Being able to definitively exclude mercury intoxication in such cases in a way the patient will accept is an important part of their care. This will help them accept the actual problem and treat it more consistently. The diagnostic methods presented later will allow you to do that, as will correctly diagnosing a real, physical problem with demonstrable abnormalities.

Discussion for physicians

---

[3] Stenman and Grans were able to definitively diagnose 8% of patients certain they had amalgam illness with something else. They found real medical problems for every single one of these patients - none of them were given psychiatric diagnoses. Engel found that 8% of patients having their amalgams removed reported no improvement one year later. Both Engel as well as Stenman and Grans found that many supposedly incurable psychiatric problems were cured by amalgam removal.

Amalgam Illness: Diagnosis and Treatment

The physician/patient relationship is an intimate relationship. Unfortunately, physicians are taught to hold themselves to impossibly high standards. This inhibits physicians from doing some of the things necessary to maintain an appropriate intimate relationship with their patients.

In any intimate relationship, both parties have needs to be met. If you are unable to meet your needs outside of the relationship, and do not express them inside the relationship, these needs will go unmet and you will resort to manipulative or inappropriate behaviors in an attempt to meet them.

The generally accepted standards for patient privacy, dignity, acceptance of the patient as they are, and lack of any sexual aspect to the doctor/patient relationship are appropriate.

The generally accepted standards for control, decisionmaking about what consitutes real conditions and appropriate therapy, and when second opinions are needed are not appropriate and will interfere with your ability to have an open and honest relationship with the patient, and thus to help them.

Control is best exercised by convincing the patient that what you propose to do makes sense, or that there is a reason you need to not do something for your own protection. If control is exercised unilaterally the patient will quite rationally withhold and manipulate information in order to get what he wants. If you want candor, you cannot exercise control.

Exercising control also undermines trust, which is the basis of any intimate relationship. If you do not wish to do something, explain why so the patient can continue to trust you. The ability to trust may be impaired in mercury toxic individuals. It is especially important to work to maintain trust. Trust also depends on keeping your word. The patient may interpret things somewhat differently than you intend. If you

say that you agree to something, do it. Do not say "yeah, sure," even under pressure, unless you mean it.

Intimacy also includes letting the patient know what your vulnerabilities are. If you are concerned that other physicians will be highly critical of you for entertaining the diagnosis of amalgam illness you should let the patient know this so she will act appropriately when she sees other physicians. Enlist the patient's aid in working WITH you. It is unreasonable to expect you to bear the entire burden of her care.

Involve the patient in decisionmaking about which tests to perform and which therapies to employ. This makes it much more likely he will comply, identify related problems, and not maintain a stable of doctors he keep in the dark about what the other ones are prescribing.

Admit imperfection. The patient is likely to be sophisticated about her condition and to have seen a large number of other physicians. She does not expect perfection from you. You cannot provide it. You will be able to act much more appropriately towards the patient if you do not feel compelled to project an attitude of certainty.

Be up front with the patient about prospective problems. I. e. the insurance plan will crucify you if you order too many tests, and it is against the law to order tests insurance pays for unless they really are medically necessary. Or you are very uncomfortable prescribing a certain drug because you are unfamiliar with it, the patient wants it for an unusual indication, and it has significant hazards. Or you are getting a hard time from a fellow physician the patient has also seen about the weird stuff you are doing, and if the patient wants you to keep doing it she is going to have to keep it confidential.

To avoid patient anger and encourage candor, write prescriptions exactly as requested immediately and let the patient check them for acceptability. If you aren't willing to write the requested prescription, explain your limitations, the reason for them, and what you are willing to do instead. The patient is asking for the best thing they know how to request. They may be very happy for your expert help in identifying something better, or in discovering reasons they weren't aware of why the requested prescription or test order isn't appropriate, won't do what they want, or in learning about possible side effects and hazards they weren't aware of. With test orders it is a good idea to tell them you will gladly write the order but you want to talk to them a bit to understand what they are trying to learn so as to make sure they get exactly the right test to find it out.

One very important note: the patient looks a lot healthier than she is. This will become apparent if adequate laboratory testing is conducted, and history is discussed in adequate detail over several visits. It is important to keep in mind that the patient may look well during appointments and yet be unable to conduct day to day activities, as well as be experiencing great discomfort on an ongoing basis. Physiological reasons for this, such as paradoxical adrenal response, will be discussed later.

Many of these patients appear excessively concerned about medications, office procedures, tests, etc., ask detailed questions, and wish to have extensive discussions of exactly what to do. The physician may find this frustrating. Though it may appear neurotic to the physician who has only seen this patient a few times, it is perfectly rational behavior on the part of a patient who has likely seen many health care providers and had many unpleasant experiences at their hands. These patients also have an unusually high rate of side effects and adverse drug reactions which makes it perfectly reasonable for them to require lots of information and insist that much thought goes into deciding what to prescribe. Anger is a perfectly natural emotional response on the part of the physician to frustration or possible feelings of hopelessness and helplessness that might arise from the feeling that the patient is

making it impossible for the physician to help. The physician must be aware of his or her feelings to avoid an angry decision that the patient is simply neurotic. This would only interfere with diagnosing and treating the patient's physical ailments.

The patient is likely to see other physicians. This is a good thing, since there is no standard treatment protocol for amalgam illness, the complications of each case are unique, and another physician may have some insight into how to help the patient that you do not. The patient may also become frustrated with the usually slow progress and want to see if someone else can speed things up. They may simply go to another physician for a test or prescription you were unwilling to provide. View your relationship with the patient as private, intimate, but not exclusive. Encourage the patient to do the same.

In seeing a variety of physicians, in wanting to be involved in therapeutic decisionmaking, and in requesting specific tests, the patients are simply trying to ensure that they receive the best care possible. The most basic aspect of this care is to reach a definitive diagnosis with high certainty. Medical textbooks discuss the need to routinely exclude even very rare but treatable conditions, such as Wilson's disease, before considering diagnoses of incurable diseases such as Parkinson's to be confirmed. Such thorough differential diagnosis of even widely accepted conditions is seldom performed in today's environment of managed care, yet it is the textbook defined standard of care. Patients who feel that "something is wrong" which significantly impairs them have a right to definitive, high certainty exclusion of rare conditions and of conditions that are not yet widely accepted enough to have medical textbook chapters describing them.

The pressures of managed care

Managed care has had a profound impact on the way medicine is practiced today. Even if you aren't on a managed care plan physicians have grown accustomed to practicing the way HMO's and PPO's want them to. The major factors are:

Time: Physicians are used to being under time pressure. Excuses are found to not pay them for their time. Thus they routinely do not read your file before appointments. This ensures a high error rate in complex or subtle cases. The remedy is that you must be familiar with your file and must retain your own personal copies of all lab results. You should also make notes of what happens and what the doctor says at each appointment. Then remind the physician of important material if it slips his or her mind in the future. The physician may wish to make a 'shoot from the hip' diagnosis to cut the appointment short and move on. Tell them to take their time and get it right. Ask them to explain in detail how they arrived at the diagnosis, how it explains everything that is going on, and what steps can be taken and tests run to confirm it. Rushing is a hard habit for physicians to break.

Testing: There is much pressure to reduce the number of tests ordered. Thus physicians routinely assume things will be normal and not worth testing for unless there is an obvious need. This means subtle problems will be missed and diagnoses like mercurialism which are difficult to establish will not be made. Instead, some of the major symptoms will be restated in Latin and that will be declared a "diagnosis." Solutions come from a keen awareness of past test results at each appointment, very careful history taking and physical examination, very careful selection of tests so the RIGHT ones are done, ordering medically necessary tests until the insurance company objects, bouncing around to several doctors to get them all to order medically necessary tests you can bring with you to your "main" doctor or your next doctor, and if worse comes to worst, paying for some tests yourself.

Remember, only medically necessary tests can legally be ordered by physicians for billing to insurance - especially medicare. Medically necessary tests have a legalistic

definition, but for practical purposes if the test will not help you make a decision as to what to do next, and is not needed to try to understand something there is reasonable reason to believe is not functioning properly so you can find a way to move forward when you are stumped, and is not needed to convince you or your physician that your diagnosis is correct (or isn't), then it is not medically necessary.

In an HMO, referrals are limited. You either have to find a primary care physician who will sign off on lots of them (rare) or one who is willing to take the time and responsibility to treat the various aspects of your problems (even rarer). The solution is to interview all available PCP's on these issues, grill them so they don't just give polite answers to make you happy, then change frequently as they get frustrated.

A warning to physicians and patients alike

The biggest problem in medicine today is dilettantes who understand just enough hard science to be a danger to themselves and others, and invent all sorts of therapies based on incomplete knowldege of how HEALTHY bodies are supposed to work, with no consideration for any specific bichemical problems a certain individual might be dealing with and how these might affect treatment outcome. Increasing specialization among physicians and symptom- rather than cause-based teaching methods and treatments have led both conventional and alternative medicine in the direction of suppressing symptoms instead of curing diseases. Thus patients are all too often forced to choose between excessively conservative treatment which does not help them, and wildly speculative treatment which is as likely to harm as it is to help.

Everyone must take the responsibility to check and re-check the fundamental concepts and basic principles behind new treatments or existing treatments adapted to new or newly recognized diseases. Indeed, much of this book is directed at explaining how to use

Medicine, controversy, and mercury

standard prescription and OTC chelating agents properly in order to help patients get well, instead of the way they are almost always used at present, which makes patients sicker.

Two currently popular protocols which do not stand up to any cursory check of efficacy and which have frequent adverse patient reactions are: DMPS injections of 3 mg/kg, or 250 mg, given iv or im monthly; and DMSA 200+ mg po qod (by mouth, every other day). These should never be used.

The most common DMPS injection adverse reactions follow from redistribution of mercury to the liver and pancreas with consequent damage. The symptoms often appear psychiatric. Anxious, agitated depression that is ameliorated by treatments for hypoglycemia are typical.

The most common DMSA every other day adverse reactions follow from mercury redistribution to the central nervous system. The symptoms may appear psychiatric or neurological. Psychosis and severe coordination problems with weakenss are typical.

There is an unfortunate trend for some physicians to describe their clinical experience with a protocol as "100% effective, without side effects," when the patients who were treated under the protocol do not think they got better, and considered the side effects so frightening they filed FDA adverse drug event reporting forms. Patients must take the responsibility of communicating to their physician and other patients what is happening to them. Physicians must take responsibility for listening and using the information to select appropriate therapy. If a physician considers therapy "helpful" when it is hurting the patient, s/he is simply not paying enough attention to help the patient. The "healing crisis" used as an excuse by some physicians, e. g. for the harmful and ineffective treatments mentioned above is more properly called an "adverse drug reaction," since it is observed not to lead to improved health when it is over.

This is not a new problem. It is the same problem conventional medicine had in handing out Valium® like candy in the '70's and passing out Prozac® indiscriminately more recently.

Why worry about mercury poisoning?

Chronic mercury poisoning is widespread

Detailed arguments using numbers and formulae to show that much of the population must be poisoned by mercury are given in an appendix. Some interesting direct measurements are discussed here.

Several individuals have been observed to have a high enough measured excretion of amalgam derived mercury that their body concentrations would exceed 10 μM if their personal elimination half life were 240 days (Barregård, Sällsten and Järvholm, 1995). Such a mercury concentration is promptly toxic to immune system cells cells in culture and in rodents. It also corresponds to a body burden of about 150 mg of mercury - a potentially lethal dose. Few medical textbooks would lead a physician to think to order mercury tests based on their symptoms.

Direct measurements of hair mercury in 133 Japanese patients with allergy, dementia[1], cerebral infarcts[2], diabetes and hypertension[3] show it to be uniformly higher than average (Nakagawa 1995). Lead and mercury have been shown to be elevated in the hair of emotionally disturbed children (Marlowe *et al*. 19xx). There is evidence that dental amalgam mercury may be an etiologic factor in manic-depression (Silberud, Motl and Kleinholtz 1998).

The manager of the corrosion section in the steel research department at Swedish company Uddeholm AB got amalgam illness, took his removed fillings to work and characterized the type and extent of corrosion. He found that they had corroded rapidly by crevice corrosion (Pleva 1983). He was able to determine that the amount of mercury corroded out of his fillings was in excess of a lethal dose. He was unable to find any dentists familiar with the different types of corrosion metallic materials may undergo, or with the basic principles of metallurgy, or any dental research literature based on such an understanding.

Any scientifically trained person would immediately realize that the correct scientific hypothesis is that some unknown number of people acquire chronic mercury poisoning from their amalgams. These poor people are all misdiagnosed because of inappropriate medical textbook guidelines and a poor understanding of the possible sources of mercury exposure among physicians. Dogmatic systems are able to maintain uniform beliefs contrary to current scientific understanding for prolonged periods of time. The "mainstream" medical position regarding amalgam illness appears to be dogmatic rather than scientific.

Clinical Studies highlight a dichotomy

In one well designed clinical study (Stenman and Grans, 1997), amalgam removal cured all patients for whom the diagnosis of mercurialism could not be excluded in favor of an alternative by the painstaking method of considering and eliminating all other possibilities by thorough examination and laboratory testing. Many patients who had diagnosed themselves with amalgam illness actually had other textbook conditions. 348 patients came forward. Sixty were found to have other identifiable conditions. Twenty six of the remainder chose to have their amalgams removed. All

---

[1] Of all types. Alzheimer's disease plus others.
[2] Strokes.
[3] High blood pressure.

16

of the amalgam removers were cured[4]. None of the possible amalgam illness cases who kept their amalgams in were cured. Some of those cured had been definitively diagnosed with serious and incurable somatic and psychiatric conditions by other doctors.

Another clinical study applied textbook criteria to laboratory result interpretation and decided that none of 1,300 patients who thought they had amalgam illness had a mercury problem (Langworth, 1997). This study also found some patients to have other unrecognized diseases that accounted for their symptoms.

One must conclude that standard diagnostic guidelines for mercury are wrong. After all, how can people be cured by treatment for a condition unless they had it? Amalgam illness and many other condition are difficult to diagnose and a proper diagnostic workup is necessary to ensure that patients are treated for the conditions they actually have - even if it is something as politically incorrect as mercury poisoning.

Flawed clinical trials[5] fail to resolve the mercury issue.

---

[4] as evidenced by disappearance of signs and symptoms.

[5] While this could all be read as highly critical of these workers, I wish to say something in their defense. First, Sandborgh-Englund *et al.* DID draw a correct conclusion in the paper, though it is not well reported by abstracting services. Grandjean et al. may have already been conducting their study by the time the work of Sandborgh-Englund et al. was available to them, though this does not excuse the later workers for drawing prima facie incorrect conclusions.

Second, I personally screwed up the first 9 sets of experiments for my doctoral dissertation. This is pretty common. I THINK I finally did it right the 10th time. Since I was working with chemicals and furnaces I could do it over and over and over until I got it right. The authors of the controlled trials papers were working with human subjects and don't have the luxury of doing it over and over. They only have "one bite at the apple." By doing their best and

Sandborgh-Englund and others (1994) correctly concluded[6] that DMSA in standard doses over a couple of weeks is not effective in treating amalgam illness while the amalgams remain in place. Unfortunately this conclusion is not reflected in the abstract available on medline, and many health care professionals do not obtain, read and analyze papers such as this before drawing their own conclusions. They just read the medline abstract and talk like they read the whole paper.

Despite being a later study and citing Sandborgh-Englund, Grandjean and others (1997) incorrectly conclude that placebo is as effective as chelation for "environmental illness" despite the fact that their figures also show that the body burden of mercury was unchanged by DMSA therapy. Thus this trial is properly characterized as a placebo versus placebo trial and did demonstrate that DMSA makes a good placebo if it is not administered properly. It does not, however, allow any conclusions to be drawn about amalgam illness due to poor study design.

Current levels of mercury exposure are known to poison people

Dentists and dental assistants with low mercury exposure levels have been found to have neurobehavioral impairments in direct relation to unchelated and chelated urinary mercury excretion (Echeverria and others 1998; Echeverria and others 1995). Similar results have been reported for university students (Aposhian and others 1992). Results from both studies have been

---

exposing themselves to criticism by publishing the results they allow science to progress.

Some advocates of not treating sick patients sometimes use these papers as "proof" that there is "nothing wrong." Thus it is unfortunately necessary to offer public criticism of these works.

[6] As is obvious from the figures in their published study.

Amalgam Illness: Diagnosis and Treatment

converted to a common basis and are shown in figure 1.

The university students have similar levels of chelated mercury excretion to the dentists. The university students must be experiencing negative health effects similar to the dentists. Results for unchelated mercury excretion by these dentists and dental assistants are compared to the known population distribution of mercury excretion in figure 2.

Figure 1. Comparative histograms of urinary mercury excretion after chelation for dentists and dental assistants with measured, mercury correlated neurobehavioral impairment, versus university students.

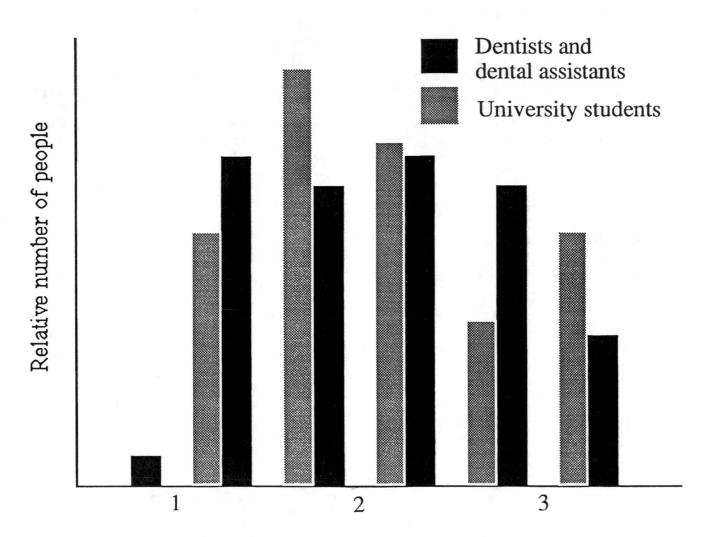

Ln (mcg Hg excreted)
Natural logarithm of the micrograms
of mercury in a urine sample

Why worry about mercury poisoning?

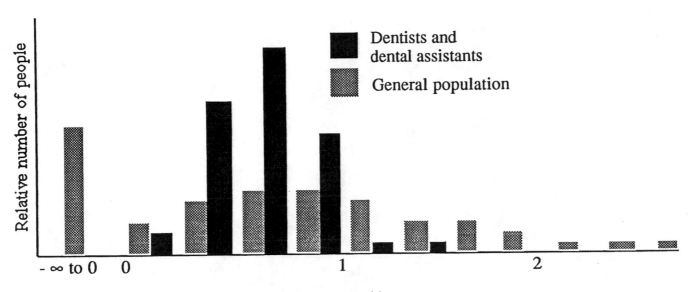

Figure 2. Comparative histograms of urinary mercury excretion for dentists and dental assistants with measured, mercury correlated neurobehavioral impairment, versus the general population.

It can be seen that much of the general population has higher mercury excretion than the dentists and dental assistants. There are a lot of people who are even more messed up by mercury than these dentists who were directly observed to be slightly poisoned by it!

Some members of the general population are experiencing neurological impairment and other adverse health effects due to mercury poisoning despite having no occupational source of exposure to mercury.

Only people who are immune to mercury work with it[7]

Figure 3 shows a graph of how fast three different kinds of people get rid of mercury; industrial workers (Ellingsen and others 1993; Roels and others 1991), rural Iraqis (Al-Shahristani and Shihab, 1974) exposed to methylmercury[8] and Germans wishing to have their amalgam fillings replaced (Begerow and others 1994) because of environmental illness or other factors.

---

[7] Apologies to physician readers for using "immune" in the popular rather than correct technical sense!

[8] Some of which is eliminated as is, and much after metabolism to mercuric ion.

Amalgam Illness: Diagnosis and Treatment

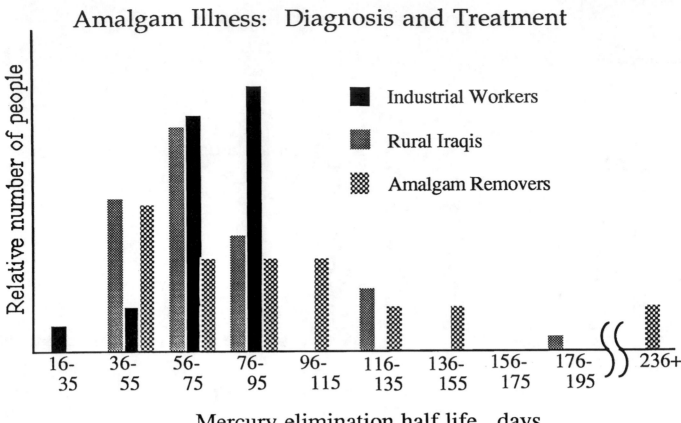

Figure 3. Comparative histograms of mercury excretion half life for three groups: industrial workers, rural Iraquis, and Germans voluntarily removing their amalgams. Half lives reported by Roels were multiplied by 0.796 to make them equivalent to the "corrected" half lives of Ellingsen.

Figure 3 implies that industrial workers are not representative of the general population - no person with a long elimination half life is found in this group. The Iraqi data[9] show three distinct distributions, and are consistent with a genetic model where a single gene[10] substantially slows elimination. The amalgam removal group clearly is distinct from the others. The readily available data represent fewer than 100 people. The large differences in distribution between groups make it impossible to generalize to the entire human species based on these measurements of a few individuals from a limited number of ethnic groups. It is common knowledge that people of northern European ancestry are more susceptible to amalgam illness, perhaps explaining the distribution of authorship on serious studies of this topic and the fact that amalgam use is sharply restricted in Sweden and Germany.

There are substantial health differences between people involuntarily exposed to mercury versus those choosing to be

---

[9] One type of US foreign aid consisted of seed grain preserved with methylmercury fungicides. This was considered perfectly safe by the US government - which now considers amalgam fillings and mercury containing vaccines perfectly safe. The seed grain was seldom properly marked and many of the people who got this grain ended up eating it. These people got methylmercury poisoning, got really sick, and a lot of them died. After this happened a number of times and thousands of people we were trying to help died, the government decided these mercury grain

preservatives might not be so safe after all and outlawed them.

[10] More properly, a single allele of a given gene with a population incidence of 0.12.

20

Why worry about mercury poisoning?

exposed. These were reported for free workers versus slave and prison labor at mercury mines in Almaden, Spain and Idrija, Slovenia in centuries past (Kussmaul, 1861). Free workers were much healthier. The simplest explanation for this is that free workers who were sensitive to the toxic effects of mercury chose not to work at chloralkali plants, fluorescent lamp factories or at mercury mines. People who are sensitive to the toxic effects of mercury didn't participate in the research studies all our government policies and medical textbooks are based on.

Industrial workers are not representative of the general population in their response to mercury. Studies at factories can't be used to come up with safe exposure levels for everyone. Unfortunately this is how the current guidelines were developed.

Sources of mercury exposure

Vaccines and other injectables preserved with thimerosal, topical antiseptics and eye care products (recently taken off the market), and amalgam fillings expose people to to mercury. There are an extremely large number of other sources of mercury exposure used in the medical industry. Sources of elemental mercury such as fluorescent lamps, thermometers, doctor's office blood pressure meters, mercury obtained for recreational use[11], etc. are in theory recognized as hazards but in practice are treated very casually and do lead to poisoning when the mercury in them is not properly collected and disposed of.

Now of course some government dweeb will try to tell you Cutler obviously doesn't know any chemistry - he must not have listened in those years and years of classes he took. Once the mercury is mixed up with silver in amalgam, it becomes perfectly safe! But in fact, it doesn't. Mercury has a certain vapor pressure. Mixing it up with another metal to make amalgam reduces the vapor

---

[11] Highly informal sources indicate that marijuana absorbs mercury from soil very efficiently.

pressure. Half mercury in the amalgam - the vapor pressure of mercury over amalgam is about half that of regular mercury. Doesn't matter if it is solid or liquid. Solids evaporate just fine. How do you think the ice cubes in your freezer go away if you leave them for a long time, or all that fluffy white frost forms? So here we have the government dweeb telling you out of one side of his mouth that you have to pay a zillion dollars to a hazardous waste disposal company to wear what amounts to spacesuits for the hour or two it takes them to clean up a mercury spill when they break a blood pressure meter in a doctor's office since it is SOOOOOOO toxic and evaporates SOOOOOOO fast, and then telling you out of the other side of his mouth that it is perfectly fine to permanently install something half that toxic in your mouth without taking any precautions at all! Which side of his mouth do you believe?

Fish mercury is a small concern

Government regulators have focussed on seafood instead of real hazards like dental amalgam. Average people get about 2 mcg / day of mercury from food. About 1.5 mcg of that is methylmercury from seafood. This corresponds to about $1.5 * 10^{-10}$ moles / kg / day for the average person, or about 0.05 μM body concentration for the 240 day slow excreter. A slow excreter eating large amounts of fish might consume 10 mcg / day of mercury from this source - about the same as the AVERAGE person gets from dental amalgam - leading to a concentration of 0.3 μM.

People who catch freshwater fish in contaminated areas, or who eat fish that accumulate a lot of mercury every day (tuna, swordfish, shellfish, shark) should have some concern - especially if they have liver problems where they don't make much bile. Very few people will have these problems, and fewer will get mercury poisoning from fish.

Amalgam Illness: Diagnosis and Treatment

Mercury exposure levels

Table 1 shows the corresponding body burdens for two people - one who excretes mercury fast and the other who excretes it slow so it builds up a lot. A small fraction of fast excreters and a substantial fraction of slow excreters are above the presently known toxic threshold. The US EPA proposes an exposure safety factor of ten (Johnson, 1998) - by which standard about 30% of the population and over half of concerned dental patients are at risk for mercury poisoning.

Table 1. Average nonoccupational mercury exposure by source

Period	Source	Exposure, μM	
		fast excreter	slow excreter
Infancy:	unrecognized domestic sources	unknown	unknown
	iatrogenic (vaccines)	0.04-0.7	0.04-0.7
Childhood:	recreational, domestic, and educational	unknown	unknown
	iatrogenic (booster shots)	0.002-0.05	0.002-0.05
	food - average fish consumption	0.015	0.05
	food - high fish consumption[a]	0.09	0.3
	dental amalgam (if used)	0.06	0.2
	topical antimicrobials[b]	0.06	0.2
Adulthood:	recreational and domestic	unknown	unknown
	food - average fish consumption	0.015	0.05
	food - high fish consumption[a]	0.09	0.3
	dental amalgam (if used)	0.1	0.3
	eye care products (if used)[e]	0.2	0.6
Adults, all sources[d]		0.06	0.19
Concerned dental patients, all sources[d]		0.13	0.43
Overt toxic effects occur at:		1	1
Exposure threshold with safety factor of 10		0.1	0.1

[a] uncommon in most populations.

[b] assuming 3 ml applied annually. Removed from market 10/19/98.

[e] assuming 4 drops daily in each eye. Mercury containing drops no longer used.

[d] calculated from measured median urinary excretion (Barregård, Sällsten and Järvholm, 1995).

Mercury poisoning doesn't get diagnosed properly

Current clinical texts instruct physicians to exclude mercury poisoning if there is no history of occupational exposure. Published cases typically resulted from unrecognized domestic or recreational exposure (e. g.

Why worry about mercury poisoning?

Henningsson and others 1993). Presumably most such cases are never caught because mercury poisoning is notoriously difficult to diagnose based on signs and symptoms alone (Gerstner and Huff 1977). Indeed, most physicians will refer a patient who asserts that she has mercury poisoning from their fillings and who has the classic symptoms of mercury poisoning for psychiatric counseling without doing any tests at all. Those who do tests just check mercury, find the patient below the occupational exposure limit - which as mentioned in *The Handbook of the Toxicology of Metals* is well known not to be a test of body burden - then refer the patient for counseling. Textbooks note that mercurialism is easily misdiagnosed as Parkinsonism, ALS or psychosis (Merritt 1995; Haddad, Shannon and Winchester 1998). The point is made very directly by Bradley (1996), "Mercury intoxication initially may be misdiagnosed as a number of psychiatric illnesses, especially since there are often no focal neurological signs or change in consciousness." Thus it is reasonable to assume that cases of mercury intoxication from nonoccupational sources will be uniformly misdiagnosed.

Typical laboratory findings alleged to go along with amalgam illness (Belsky 1998) are reduced CD8 T suppressor cell number, reduced NK cell number, aberrations in liver phase 1 and 2 metabolism of xenobiotics, toxic porphyria, elevated hair calcium and reduced HDL cholesterol. More are given in the diagnosis section of this book. Most of these findings have been demonstrated to be caused in laboratory animals (and a few in humans) by mercury exposure. Few physicians would think to order these tests in a prospective case of amalgam illness, nor would many accept abnormal results as suggestive of the diagnosis.

It is worth recalling that endocrinology textbooks make a point about misdiagnosis of adrenal insufficiency - especially since adrenal insufficiency is often one of the major factors in mercury poisoning. The early symptoms of adrenal insufficiency are fairly vague things like weakness, fatigue, inability to concentrate, irritability, periods of depression, and a sense that "something is wrong." The physician often decides that the patient is neurotic, and then chalks up later, more definitive symptoms to more neurotic behavior rather than thinking about their implications and ordering appropriate testing. Given that physicians frequently misdiagnose a common, well understood condition described in several textbooks as being all in the patient's head, then proceed to ignore further key complaints it is no wonder so few physicians respond appropriately to cases of chronic mercury poisoning.

Most side effects and adverse reactions are not found in controlled clinical trials. They are reported anecdotally after the materials are approved for general use. Indeed, the FDA makes forms to report adverse reactions widely available and encourages both physicians and patients to use them. The difficulty in identifying adverse reactions in controlled trials is the reason many drugs are approved and later withdrawn from the market.

People at risk for mercury poisoning - but not from amalgam

Hospital workers such as nurses (from thimerosal preserved solutions and antiseptics widely distributed through October 19th, 1998).

Doctors and nurses who work in an office where the mercury from a blood pressure meter was spilled in an exam room - especially a carpeted one.

Optometrists (from thimerosal preserved contact lens solutions widely used in the '80's).

Clinical laboratory workers (from thimerosal preserved reagents and solutions).

Dentists and dental assistants (vapor from amalgam and mercury used in the office and dropped in the office).

23

The janitor who vacuums the carpet at dental offices - especially ones with carpeted exam rooms.

Recipients of prolonged series of allergy shots (from thimerosal preservative).
Anyone who had a lot of topical antiseptic put on them (many hospital and medical office antiseptics other than alcohol also contained mercury).

People having spilled mercury (e. g. from broken thermometers or broken fluorescent light tubes) on their carpets at home or at work.

People having used merbromin (mercurochrome®) or merthiolate extensively.

People exposed to mercury obtained by children or adults to play with.

People who vacuum up broken thermometers, fluorescent light tubes, etc.

People exposed to mercury in their work.

People who work or live at the site of a former dental office or other mercury using facility if it was not properly decontaminated (which seldom occurs).

Factors contributing significant amounts of mercury in addition to amalgam:

Use of contact lens solutions containing thimerosal (most popular in the '80's, some continued well into the '90's).

Use of vaginal contraceptives preserved with thimerosal (manufactured and distributed through October 19th, 1998).

Thimerosal preserved hemmhoroid creams.

Thimerosal preserved lubricating gels.

Red tatoos (mercury sulfide is the red coloring agent).

Many additional health care products available at various times past which contained calomel, thimerosal, or other forms of mercury compounds.

What not to worry about

I discuss a wide variety of symtpoms, diseases, and frightening problems in this book. Don't worry that you will experience all of them! No matter how sick you get, you will in fact only experience a few of them. The ones that seem totally unrelated to what is happening to you actually ARE unrelated to what is happening to you. They are related to what is happening to SOMEONE ELSE, who has different genes and a different biochemistry. The book is full of ALL the things I know that can happen to ANYONE who gets mercury toxic. Nobody gets everything! Just pay attention to the parts that are relevant to you. Don't let the other parts scare you.

What mercury poisoning does to you

Description of chronic mercury poisoning

All of the following symptoms come and go. None of them are constant. The more poisoned someone is, the more frequently they will have the symptoms their own personal physiology makes them prone to. Due to individual variability different people will exhibit different symptoms, and any particular person may or may not ever have a specific symptom.

In an overall lifestyle sense, the fact that symptoms come and go leads to the victim having periods of weeks to years of being highly functional and productive, interspersed with periods of being nonproductive and having a hard time getting anything done. Life seems to progress in fits and starts. Great progress is made on projects which later get shelved for long periods. As the disease continues, the productive periods become shorter, fewer, and farther between.

The symptoms of chronic mercury poisoning mainly originate in the central nervous system. Immune dysfunction and gastrointestinal problems appear later with deranged liver metabolism. There may also be endocrine problems. There is seldom any evidence of the kidney problems which are present in acute poisoning.

There is no typical presentation - the clinical spectrum spans the range from imperceptible disturbance to complete incapacitation. Poisoning sets in slowly, and progresses as an ever changing picture of increasing dysfunction.

There are emotional changes in mercury poisoning. Depression slowly sets in. Victims feel fatigued and listless. They lack motivation - even for crucial tasks. They lose interest in their surroundings and in their own life. They do not enjoy life, or experience happiness or joy. They experience constant fear e. g. of losing their job. They may be very tense. They feel hopeless. They have a sense of impending doom. Every small problem is discouraging. Minor difficulties seem overwhelming and insurmountable.

The altered emotional state of a mercury intoxicated person leads to impaired interpersonal relationships. They become increasingly irritable and sensitive, reacting strongly to relatively innocent remarks. They may not be able to take orders, instructions, or suggestions without losing their temper. They resent criticism and may interpret innocent remarks critically. They may have an exaggerated response to stimulation and become fearful or anxious and nervous. They may project their fears and anxieties onto others, making inappropriate criticisms or attacks. They become shy and avoid dealing with strangers. While timid, they may unexpectedly lose self control with strangers. They may wish to visit with friends and family extensively, often wishing to engage in long, repetitive conversations, then withdraw for prolonged periods of time. They withdraw more and more from social contacts.

The emotional changes reduce the victim's ability to function day to day. The victims are often restless. They lack self control and have poor judgement. They are easily upset and embarrassed. They may become quarrelsome and neglect work and family. They have little patience. They lose their self confidence and become indecisive. Euphoria or manic-depressive type behavior sometimes occurs. Obsessive or compulsive behavior or thought patterns are common at later stages of intoxication. Delusions and even hallucinations are possible in severe cases.

Intelligence gradually deteriorates. Previously bright persons become dull and slow in thinking. They suffer from a progressive decline specifically affecting short term memory as well as the faculties for logical reasoning. Thus their ability to do things like balance the checkbook, do math, or play chess suffers. They lose the ability to concentrate. Memory problems may be more from distractability and inability to concentrate and pay enough attention to get things INTO their memory than an actual failure to remember things (thus they may complain of memory problems but do well on memory tests). They cease being motivated towards their work or other tasks. Thoughts become heavy, repetitive and pedantic. Creative thinking becomes progressively more difficult, eventually becoming impossible. They become unable to select the right words to convey their meaning, and make stylistic and grammatical errors. Their ability to express themselves declines progressively.

There is a distinctive cognitive symptom of being unable to think clearly without great effort. The best description for people who have not experienced it is of a hangover without pain. People who have experienced it will recognize the term "brain fog" as entirely descriptive.

As the victim's level of intoxication waxes and wanes they go through periods of life when they do or do not dream. Dreaming may be in black and white.

The victim's subjective experience of chronic mercury intoxication consists of irritability, excitability, fearfulness, restlessness, melancholy, depression, weakness, timidity, fatigue, indecisiveness and headache. Feelings of hopelessness, depression and futility are a part of the intoxication syndrome. The victim generally feel that their behavior patterns are rational, appropriate and well justified. The mental effects of mercury poisoning are distressing and frightening.

Early physical symptoms include dizziness, tinnitus (ringing in the ears), insomnia, daytime drowsiness, loss of appetite, a tendency towards diarrhea - often alternating with constipation, cold hands and feet, a tendency towards sweating (some people have the opposite symptom and do not sweat at all), flushing or reddening of the skin - particularly on the face and neck. Some people blush frequently, but others do not blush at all. Asthma is a symptom of chronic mercury poisoning. Digestive disturbances are also common.

The skin becomes dry, athlete's foot and toenail fungus progress, and the insides of the ankles, particularly behind the ankle bone and a bit above it become dry, itchy, flaky and peel. This often becomes painful and annoying enough to keep the victim up at night. Even after fungus and yeast infection has been eliminated hyperkeratosis, often with papular erythema and itching are common.

The hair becomes thinner, dryer, duller, less strongly colored, slower growing, and more brittle.

The biological clock is disturbed. Waking up late and staying up late is more common than being an "early bird." Try as they might, the mercury poisoned person simply cannot control their circadian rhythm.

Victims may become photophobic and find bright light uncomfortable and unpleasant.   There may be visual disturbances, including alterations in color perception leading to reduced sensitivity to the color red, or color blindness. The ability to focus on distant objects may be sporadically impaired. Peripheral vision may be reduced in the most severe cases.

The hands and feet often become distinctly cold. This can occur suddenly and is most distinctive when combined with sweating. Later in more severe poisoning they may also tingle or lose feeling.

The effects of mercury on the mouth are receding, sometimes spongy gums that bleed easily and teeth that are 'loose' in their sockets and can be wiggled very slightly. It also causes excessive salivation and unusually bad breath.

What mercury poisoning does to you

Mercury interferes with the sense of smell which becomes less acute, and later with hearing, in which perception of sounds does not diminish as notably as the patient's ability to understand and interpret them - e. g. to understand speech directed at them even though they hear it clearly.

Victims often experience discomfort that feels like a "tight band around their head." They may also experience sharp points of discomfort in their ear canals at bedtime.

Mercury also interferes with the body's ability to regulate temperature. Victims may alternate between being hot and cold when the temperature isn't changing, or have to wear more clothes than other people, or have more difficulty than other people in staying comfortable while the temperature changes. Temperature disregulation also leads to 'night sweats.'

There is also profuse sweating in most individuals, who then generally have moist skin. Some individuals (most often females) do not sweat much, or at all. In these people sweating will not be induced appropriately by heat or exercise.

Heart racing (tachycardia) is quite common. The heart rate may vary dramatically over a period of a few minutes for no apparent reason. Heart pain (angina) may occur. Doctors may hear intermittent heart murmurs and may find a flattened T wave or a prolonged QT interval on an EKG.

Women may have profuse menses with abdominal pains, may experience stinging pain in their ovaries, and may experience a sensation of rawness in their female parts.

An unusual edema (puffiness) of the face and legs may occur.

Mercury interferes with the endocrine system. The thyroid may be underperforming, which is most easily tested by taking the temperature in the morning before arising (for menstruating females, days 2, 3, and 4 of their period). Leave the thermometer in place for a long time (5 minutes or so) either under the arm or tongue. If the average temperature is less than 97.5 there are problems with thyroid hormone metabolism regardless of blood test results. Women also get a periodic check on their thyroid levels since their menstrual flow should be bright red if thyroid levels are normal and brownish if levels are low.

Another often unrecognized endocrine problem is excessive urination. More than 2.5 liters of urine per day - urinating more than 5 or 6 times per day - is abnormal. Awakening every night to urinate is also abnormal.

Subclinical adrenal hypofunction with symptoms suggestive of Addison's disease is common. These consist of weakness, fatigue, depression, weight loss, hypoglycemia, anxiety and low blood pressure.

If baseline adrenal function is adequate, high blood pressure may be part of the symptom complex, and the victim may experience continuous hunger.

Mercury also directly interferes with the body's ability to regulate glucose. Feeling tired 2-3 hours after meals, and craving a sweet which fixes the problem for a while are signs of hypoglycemia (whether it is due to adrenal problems or not).

Occasional hypogonadism is known and may be difficult to recognize in males.

Mercury causes immune disregulation. Victims often have difficulty fighting off minor illnesses, get sick more often, and have a more serious and prolonged illness than others who get the same thing (e. g. recurrent bouts of bronchitis). Immune disregulation can also lead to increased allergy, asthma and other respiratory complaints.

Allergy commonly expresses itself with asthma, sinus pain, itchy skin and fatigue, but not a runny nose. A nonliquid discharge slowly builds up in the nose. Itching is on exposed areas of skin and may be relieved by washing, which will also reduce fatigue.

Victims of chronic mercury poisoning have difficulty metabolizing alcohol and often give up drinking because they do not enjoy it, or feel terrible after a drink or two. If metabolic problems become severe, chemical sensitivity sets in.

Mercury (and other heavy metals) have their effects by taking up residence in the active site of certain enzymes where some other metal is supposed to be sitting. Thus these enzymes stop detoxifying pollutants and naturally occurring toxins and the victim becomes more sensitive to air quality, foods and chemicals. The victim may become a 'picky eater;' feel tired or depressed during periods of significant air pollution; feel bad after routine exposure to chemicals such as during photocopying, using bleach or chlorine containing scouring powders, or after painting, carpet, insulation or tile installation; and may experience skin irritation from clothes washed in many detergents, or from washing themselves with some soaps or lotions. Ultimately victims may develop "multiple chemical sensitivities" or "environmental illness." The most typical sensitivity is anxiety on exposure to hydrocarbons as in paint fumes, exhaust, etc.

Mercury interferes with oxygenation of the blood. Rapid breathing and achiness as if exhausted will often occur when there has been no recent exertion. Being unusually cold and unable to generate body heat to warm up often goes along with this panting. Supplementary thyroid hormone will relieve this muscle aching, fatigue, and being out of breath even when all laboratory tests for thyroid function are normal.

Mercury affects the blood coagulation mechanism and leads to easy bruising and bleeding in some people.

Mercury poisoned people may acquire a distinctive body odor which can be described as colostrumlike or as milky sweet.

On defecation, mercury toxic people may feel they are not done and have not passed the whole stool when they have.

A feeling of weakness occurs in the upper arms. It occurs on that part of the upper arm and shoulder that is on top if the arms are held out to the sides. The feeling of weakness actually occurs on the part of the upper arm between the biceps and triceps - there is no muscle there to BE weak, but the feeling is very distinctly localized in that area. The actual muscle that causes the weak feeling movements is the top portion of the deltoid on the shoulder.

Fine muscle tremors eventually appear. These can include twitching of the eyelids, as well as poor coordination of the lips and tongue rendering speech indistinct, unclear and more difficult to understand. Speech may also be tremulous and halting. Tremors in the fingers, eyelids, and lips appear before tremors elsewhere. Tremors in the arms interfere with tasks requiring good finger coordination - handwriting becomes unsteady and ultimately illegible, straight lines cannot be drawn, and the execution of other precision work deteriorates. Tremors occur in the legs last. These are 'intention' tremors which disappear during sleep and become more pronounced during stress as the victim tries to control them. These tremors are coarser and less regular than those observed in hyperthyroidism. They consist of fine tremors which may be interrupted every few minutes by coarse, jerky movements. The tremors begin in the fingers, with the ring and middle finger first, and are less severe when familiar tasks are performed. Tremors eventually cause muscle spasms and difficulty in walking. Seizures eventually occur.

Coordination affects the eyes as well. The ability to focus the eyes and to control the iris progressively deteriorates, as does convergence - the ability to bring both eyes to bear on nearby objects so as to see one of them with depth perception rather than to have double vision. Eventually the muscles that move the eye become weak and the victim turns their head to see up, down, or side to side instead of turning the eyes.

One sign of this coordination loss is difficulty dialing phone numbers accurately, or repeated errors when entering long strings of numbers on the keypad, or reduced typing skills.

Acrodynia is a rare syndrome found in children exposed to elemental mercury or inorganic mercury compounds. It is characterized by severe leg cramps, irritability, paresthesia (a sensation of prickling on the skin), and painful pink fingers and peeling hands, feet, and nose. Similar symptoms are seen in some adults, particularly those who are chemically sensitive.

Mercury poisoning has a sexually dimorphic effect. Men more frequently become quietly depressive and withdrawn, while women more often become anxious, shy, fearful and high strung.

In certain circumstances mercury poisoning may be recognized in the earlier 'acute' phase. For example, after placement of fillings which extend below the gumline, after placement or replacement of several fillings, after placement of a dissimilar metal crown or bridge over or against amalgam. Of course, other occult exposures may also cause acute mercury poisoning. In this earlier phase there may be blood cells in urine, greatly elevated urinary porphyrins leading to pink - not red-tinged - urine, burning urination, as well as the above symptoms. Very high exposure levels cause nausea, loss of appetite and diarrhoea. In general acute poisoning leads to much more pronounced physical symptoms and much less pronounced mental and emotional symptoms or endocrine changes.

Complication by other toxins

Mercury intoxication is often complicated by lead or arsenic. Nickel is usually elevated in hair samples from amalgam illness victims but does not appear to be a toxin in most of them. However, exposure is ubiquitous. Some symptoms more characteristic of these may help determine whether they are involved, or are the primary toxin.

ARSENIC:

Behavioral symptoms: The victim experiences great anguish, and often has an agonized expression on their face. Restlessness leads the victim to change locations frequently. There is much generalized fear - most notably of death and of being alone. Victims are frightened, worried, and selfish. They may curse, rave, and act viciously. They may be self injurious and suicidal.

The victim has fearful dreams. The victim sleeps with their hands laid beyond the pillow, "above" the head, rather than on or under the pillow cradling their head, or by their body.

Victims drink burning hot liquids. They crave acids and coffee, as well as milk. They need a high protein diet. Women may have an unusually short menstrual cycle. Victims tend to be sleepy a lot, and to have gastrointestinal problems that eventually lead to malabsorption and food allergies. They also suffer a lot of headaches.

Specific symptoms that have been observed in severe chronic arsenic poisoning at a substantially greater incidence than in other ill populations are: tender or painful feet, pins and needles in the toes and feet, numbness and tingling of the legs and feet, pain in the hands, weakness of the fingers, periods of being unable to stand, and peeling skin.

There are no distinctive laboratory test abnormalities for arsenic. It does not appear in urine or blood once exposure has ended, nor in hair for more than a few months thereafter. The most relevant test is a lipoic acid challenge, which does not have well standardized results to interpret it. Thus the diagnosis of arsenic versus mercury or arsenic plus mercury versus mercury alone must be made on the basis of signs and symptoms.

LEAD:

Gout, glaucoma, paleness, weakness and drooping of the wrists and ankles, wasting of the shoulder girdle muscles, low sex hormones (with the corresponding pituitary hormones elevated, unlike for mercury where both pituitary factors and hormones are relatively low), fear of being murdered. The victim will feel worse at night, and better during exercise.

The victims will also have a lot of gastrointestinal pain (colic) and gas.

There are many laboratory test abnormalities that are distinctive for lead poisoning that can be used to see how much of a problem lead is versus mercury for a particular person. Results in the high end of the normal range are significant for a person who also has some mercury in them because lead and mercury are synergistic in their effects.

COPPER:

The behavioral effects of copper poisoning are indistinguishable from those of mercury. The symptoms of copper poisoning are readily confused with those of mercury and there are no distinctive differences. Blood, hair or urine elements distinctively show high copper in the presence of poisoning, and do NOT show other patterns characteristic of mercury.

How mercury hurts you

Mercury catalyzes oxidation of important parts of your body. The part it messes up the most is the membranes around and inside cells. It sticks to sulfhydryl groups that are present on membranes. Then it catalyzes oxidation of the unsaturated compounds in the membranes. This destroys the essential fatty acids that your body can't replace. It also destroys the phospholipids (like phosphatidylcholine and phosphatidylserine)

that hold the membrane together. Since the membrane is damaged, it does not perform its function of passing signals along properly so lots and lots of messages your body needs to pass around become garbled. This is why it affects the brain so severely - the message center of your body is the most sensitive to garbled messages. This is also why it affects the endocrine system so much - your hormones are really part of a complicated communications system that carries messages around to make your body do the appropriate physiological thing.

Mercury also oxidizes the proteins inside your cells. These hold the cell together, keeping things like your DNA in the right place, they are enzymes that catalyze reactions, and they are receptors that receive signals. Many enzymes work because they hold a particular metal atom in their "active site" so that it is in just the right place to catalyze the particular reaction that enzyme causes. Mercury likes to sit in these active sites, so it kicks the proper metal atom out and deactivates the enzyme.

By catalyzing oxidation, mercury also creates free radicals that attack your DNA and mutate it. These mutations make your cells work less efficiently, and if enough happen, the cells die, or worse yet turn cancerous.

Mercury concentrates in and near a part of your brain called the hypothalamus. The hypothalamus is responsible for your memory, moods and emotions, and how your hormones, breathing and heartbeat work. It also concentrates in your liver, which is responsible for getting rid of natural and synthetic chemicals in the food you eat and from other sources. Mercury is also absorbed by the immune system, and makes it attack innocent bystanders like pollen or your body parts instead of the bacteria and viruses it is supposed to fight.

You can protect yourself against mercury by taking antioxidants to prevent the damage it is doing, essential fatty acids and other things that sit in membranes to repair the damage, and chemicals with lots of

What mercury poisoning does to you

sulfhydryl groups for the mercury to hold on to so it can be excreted from your body.

Mercury does its damage when it gets inside cells - particularly the cells of your brain. Your cells have membranes that are good at keeping the mercury out - or in. So when you are exposed to it for a short while, nothing happens. Most of it stays outside your cells. When you are exposed for a long time, it slowly leaks into your cells and fills them up. Then you are in trouble. But it doesn't come out very fast, so a physician who checks for mercury in your blood or urine without understanding the physiology of mercury will think you are just crazy - after all, there isn't much mercury there and he knows that people get exposed to much more mercury for short periods of time and are fine!

How your body handles mercury

Let me describe the various forms of mercury. There are a lot of them and they interchange a lot.

Inorganic mercury is the nasty stuff that actually hurts you. It is Hg^{++}.

If you swallow inorganic mercury, you don't absorb it very well.

Metallic mercury is Hg^{o}. The liquid metal, which is not dangerous if swallowed (amazingly). Metallic mercury is also the vapor form.

The vapor is dangerous because your lungs absorb it and it goes all over your body where your metabolism oxidizes it to the nasty, dangerous Hg^{++} inorganic stuff that hurts you. Even though this oxidation happens fast, a lot of the mercury gets into your brain before it gets turned into Hg^{++}.

Organic mercury is RHg^{+} where R is some carbon thingie like a methyl group (-CH_3). So methylmercury is CH_3Hg^{+}. Your intestines absorb this form of mercury really well.

As long as it STAYS in organic form, mercury is actually not toxic!

Unfortunately, your body slowly converts it to the nasty toxic inorganic form and there is nothing you can do to stop that. So once you eat some organic mercury you get mercury poisoning from it.

The inorganic form has a hard time getting from your body into your brain.

The vapor form and the organic form get into your brain easily. Then they can be oxidized to the inorganic form and mess your brain up.

You pee out Hg^{++} but not RHg^{+}.

You poop both of them out.

Fish protect themselves from mercury by having enzymes that methylate it. That is why fish can have lots of mercury in them and be healthy. But mammals don't do this, so if they get any form of mercury in them it is bad.

If mammals like us end up with organic (e. g. methyl) mercury inside they get poisoned, but they don't have problems right away because the organic mercury is safe - the problems start when their bodies turn it into poisonous inorganic mercury.

Mercury shows up in sick people

Here are a few examples of mercury showing up where physicians never thought it would:

Mercury reduces thyroid function (Barregård et al. 1994) and is concentrated in thyroid cancer tumors (Zuichik, Tsyb and Vtyurin).

Mercury is concentrated in heart tissue from people with heart disease (Fruscati et al.)

31

Amalgam Illness: Diagnosis and Treatment

Nakagawa found that hair mercury was vastly elevated compared to the general population in people with a wide variety of diseases, strokes, diabetes, high blood pressure and senile dementia.

Mercury lowers the intelligence of children and makes them emotionally disturbed (Marlowe *et al.*).

Physiology in outline

This section gives you a VERY brief and VERY abbreviated outline of a few physiological concepts that are helpful in understanding the rest of the book. A little knowledge is a dangerous thing - more complete information can be found in other sources.

Hormones tell your body to do a whole set of things that all go together. Be a man (testosterone). Be energetic (thyroid). Mobilize resources that can be used to fix things up (cortisol - by breaking down certain tissues). Etc.

Figure 4 shows you what the various hormones do, and how they are controlled by the brain and interact with each other. This is described in words below.

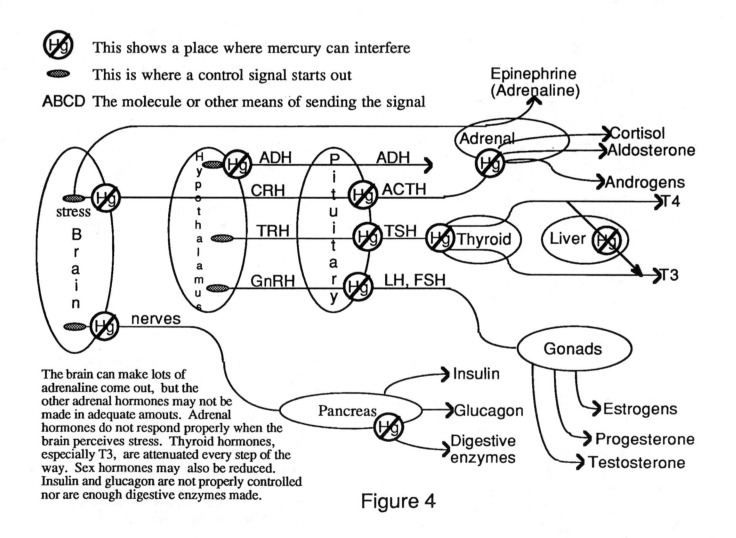

(Hg⃠) This shows a place where mercury can interfere

⬭ This is where a control signal starts out

ABCD The molecule or other means of sending the signal

The brain can make lots of adrenaline come out, but the other adrenal hormones may not be made in adequate amounts. Adrenal hormones do not respond properly when the brain perceives stress. Thyroid hormones, especially T3, are attenuated every step of the way. Sex hormones may also be reduced. Insulin and glucagon are not properly controlled nor are enough digestive enzymes made.

Figure 4

What mercury poisoning does to you

Hormone	Effect on: Mood	Muscles	Immunity	Heart	Liver	Appetite
cortisol	be cheerful, clear headed, able to concentrate	increase epinephrine sensitivity, send amino acids to liver	turn inflammation and allergy down	increase epinephrine sensitivity	increase epinephrine sensitivity, make sugar from amino acids	+
(nor)epinephrine	anxiety, fear or aggression	be strong now!	Don't do anything!	beat fast!	make sugar now!	-
thyroid T3	have a happy bright outlook	build up, be energetic			speed up phase 1 and 2	+
thyroid T4	none			beat hard, fast		+
androgens	feel good, confident, sexy	get BIG and STRONG	calm down	be strong	make taurine	+
estrogens	PMS	make fat instead	increase inflammation	be sensitive	speed up phase 1	
progesterone	feel good	build up	reduce inflammation			
insulin	take up sugar for energy	take up sugar for energy		be sensitive	store sugar	
glucagon		have energy			release sugar	
digestive enzymes		Digest protein to make muscles with	destroy food antigens - no allergies			+

Some hormones work by attaching to special proteins on the surface of cells to deliver their message. Others go into the cell, bind to special hormone receptor proteins, then these proteins go into the nucleus and activate DNA so it makes more of the right proteins (or less of the wrong ones). Hormones that go through the receptor-DNA-protein route are steroids like the sex hormones and cortisol, as well as thyroid hormone. Most other hormones use cell surface receptors, for example, growth hormone, IGF1 and 2, insulin, adrenalin, antidiuretic hormone, and all the hypothalamic and pituitary factors.

Mercury can interfere with the production of a hormone, the way it interacts with its receptor, or the way the receptor makes things happen in the cell. Lab tests usually determine the amount of hormone present but do not check whether the receptors are OK and whether things respond properly to the presence of the hormone. Sometimes you will have low hormone function, or excess function, even when the few parts of the cycle the lab can measure look fine. Because of this, good doctors will sometimes have you try a medicine for a while and see how you respond even if the lab tests don't show you need it.

Thyroid hormone tells your body to make more proteins, burn up more energy, be more sensitive to the signals of OTHER hormones, and get things done! Too little and you slow down until you sit there like a bump on a log. Too much and you burn energy until you are as thin as a scarecrow by bouncing around like the ball in a pinball machine.

Androgens are the "male sex hormones," such as testosterone or androstenedione. They are steroid hormones. These actually are very important for women, too, though in smaller amounts. Androgens make both men and women have muscles, want sex, and have other functions. Androgens are mildly immunosuppressive and cause tissue growth and healing.

There are two kinds of "female hormones." Estrogens and progesterone. These are steroid hormones. They have different functions in women's menstrual and reproductive cycle. Estrogens make women's skin fuller and make women have more fat - mostly in appropriate locations. Progesterone relaxes smooth muscle - low levels lead to cramping, irritable bowel syndrome, asthma and hypertension.

The adrenal glands make the steroid hormone cortisol (also known as hydrocortisone). This tells the body to break tissue down, make more blood sugar and amino acids available, raises cAMP levels by inhibiting the enzyme that breaks it down, reduces inflammatory immune reaction, increases blood pressure, elevates mood and causes weight gain. These types of hormones are called glucocorticoids. There are many synthetic ones used as medicines, such as prednisolone, which is stronger than the natural ones.

Cortisol is released in response to signalling from the brain by the messenger hormone ACTH. Cortisol can be released in the wrong amounts if the adrenal gland is diseased or if the pituitary does not release the right amount of ACTH, or if the hypothalamus does not release the proper amount of CRH which is what tells the pituitary to release ACTH. The pituitary and hypothalamus are parts of the brain, and the hypothalamus is where all the nerve (e. g. emotional) signals are turned into chemical signals. It is difficult to test for whether the right amount of cortisol is being released because the body has such varying needs for it and the "normal range" for lab measurements is quite wide. To make matters worse, cortisol naturally goes up and down quite a lot during the day - high in the morning, falling in the afternoon to low values in the evening.

Another steroid hormone the adrenal gland makes is aldosterone. It is a mineralocorticoid. It regulates the balance of sodium and potassium (and to some extent magnesium) in the body. This balance is messed up if the adrenal gland or the kidney are diseased.

Figures 5 and 6 show the steroid hormones that are made by your adrenal glands and gonads. Figure 5 is the easy to follow figure since I have only put the steroids on it that do something important or that you can buy. Figure 6 has all the steroids named on it with more detail of what they do in case you run into them in other things you read.

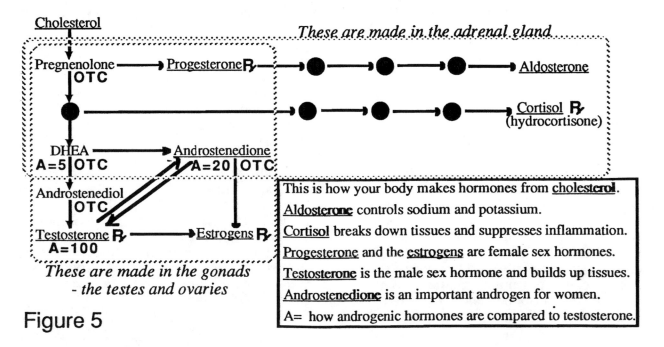

Figure 5

These are made in the gonads - the testes and ovaries

This is how your body makes hormones from cholesterol.
Aldosterone controls sodium and potassium.
Cortisol breaks down tissues and suppresses inflammation.
Progesterone and the estrogens are female sex hormones.
Testosterone is the male sex hormone and builds up tissues.
Androstenedione is an important androgen for women.
A= how androgenic hormones are compared to testosterone.

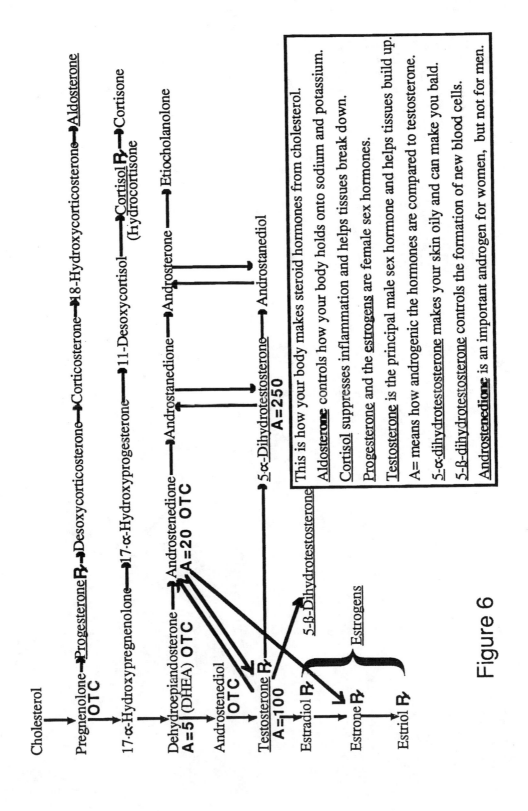

Figure 6

Growth hormone tells the liver to make insulin like growth factors 1 and 2 (IGF-1 and IGF-2). These tell the rest of the body to make or repair tissue. IGF-1 is also called Somatomedin C, or SM-C.

Amino acids are the building blocks proteins are made from. They have other uses as well. They can be turned into glucose for energy or neurotransmitters to run the brain or nervous system.

There is a family of amino acids called the "sulfur amino acids." Some are available in the diet. The body has enzymes that turn one into another in a specific sequence. These amino acids and their later products are used in the body (and sulfite is fairly toxic). The different enzymes can get blocked by mercury causing a 'logjam' at some step of the process. The metabolism of the SAA's is shown in figure 7 below:

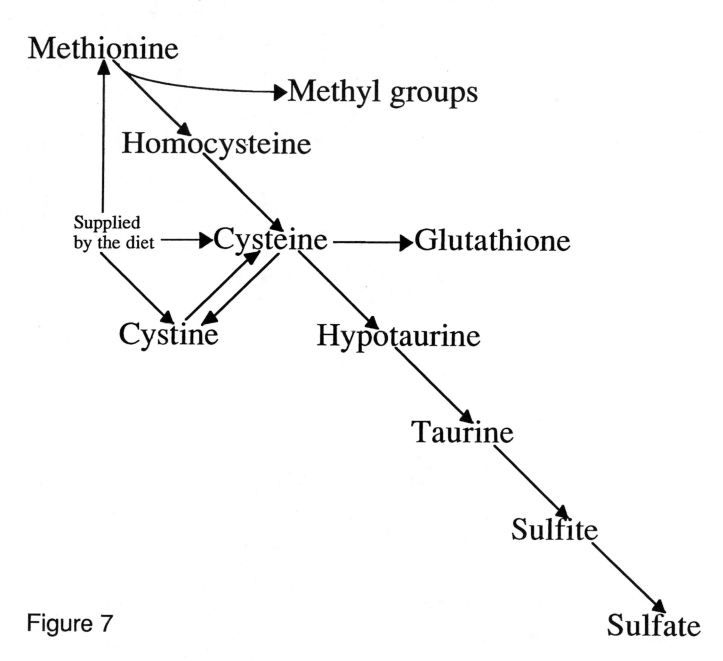

Figure 7

What mercury poisoning does to you

Essential fatty acids help keep cell membranes working properly, and are also used to make some special signalling molecules used by the immune system to create and control inflammation. Some EFA's are precursors to signalling molecules for MORE inflammation, while other ones are precursors to signalling molecules for LESS inflammation.

The metabolism of the fatty acids is shown below. Figure 8 gives a simple explanation suitable for most purposes. Figure 9 provides a more complete description in case you want to read up on the technical details yourself.

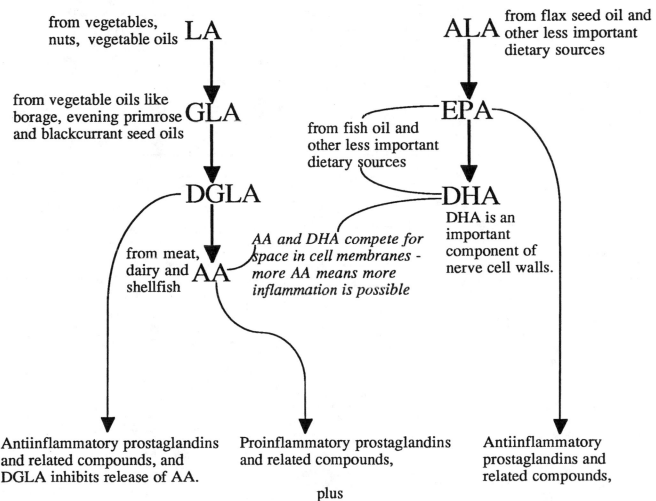

from vegetables, nuts, vegetable oils **LA**

ALA from flax seed oil and other less important dietary sources

from vegetable oils like borage, evening primrose and blackcurrant seed oils **GLA**

EPA

from fish oil and other less important dietary sources

DGLA

DHA

AA and DHA compete for space in cell membranes - more AA means more inflammation is possible

from meat, dairy and shellfish **AA**

DHA is an important component of nerve cell walls.

Antiinflammatory prostaglandins and related compounds, and DGLA inhibits release of AA.

Proinflammatory prostaglandins and related compounds,

plus

Prostaglandin I2 which induces formation of thyroid and adrenal hormones and also prevents heart attacks, strokes, and lowers blood pressure. The formation of this is reduced by lipid peroxides which mercury catalyzes the formation of.

Antiinflammatory prostaglandins and related compounds,

plus

a prostaglandin which inhibits the conversion of AA to proinflammatory compounds

Figure 8

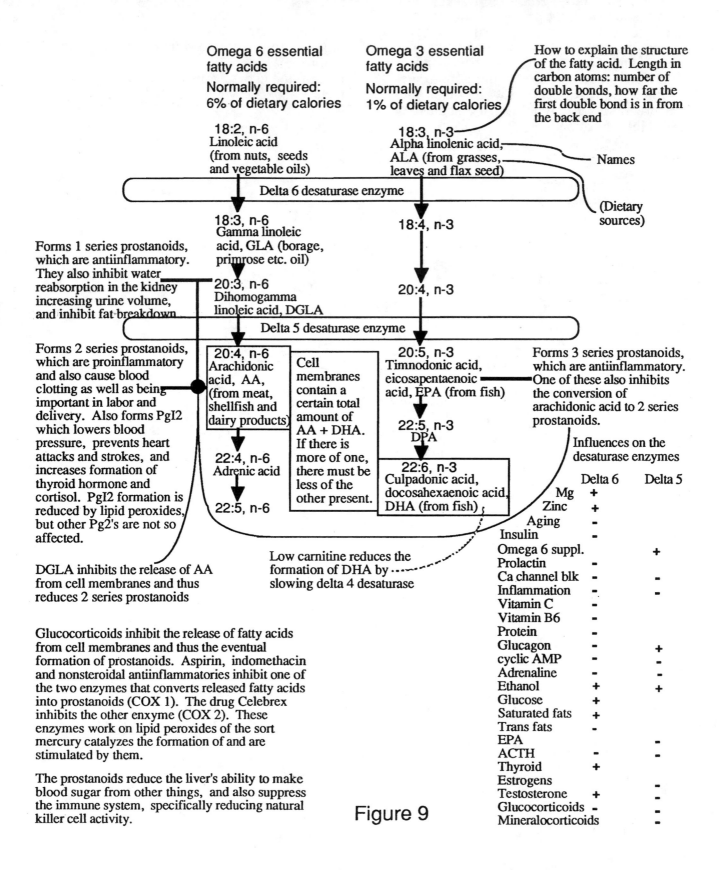

Omega 6 essential fatty acids

Normally required: 6% of dietary calories

Omega 3 essential fatty acids

Normally required: 1% of dietary calories

How to explain the structure of the fatty acid. Length in carbon atoms: number of double bonds, how far the first double bond is in from the back end

18:2, n-6
Linoleic acid
(from nuts, seeds and vegetable oils)

18:3, n-3
Alpha linolenic acid, ALA (from grasses, leaves and flax seed)

Names

Delta 6 desaturase enzyme

(Dietary sources)

18:3, n-6
Gamma linoleic acid, GLA (borage, primrose etc. oil)

18:4, n-3

Forms 1 series prostanoids, which are antiinflammatory. They also inhibit water reabsorption in the kidney increasing urine volume, and inhibit fat breakdown

20:3, n-6
Dihomogamma linoleic acid, DGLA

20:4, n-3

Delta 5 desaturase enzyme

Forms 2 series prostanoids, which are proinflammatory and also cause blood clotting as well as being important in labor and delivery. Also forms PgI2 which lowers blood pressure, prevents heart attacks and strokes, and increases formation of thyroid hormone and cortisol. PgI2 formation is reduced by lipid peroxides, but other Pg2's are not so affected.

20:4, n-6
Arachidonic acid, AA, (from meat, shellfish and dairy products)

Cell membranes contain a certain total amount of AA + DHA. If there is more of one, there must be less of the other present.

20:5, n-3
Timnodonic acid, eicosapentaenoic acid, EPA (from fish)

Forms 3 series prostanoids, which are antiinflammatory. One of these also inhibits the conversion of arachidonic acid to 2 series prostanoids.

22:4, n-6
Adrenic acid

22:5, n-3
DPA

22:6, n-3
Culpadonic acid, docosahexaenoic acid, DHA (from fish)

Influences on the desaturase enzymes

22:5, n-6

DGLA inhibits the release of AA from cell membranes and thus reduces 2 series prostanoids

Low carnitine reduces the formation of DHA by slowing delta 4 desaturase

	Delta 6	Delta 5
Mg	+	
Zinc	+	
Aging	-	
Insulin	-	
Omega 6 suppl.		+
Prolactin	-	
Ca channel blk	-	-
Inflammation	-	-
Vitamin C	-	
Vitamin B6	-	
Protein	-	
Glucagon	-	+
cyclic AMP	-	-
Adrenaline	-	-
Ethanol	+	+
Glucose	+	
Saturated fats	+	
Trans fats	-	
EPA		-
ACTH	-	-
Thyroid	+	
Estrogens		-
Testosterone	+	-
Glucocorticoids	-	-
Mineralocorticoids		-

Glucocorticoids inhibit the release of fatty acids from cell membranes and thus the eventual formation of prostanoids. Aspirin, indomethacin and nonsteroidal antiinflammatories inhibit one of the two enzymes that converts released fatty acids into prostanoids (COX 1). The drug Celebrex inhibits the other enzyme (COX 2). These enzymes work on lipid peroxides of the sort mercury catalyzes the formation of and are stimulated by them.

The prostanoids reduce the liver's ability to make blood sugar from other things, and also suppress the immune system, specifically reducing natural killer cell activity.

Figure 9

What mercury poisoning does to you

Cell membranes have all kinds of receptors on them for signalling molecules and also control the flow of things into and out of cells. There are also membranes INSIDE the cell that control how things get passed between different compartments. Cell membranes are made out of special fat molecules the body builds up out of phosphate or amino acids, glycerol, and various fatty acids. The way cell membranes do various things is shown in figure 10.

Neurotransmitters are substances that the brain and nervous system uses to convey messages. There are many different kinds of neurotransmitters and each has one general kind of message it conveys. Acetylcholine: lets you pay attention. Adrenaline: Makes you alert! Serotonin: calms you down. GABA: relaxes you. These neurotransmitters are also released into the body to talk to the different immune system cells. A few are also used as hormones - most notably adrenalin, which comes from the adrenal glands. Adrenaline makes you excited, alert, anxious, etc. and also increases blood sugar and does some (but not all) of the other things cortisol does. Most neurotransmitters increase a basic physiological response but the exact effect can be situational. Alertness due to adrenaline usually causes anxiety but might cause excitement, e. g. during sporting competition.

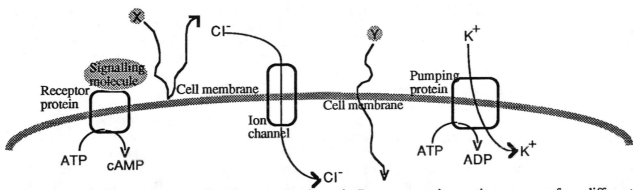

ATP is an energy providing molecule cells can use to do work. Receptor proteins receive messages from different signalling molecules in the blood and make second messenger molecules inside the cell to tell it what to do. cAMP is a second messenger. Many different external signalling molecules might make the same second messenger. Ion channels let certain ions diffuse in and out of the cell. Pumping proteins use energy to move molecules into or out of the cell as desired. Some molecules, like X, cannot diffuse through the cell membrane on their own. Others, like Y, can.

Figure 10

Adrenaline is made by methylation of noradrenaline, which is made from dopamine (another neurotransmitter), which is made from the amino acid tyrosine, which is in turn made from the amino acid phenylalanine. Dopamine adrenaline and noradrenaline are destroyed after use either by methylation or by the enzyme monoamine oxidase (MAO).

Adrenaline and noradrenaline are "popular" or old fashioned names. The current correct names are epinephrine and norepinephrine.

Melatonin (the sleepy time hormone) is made from serotonin, which is made from 5 hydroxytryptophan (available as a nutritional supplement), which is made by the body from the amino acid tryptophan.

Water balance is controlled by how much you drink and how much you urinate. There is a hormone, called antidiuretic hormone, ADH, or sometimes vasopressin, that controls how much you urinate. It is released by the pituitary gland after being made in the hypothalamus. How much you drink is controlled by the hypothalamus.

Most hormones are controlled by the hypothalamus and pituitary. These are a part of your brain. The hypothalamus puts together the signals from your brain with how much hormone it remembers being around recently and sends special releasing factors to the pituitary, which combines how much of these releasing factors it receives with how much hormones it has been exposed to recently and releases stimulating factors. The stimulating factors from the pituitary make the endocrine glands let out appropriate amounts of hormones. If the glands don't work, the stimulating factors become very high, lab tests show this and it is easy to diagnose the problem. If the pituitary or hypothalamus doesn't work well it is very difficult to figure out what is going on and how much hormone your body really needs.

The liver converts all the millions of different poisonous things in the food we eat into a few chemicals the body likes. It also stores up sugar and amino acids to let out into the blood when you haven't eaten for a while. It also makes bile, which helps you digest fats. The liver excretes some toxic compounds into the bile to get rid of them, since they go into the intestine and the toxins then go out with the feces.

Both phase 1 and phase 2 consist of a number of parallel paths. There is significant crossover between what goes down which paths among the phase 1 enzymes and limited crossover among the phase 2 enzymes.

Premenopausal and, in particular, pregnant women have on average about 1/3 faster phase 1 metabolism by one of the families of enzymes (CYP3A, especially CYP3A4) than do men or postmenopausal women. This may account for the apparent greater likelihood for women to develop multiple chemical sensitivities. Age, health, individual genetics and many other unknown factors also influence the rate and manner with which phase 1 and 2 metabolism occurs in any particular person.

Certain drugs induce or inhibit phase 1 metabolism. Also, there are drugs which are metabolized by phase 1 reactions (or certain phase 2 reactions) which produce much higher or lower than expected blood levels in people with abnormal phase 1 metabolism. E. g. carbamazepine induces phase 1 enzymes which clears it faster. Valium and Klonopin are cleared by phase 1 enzymes but don't induce them. Supplements and drugs can be used to speed up or slow down phase 1 metabolism, providing great benefit to the patient.

Figures showing phase 1 and phase 2 metabolism for some pathways are shown in figures 10 and 11.

There are a number of things that induce, inhibit or are metabolized by phase 1 enzymes but it has not yet been determined exactly WHICH of the isozymes is involved:

Phase 1 inducers:

Acetate, carbon tetrachloride, BHT, BHA, sulfonamides, dioxin, exhaust fumes, high protein diets, niacin, oranges, organophosphorus pesticides, paint fumes, riboflavin, sassafras, saturated fats, tangerines, cisplatin, doxorubicin HCl, felbamate, primidone, broiled foods, the amino acid histidine (in large amounts), schizandra, ginseng, licorice.

Phase 1 inhibitors:

omeprazole, oral contraceptives, amphetamines, bacterial endotoxins, iron deficiency, naringenin, quercetin, heavy metal toxicity, clarithromycin, danazol, dilitazem, troleandomycin, lorstatidine, terfenadine, niacinamide, valproate, verspanol, sugar excess, partially hydrogenated fats, the amino acid tyrosine (in substantial amounts), stirpentol, remacidine, acetazolamide, macrolide antibiotics, metronidazole, verpramil, danazol, dextropropoxyphene.

These are not complete lists.

What mercury poisoning does to you

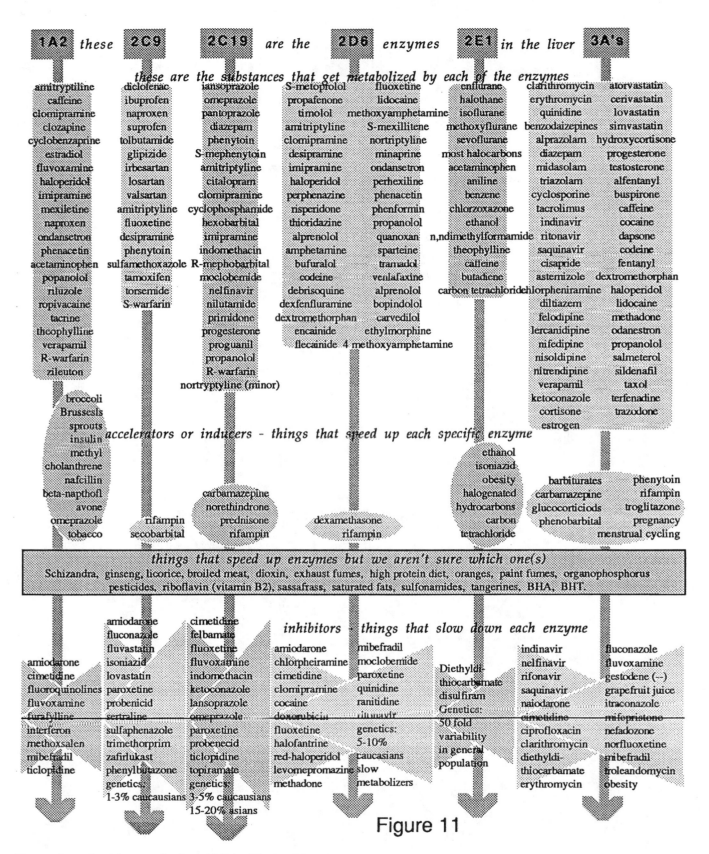

Figure 11

Reproduced with permission of David Flockhard, MD

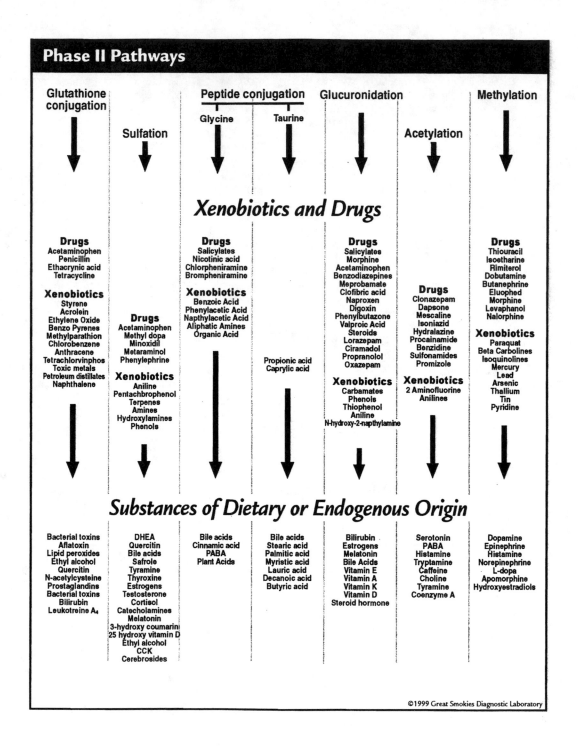

Reproduced with permission of Great Smokies Diagnostic Laboratories

What mercury poisoning does to you

If any of the phase 2 pathways is slow the compounds that pass through it can build up to toxic levels in you. Phase 2 pathways can be speeded up by supplementing the substrates or by other means.

Phase two pathway	How to increase phase two rate
Glutathione conjugation (mercapturation)	Increase glutathione levels[1], provide cofactors with supplements[2].
Sulfation	Increase sulfate availability via supplementation of sulfate and molybdenum.
Glucuronidation	Reduce insulin resistance with chromium, provide cofactor supplements[2], increase thyroid levels, reduce inflammation (inflammation lowers rate).
Glycination and taurine conjugation	Supplement glycine or taurine and cofactors[2].
Methylation	Supplement methyl donors[3].
Acetylation	Primarily genetic control.
Hydrolysis of epoxides	Primarily genetic control.

[1] Take 4 parts NAC to 2 parts glutamine or glutamate to 1 part glycine between meals.

[2] Any mercury relevant supplement program will do this.

[3] Trimethylglycine (TMG), choline, lecithin, SAMe, (methionine not recommended due to homocysteine formation and the need to restrict sulfur foods in some individuals) and to mobilize the methyl groups vitamin B-12 and folate.

The digestive tract breaks down food into its components, absorbs them, but leaves all the useless stuff and all the bad nasty stuff like bacteria behind, and sends the good stuff to the liver in the bloodstream.

The way the liver controls amino acids and blood sugar is shown in figures 12 and 13 - one is for about 2-3 hours after you ate a meal, and the other is for the rest of the time.

The mitochondria are special compartments inside each cell (except red blood cells) that convert blood sugar or fat into energy by burning them with oxygen.

The blood is an organ. It carries oxygen, nutrients, and the immune system around. All those different kinds of white blood cells are a big part of your immune system. The blood also makes clots to keep everything from leaking out of holes that accidentally get made in you.

As well as controlling all the hormones, the hypothalamus also controls mood, emotion, remembering, eating, and sleeping.

There are many different metabolic transformations that require methyl groups. Some of these get rid of bad chemicals, some turn one useful chemical into another, and some control how DNA is used by marking portions of it. We can't synthesize methyl groups from anything else so we have to get them from things in the diet, such as methionine, choline, etc.

Enzymes are proteins that our body uses to catalyze chemical reactions it needs to perform. Many enzymes have a metal in a special place that is needed to make the reactions go. If a metal gets stuck in there that doesn't belong, then the enzyme doesn't work. Many heavy metals are poisonous because they stick to enzymes this way and prevent essential metabolic processes from being catalyzed.

Eating enzymes doesn't do any good if we need them in our body instead of in our stomach and intestines. The digestive tract exists to make sure that proteins like enzymes get destroyed and don't make it into our bloodstream.

Figure 13: metabolic energy transfer right after eating

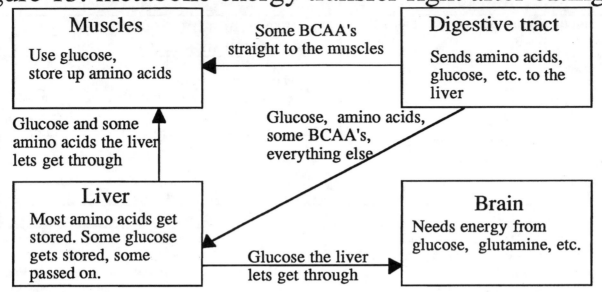

Figure 14: metabolic energy transfer after digestion

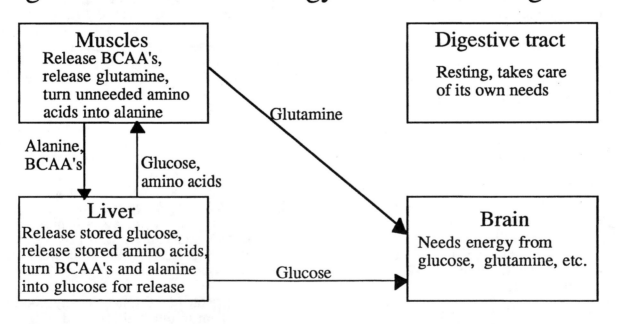

Cortisol is needed to release amino acids and convert them to blood sugar.

BCAA's are Branched Chain Amino Acids. These are leucine, isoleucine and valine.

Free radicals are produced in the mitochondria by burning oxygen to make energy. They are produced by certain immune system cells to destroy invaders. They are toxic and destroy the basic chemicals that compose our cells by oxidizing them - for example, messing up essential fatty acids in cell membranes. Free radicals are carefully controlled in our body and we have lots of natural antioxidants to keep them in control. Many toxins, mercury being one, catalyze the formation of extra free radicals.

The immune system has a fascinating variety of ways to recognize and kill harmful cells and viruses. One of them is to make antibodies. Another is to have special cells go around to fight invaders. There is a bunch of very sophisticated but poorly understood signalling that happens in the body to tell the immune system what to do.

Your immune system has a large number of different kinds of cells. Some of them are: CD4+ or T helper cells which activate macrophages and control the proliferation of T and B cells, CD8+ or T suppressor cells which go out and kill cells they are sensitized to, CD19 or B cells which make antibodies and attack bacteria, NK or natural killer cells which kill virus infected or cancer cells without having to be sensitized first, neutrophils which kill yeast[1] and other "bad" cells, macrophages which activate T cells by presenting antigens to them and also go attack "bad" cells. These kinds of cells are the white blood cells that get counted in a complete blood count. If you don't have enough NK cells you will suffer recurrent viral infections because cells that harbor viruses don't get killed. If you don't have enough CD4+ T cells you become susceptible to all kinds of infections as is seen in AIDS. Antigens are the parts of the invading cells that the immune system recognizes, and that antibodies bind to. The immunoglobulins, IgA, IgE IgG and IgM are antibodies. They neutralize enemies or target them for attack. The effects of mercury on the immune system

---

[1] Mercury directly interferes with neutrophils killing yeast.

have been reviewed by Pollard and Hultman as well as Eneström and Hultman.

The physiological effects of mercury intoxication

This is my outline of ways mercury can affect the metabolism. It is intended to provide an overview so that people can get a perspective on what may be going on in order to facilitate supportive diagnosis and treatment during the rather prolonged detox period. This is intended as an OUTLINE, which simply MENTIONS and CATALOGS things.

BRAIN

Chronic mercury intoxication affects the hypothalamus, and through it the endocrine system, mood, hunger, memory, autonomic nervous system, the heartbeat, sweating, temperature regulation and circadian rhythm. In more serious cases the pituitary may also be affected and hormone releasing factor levels reduced.

The third cranial nerve which controls most of the muscles in the eye comes out of the brain just at the hypothalamus and becomes poisoned too.

Senses:

Sight - light sensitivity and focus difficulties, difficulty converging both eyes on close objects, difficulty moving the eyes to track things. Color sensitivity also impaired.

Smell - impaired.

Taste - impaired.

Hearing - tinnitus. Difficulty parsing words. Difficulty picking things out of background noise.

Balance - significantly impaired.
Emotion - emotions both change in nature and are somewhat flattened. This leads to impaired interpersonal relationships,

emotional volatility, sensitivity to innocent remarks, difficulty trusting people, difficulty understanding what people really intend to do, shyness, timidity, withdrawal, and extreme procrastination.

Intellect - slower, duller, impaired memory. Short term memory is by far the worst hit, leading to absent-mindedness.

Dopamine is elevated, and the dopamine D_2 receptor is also stimulated by mercury. Schizophrenia like behaviors are reasonably expected. Pituitary TSH secretion is stimulated and may for a while make up for thyroid gland poisoning.

Endocrine - central control of endocrine functions is impaired (e. g. CRH and thus ACTH and thus cortisol falls in response to stress instead of rising like it is supposed to). Temperature regulation is also impaired. Hunger may not match physiological requirements. Urine output may be excessive because of low vasopressin release.

Autonomic nervous system - inappropriate sweating or lack of sweating, cold hands and feet with eventual tingling pain and numbness due to blood vessel spasms leading to Raynaud's phenomenon, heart racing, etc.

ENDOCRINE GLANDS

Mercury concentrates selectively in endocrine and nervous tissue.

Thyroid - Affected by direct mercury concentration, reduction in PgI_2 synthesis because of unsaturated fatty acid peroxides (PgI_2 is a signalling molecule used by the thyroid). Dopamine D_2 receptor stimulation lowers TSH response to TRH slightly. Peripheral conversion of T4 to T3 is also impaired. Since the pituitary uses its own enzyme for this conversion, TSH may be normal in the face of overt peripheral hypothyroidism which must then be diagnosed on the basis of physical signs and symptoms.

Adrenals[1] - Affected both by direct mercury concentration, reduction in PgI_2 synthesis due to unsaturated fatty acid peroxides (PgI_2 is a signalling molecule used by the adrenal), and by aberrations in steroid synthesis. People with hypoadrenalism will have low blood pressure. Those with a paradoxical adrenal stress response but high average levels of cortisol have normal or high blood pressure but respond poorly to stress. In adrenal insufficiency, the senses of smell, taste, touch, and pain sensitivity are substantially increased.

Gonads-Affected by reduced pituitary output of LH/FSH, as well as by direct concentration of mercury, and by aberrations in steroid synthesis. Androgens affect immune function. NB, in females, about half of androgens are formed in the adrenal in response to ACTH, so hypoadrenal females will also be hypoandrogenized.

Adrenal and gonadal steroids are made from cholesterol, and these problems may be worse if cholesterol is low due to liver problems.

Pancreas - exocrine. Insufficiency of pancreatic digestive enzymes is common. This may also lead to food allergy, malabsorption, etc.

Pancreas - endocrine. Aberrations in insulin and glucagon metabolism may cause hyperglycemia, hypoglycemia, reactive hypoglycemia, etc. as well as overall weight gain in some individuals.

ENDOCRINE INTERACTIONS

The endocrine system has many sophisticated feedback loops which must be

---

[1] Cortisol has a wide dynamic range and substantial circadian variability, so the standard tests of adrenal function miss most of the problems mercury toxic people have. Discussion of how to use cortisol profiles (4 samples in a day) or stress tests is given later in the book. Physical signs and symptoms must be the ultimate guide since laboratory tests are not completely reliable.

kept in mind to understand its response to disease and therapy.

Low thyroid levels lead to low overall cortisol levels plus ACTH hyperresponsiveness to stimuli. When coupled with an ACTH fall on stress, this leads to an extremely difficult to control circadian rhythm with a base level of poor overall physical and social performance with unpredictable miraculous accomplishments, and subsequent withdrawal or collapse.

Adrenal insufficiency can also downregulate thyroid hormone production, possibly due to a lack of beta adrenergic receptors which are made in response to cortisol.

As thyroid levels rise, serum binding of cortisol increases and cortisol requirements rise. Thus, in mixed hormone deficiency, replacing thyroid first (or alone) can worsen adrenal insufficiency.

Cortisol increases beta adrenergic sensitivity in all tissues. This increases heart rate, relaxes the lungs, releases lipids from fat cells, amino acids from muscle, and blood sugar from the liver when adrenaline is released.

Cortisol causes the enzyme glutamine synthetase to be made. This enzyme is necessary to clear ammonia from the brain.

Thyroid hormone increases overall sensitivity to catecholamines, which includes beta adrenergic sensitivity. It also increases the general rate at which all neurotransmitters are produced.

Estrogens increase sex hormone binding globulin and thus decrease free androgen levels.

Thyroid increases sex hormone binding globulin, and androgens increase thyroid binding globulin. Thus increasing one decreases levels of the free form of the other.

Growth hormone increases the conversion of T4 to T3, the active form of thyroid hormone.

The beta blocker propanolol reduces the conversion of T4 to T3. Increased beta adrenergic sensitivity (e. g. from cortisol, thyroid) increases conversion of T4 to T3. Beta agonist medicines (asthma medicines) increase the conversion of T4 to T3.

Carbamazepine increases the conversion of T4 to T3.

These must be kept in mind to understand both the expected response of an individual to the primary effects of mercury intoxication on their personal physiology and to understand the multiple changes that may take place in response to hormone therapy.

ORGANS

Liver - phase 1 and 2 metabolism of xenobiotics (foods and drugs) may be impaired. Liver inflammation and damage may result, as well as intoxication by poorly metabolized compounds.

Heart - reduction in co-q-10 content leads to poor energy production and utilization. Enhanced radical generation leads to ischemia and atherosclerosis. These lead to angina and increased risk of heart disease.

Gastrointestinal tract - has a high affinity for mercury. Acute toxicity (e. g. caused by inappropriate administration of chelating agents) concentrates mercury in the GI tissues and may lead to digestive disturbances, yeast overgrowth, malabsorption, etc.

Malabsorption - has systemic consequences. Appropriate supplementation may be difficult. Low serum triglycerides and cholesterol are signs of malabsorption.

Leaky gut - causes immune sensitization to food components.

Kidneys - targets of acute toxicity. Lower back pain in the area of the kidneys is highly unlikely to be due to kidney problems.

Muscles - primarily affected by impaired oxidative phosphorylation.
May be weak from adrenal insufficiency (a good test for chronic adrenal insufficiency), and may waste due to malabsorption. Muscle protein may be mobilized to provide energy in hypoglycemia. Cortisol is needed to allow muscle protein to be broken down to provide energy, so adrenally insufficient people are often very thin, weak, but appear muscular.

Connective tissue - target of certain autoimmune problems mercury may cause, such as rheumatoid arthritis, lupus, etc.

Skin - will typically be dry and prone to infection and inflammation due to mercury induced oxidation of cell membrane EFA's. Hypothyroidism also makes the skin thin and weak. Elevated cortisol (as seen in people with elevated average cortisol but paradoxical stress response) also thins the skin.

Lungs - Prone to inflammatory response from mercury induced oxidation of EFA's. Intractable or frequent respiratory infections are common in the earlier phases of mercury poisoning because of immune suppression. Asthma may be induced directly by alternations in signalling molecule function or indirectly by allergy induction. Bronchial spasms may also be due to low progesterone.

Circulatory system - mercury favors arteriosclerosis.

Blood - Mercury interferes with red blood cell oxygenation. This may be partially corrected by epinephrine and its analogs. Mercury also interferes with clotting, leading to easy bleeding and bruising.

CELLULAR SIGNALLING

Excess lipid peroxides interfere with the formation of PgI_2, which is used by the adrenal and thyroid to make more of their respective hormones in response to appropriate signals. Thus these two glands will be more suppressed than the other endocrine glands. PgI_2 is also known to be helpful in ameliorating strokes and heart attacks, so one may presume that reduced PgI_2 because of mercury increases the risk and severity of these. PgI_2 causes vasodilation, reduces blood pressure, and is part of tonic blood pressure control.

Mercury stimulates the dopamine D_2 receptor, which is involved in psychotic disorders. This stimulation probably causes some of the emotional changes associated with mercury intoxication. It is also reasonably expected to specifically suppress pituitary secretion of PRL and TSH, and to generally lower pituitary function.

This excessive stimulation causes headache, increased appetite and stomach upset (dopamine is what signals that the stomach is full). The body deals with this excessive stimulation in one of two ways: receptor downregulation or dopamine decrease, which causes receptor upregulation.

Downregulated people need large amounts of stimulants to function, can take supplements in large quantities, must take care to taper off supplements and medicines when stopping them.

Upregulated people become allergic and sensitive to everything, often need high amounts of supplements but must start at low levels and increase them slowly.

While all this upregulation and downregulation happens, TSH and prolactin bounce all over the place.

Mercury directly interferes with the enzyme adenlyate cyclase, which forms the second messenger cyclic AMP, used in perhaps half of all cellular signalling pathways to transduce the signal. Thus the "gain" is turned down in the nervous and endocrine systems and everything has a reduced and "flatter" response to stimulation.

What mercury poisoning does to you

By reducing membrane essential fatty acids, mercury reduces the amount of material available to form the prostaglandins, thromboxanes, leukotrienes, etc. which are important anti and pro inflammatory signalling molecules. Prostaglandins are important in the regulation of smooth muscle contraction. Hence asthma, blood pressure disturbances and dysmennhorea occur due to disturbances in their metabolism. Fibromyalgia may be due to an imbalance in the different kind of prostaglandins formed. Prostaglandins also increase body temperature in fever, and their lack is implicated in certain cases of schizophrenia, so low EFA's might result in reduced body temperature and schizophrenia like behaviors.

Acetylcholine levels are reduced (possibly due to D_2 receptor stimulation). This causes difficulty in voluntary muscle contraction, vagus nerve reduction of heart rate, memory and cognition (cholinergic agents help in alzheimer's disease), regulation of mucus secretion, and regulating the iris of the eye.

Some people respond to reduced acetylcholine levels by upregulating their M1 muscarinic acetylcholine receptors. This makes the processes that particular receptor participates in adequately sensitive to the small amounts of remaining acetylcholine to continue to function. These people will react poorly to acetylcholine boosters like DMAE. They will usually benefit greatly from methylating agents like SAMe. Thiamine desensitizes the M1 acetylcholine receptors and brings them back into balance with the other receptors. One of the things the M1 receptors do is inhibit sweating, so such people often will not sweat (the proper medical term is anhydrosis). It also causes arachidonic acid release, so such people will have high levels of leukotrienes and proinflammatory prostaglandins. Arachidonic acid in turn increases acetylcholine levels, so such people can end up in a positive feedback loop which renders them hypersensitive. They often have multiple chemical sensitivities, and are sensitive to supplements at extremely low doses.

Metabolism to form dopamine, epinephrine, and norepinephrine is often deranged one way or the other, so emotional and sometimes somatic disturbances related to these are common. Men and women use norepinephrine quite differently[1] and this difference may relate to the apparent greater prevalence of anxiety and fear in mercury toxic women.

Tryptophan metabolism may be affected, making serotonin and melatonin levels inappropriately high or low.

Steroid synthesis is affected, changing the ratios of the various steroids made in the body. Steroids are involved in cognition and mood as well as controlling anabolism, catabolism, and secondary sexual characteristics in the body.

Glucose uptake is enhanced by mercury, leading to hypoglycemia and sometimes weight gain. Chromium supplementation[2] appears to correct this for unknown reasons.

MITOCHONDRIA

The effects of mercury on the mitochondria are not understood in detail. However it appears that chronic mercury intoxication has much of its effect by poisoning the mitochondria and inhibiting their ability to perform oxidative phosphorylation appropriately coupled to the body's needs. Partly this is overall poisoning, partly it is poisoning of specific pathways which then become sensitive to common dietary components (e. g. partially hydrogenated fats), and partly it may be due to ineffective intracellular signalling.

---

[1] the details of these differences are not well understood. However it is known that men make a lot more NE than women, and that fat mobilization in men depends slightly on E and strongly on NE, but in women it is entirely controlled by E and NE has no effect.

[2] as given in the treatment discussion. The dose is about 200 mcg of chromium picolinate with each meal, plus some extra for about 1,000 mcg per day.

Amalgam Illness: Diagnosis and Treatment

MOLECULAR PATHOLOGIES

Glucose (blood sugar) transport and metabolism is impaired by a number of mechanisms.

ATP formation is impaired.

Essential fatty acids (EFA's) are oxidized excessively rapidly.

Cholesterol is elevated early in the disease process, and later falls.

Metabolic use of many vitamins is impaired, requiring supplementation at high levels.

The conversion of the thyroid hormone T4 to the active form T3 is impaired because the enzyme which performs this transformation has selenium at its active site. Mercury has an exceptionally high affinity for selenium. Some tissues use circulating T3 and some make their own, so some tissues will be hypothyroid in the face of apparently normal circulating levels of T3.

The synthesis of porphyrins is impaired, resulting in difficulties making enough hemoglobin for red blood cells, the enzymes that make energy in mitochondria, and the enzymes that detoxify chemicals in the liver.

Phase 1 and 2 metabolism in the liver are impaired. Fast phase 1 leads to multiple chemical sensitivities (MCS). Fast phase 1 and slow phase 2 is very dangerous and leads to severe MCS.

Amino acids - plasma levels of assorted amino acids may deviate from what is expected due to mercury affects on many parts of the metabolism. This may affect the downstream parts of the metabolism that use that amino acid. Taurine may be high or low (low leads to anxiety plus reduced bile secretion which impairs digestion plus poor kidney health). Phenylalanine and tyrosine may be low (or possibly high) affecting melanin, thyroid hormone, and the neurotransmitters dopamine, norepinephrine and epinephrine. Tryptophan may be high or low affecting melatonin and serotonin. Glutamine may be low leading to "crazy thoughts." Histidine may be low, leading to low histamine, which may lead to psychotic thought processes in some individuals, and means that the immune system's inflammatory response will be impaired leading to chronic activation of other parts of the immune system. High histamine (via high histidine) may lead to excessive inflammation, anaphylaxis, and also to psychotic thought processes. Low GABA may lead to agitation or impaired sleep. GABA elevates dopamine. In this context, "high" and "low" must be interpreted relative to the average of all other amino acids in their "normal ranges," rather than only in the literal sense of being outside the normal range. It is important to remember that everyone is different in a basic biochemical sense, and some people's bodies may actually be in proper balance with a surprisingly high or low level of a particular amino acid - but most people aren't, and if everything is all over the place, something is definitely wrong.

Mineral balance may be impaired. Hypomagnesemia, hypo or hyperkalemia and sometimes hyponatremia are seen.

Fat mobilization and deposition - mercury can interfere both directly with fat mobilization by inhibiting cAMP formation, and indirectly with it by stimulating insulin receptors. Some mercury toxic individuals gain weight easily on reasonable diets. These may be the ones with adequate day to day levels of adrenal hormones.

Enzyme inhibition - many enzymes are inhibited by mercury. This is the root of the pathological process. Since it interferes in a fundamental chemical way with a wide variety of enzymes, the effects of mercury on a given individual are highly variable since they depend on the sensitivity of the specific allele of each enzyme that particular person has in his or her genes.

Sulfite oxidase and related enzymes are often impaired. Can lead to sulfite sensitivity, sulfite-like reactions to sulfur containing foods if the enzymatic bottleneck is at this particular enzyme, and also may limit the amount of sulfate available for phase 2 metabolism of xenobiotics.

Cytochrome P450 system - the heart of the phase 1 metabolic processes, oxidative phosphorylation, and also of steroid biosynthesis. Mercury inhibits the different enzymes in this system to different extents.

Cysteine dioxygenase is one of the CYP450 enzymes that makes hypotaurine (which becomes taurine) from cysteine. Mercury inhibition of this enzyme will lead to low taurine which can only be corrected with taurine supplementation, as well as high cysteine which must be controlled by dietary restriction.

Taurine elevates dopamine which elevates insulin and can cause reactive hypoglycemia.

Mercury inhibits several enzymes which metabolize acetylcholine.

Methylation is usually inhibited by mercury. It is responsible for handling of fats and cholesterol as well as for many other important biochemical reactions. Methylation is accelerated by folate, B6, B-12 and methyl donors. Methionine is the natural methyl donor, but in those who have elevated cysteine methionine must be restricted because it metabolizes to cysteine via homocysteine. Choline, trimethylglycine, etc. are also methyl donors and can be substituted for methionine. Elevated homocysteine due to dietary methionine intake without other methyl donors and with blocked cysteine metabolism can lead to vastly accelerated atheroschlerosis.

The catecholamine neurotransmitter pathway is phenylalanine ---> tyrosine ---> dopamine ---> norepinephrine ---> epinephrine is the metabolic pathway to make neurotransmitters from the amino acids phenylalanine and tyrosine. The conversion of norepinephrine to epinephrine requires methylation.

Tryptophan --> 5 hydroxytryptophan (5HTP) --> serotonin --> melatonin is the metabolic pathway to these neurotransmitters.

Steroid synthesis can be deranged in mercury intoxication.

Mercury selectively catalyzes the oxidation of cell membranes. This destroys essential fatty acids and membrane constituents like phospatidylserine and phosphatidylcholine at an accelerated rate. The alteration in membrane components interferes with cellular signalling, interferes with cell function, renders the cells more susceptible to oxidative stress, and favors other pathological processes. Phosphatidylserine deficiency in particular impairs short term memory and when severe causes depression.

IMMUNE SYSTEM

Mercury at "acute" or 1 year post dental work levels can lead to overall immune suppression which causes recurring respiratory infections, etc.

Mercury changes the ratio of T helper to T suppressor cells so as to increase sensitization to antigens. This causes allergies to develop.

Mercury interferes with cellular immunity, so that virus infected cells are not killed - hence viral infections are hard to clear and go on for long periods. Natural killer (NK) cells are reduced and it is these cells that kill cancer cells, so mercury presumably increases susceptibility to cancer.

Mercury changes the ratios of the various kinds of antibodies produced. Thus there may be excessive production of some classes and underproduction of others (IgG 1 and 3, and sIgA often being underproduced) leading to susceptibility to certain infections.

MERCURY METABOLISM DURING TREATMENT

It is observed that your body handles mercury in the following manner when you are being treated for amalgam illness. When you became poisoned, all of your organs got filled up with mercury. Your blood was also filled up with mercury. But the cell membranes keep mercury from going back and forth between the blood and organs very rapidly.

Once your source of mercury exposure is removed, e. g. your amalgam fillings get replaced, your bloodstream clears of mercury and your urine and blood mercury decline during the first several months. Then your organs start to dump their mercury out. Your blood and urine mercury go back up again. This is in contrast to what is seen with most people in research papers that studied subjects who were tolerant of mercury and worked in mercury using businesses. Your subjective symptoms also track this process, declining at first and then getting worse again. Using chelating agents properly can greatly reduce this second phase of suffering and leave you much more able to get on with your life. This is shown in figure 15 below. Note that you will be at your worst about 6 months after amalgam removal if you stop using chelating agents after you start to feel good 2-3 months out.

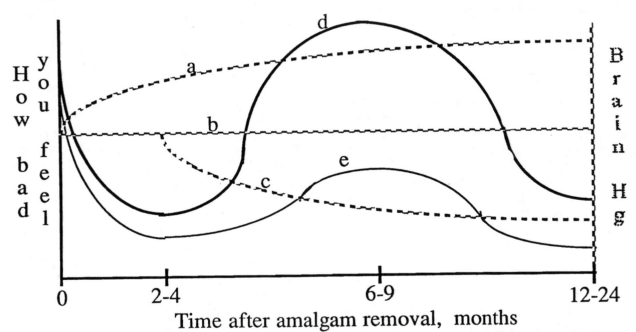

a) brain mercury using DMSA every other day chelation schedule, or large amounts of chlorella or "sulfur foods." b) brain mercury using no chelation or DMPS injections every month. c) brain mercury using DMSA every 4 hours on alternate weeks for 3 months, then DMSA + LA every 3-4 hours for 3 days per week. d) subjective sensation of sickness not chelating or using DMSA every other day or monthly DMPS injections or chlorella or "sulfur foods." e) subjective sensation of sickness using DMSA then DMSA+LA.

Figure 15

COPPER METABOLISM

Copper is mentioned here because there are a variety of poorly described abnormalities of copper metabolism that appear very similar to amalgam illness, and also because copper interacts with mercury - in amalgam illness it is best to keep copper somewhat low.

Absorption: copper is absorbed from the intestines. Zinc and molybdenum reduce absorption.

Excretion: in normal individuals 96% of copper is excreted in the bile and 4% is excreted in the urine. In the rare condition Wilson's disease, there is no biliary copper excretion and individuals eventually become copper toxic on a normal dietary intake. Biliary excretion may be deranged in other uncharacterized syndromes. Lipoic acid dramatically reduces the biliary excretion of copper, and increases urinary excretion. The transport protein ceruloplasmin is involved in some not understood manner in the biliary excretion of copper.

The protein metallothionein is involved in the storage, handling and excretion of copper. Metallothionein production is increased by vitamin D and cortisol, and is intimately tied in with zinc metabolism - zinc takes up sites in the metallothionein as well as causing more of it to be produced, so more zinc will help most but not all people. Selenium often creates more free sites in the metallothionein that hold onto copper.

Transport: copper is bound in serum to the transport protein ceruloplasmin. Low levels of ceruloplasmin are found in Wilson's disease. Nonfunctional forms of this protein may be involved in uncharacterized syndromes.

Distribution: in copper intoxication syndromes, copper will be elevated in red blood cells, in other tissues not generally accessible for analysis (e. g. liver and brain), in hair and possibly in urine. It may be normal in serum. There may or may not be some copper excretion in the feces via the bile.

Do you have it? How to diagnose mercury poisoning

What to do if you can't get medical help

You may find a chiropractor, naturopath, acupuncturist, etc. who is more than able to help you. Indeed, in some states standard allopathic medical tests like blood tests and urine tests can be ordered by people other than physicians. And remember, I wrote a book about ALLOPATHIC medicine. Many people practice OTHER kinds of medicine (acupuncturists, chiropractors, doctors of oriental medicine) and have OTHER kinds of tests that I don't discuss here because I am not familiar with them. The most important thing to use these tests for is to make sure you don't have a copper problem instead of amalgam illness.

Assuming you either can't get such help, or want to make your own decision anyway:

The best place to start is to read the description of mercury poisoning thoroughly. Does it describe you?

Next, spend some time making a lifetime health and dental history and getting all the possible sources of mercury exposure into it. Revisit it several times until you are sure it is complete. Do new problems start in the year or two after a lot of dental work?

You can do your own "physical exam."

You can take certain measurements, like span to height and 24 hour urine volume and basal body temperature.

You can try a 'sulfur food' exclusion diet for a week and see how you feel.

You can do the diagnostic checklists for symptoms.

You can get old medical records and see if there are any relevant test results in those which can be used on the diagnostic checklist.

With all of these you can get about as good an idea as any physician would have of whether you are mercury poisoned. It will take you somewhat longer and you will have to think harder, but it won't cost any money. Unlike you, however, a physician will have a good idea of what ELSE you might have. S/he may also be able to guess which tests will be very informative to run.

First, do no harm.

Note: the "DMPS challenge" is not a legitimate diagnostic test since over half the population will give a positive result but most of them do not appear to have amalgam illness. In addition there is a high incidence of adverse drug reactions during it, including permanent disability and death. It should never be used. DMSA challenge tests that involve the administration of 500mg - 3g of DMSA as a single dose are also dangerous and not diagnostic. More appropriate challenge tests are described elsewhere in this book for certain very specific, limited indications. No challenge test is truly diagnostic or truly safe. DMPS and DMSA challenge tests measure the amount of mercury in the kidneys. The amount of mercury in the brain is the important quantity - but of course you can't determine it using a DMPS challenge test or any other way. The best you can do is check everywhere else in

Do you have mercury poisoning?

the body and make the best guess you can using the diagnostic procedure below.

For the cost of one "DMPS challenge," several tests which actually are diagnostic can be run, such as hair element analysis, fractionated urine porphyrins (through a reputable laboratory such as MetaMetrix) and an appropriate blood chemistry panel or a blood count.

The "DMPS challenge" is sometimes referred to as the "Dimaval® challenge." Dimaval® is the trade name of Heyl brand DMPS in capsules for oral administration, sold in Europe but not available in North America. Most "Dimaval® challenges" are not in fact conducted with Heyl brand Dimaval or the equivalent parenteral formula, DMPS-Heyl®.

Note that as of May 1999, DMSA is an FDA approved drug in the United States and DMPS is an investigational new drug, not yet fully approved.

How to diagnose chronic mercury poisoning

As discussed in greater detail above, urine and blood levels of mercury are not diagnostic for chronic mercury intoxication[1] since they do not correlate with the amount of mercury in the internal organs - especially the brain. Thus other, less direct tests must be used to measure the effects of mercury on the physiology and metabolism to determine if a person has chronic mercury poisoning. High

[1] They are diagnostic for, and are intended to be diagnostic for, acute intoxication where there was a single recent exposure. In that case the target organ is the kidney and it will not suffer damage if blood and urine levels are below those given in standard toxicology textbooks. As discussed in the most recent editions of Cecil, Harrison's and Merrit's these levels are not diagnostic in all cases. Indeed perusal of clinical papers describing mass poisonings typically shows that even in acute cases some people may suffer serious morbidity who are known to have ingested large amounts of mercury, yet who have blood or urine mercury levels below the "toxic" cutoffs.

levels of blood or urine mercury (they correlate well, there is no need to measure both) definitively establish that the person is mercury poisoned and something must be done, but this is rare. Low levels do not exclude mercury poisoning and should not be relied upon to do so.

In an acutely poisoned person, once blood and urine mercury levels have been reduced to reasonable levels, the problem still remains as to whether they were acutely poisoned long enough to have CHRONIC poisoning where their internal organs are affected. Thus the following diagnostic procedure comes into play in acute intoxication as well.

Any diagnosis starts with a thorough understanding of the symptoms of the condition in question, and of related conditions. These have been given earlier. A practitioner very familiar with chronic mercury poisoning and related conditions may be able to make an accurate diagnosis based on observations at two or three appointments. Such a clinical approach may be appropriate for some patients, though it is difficult to conclusively exclude copper poisoning without at least one test. For other patients laboratory testing is appropriate both to document the condition and to identify exactly what physiological problems exist so they can be corrected promptly.

Most patients who believe they have amalgam illness will have had some other diagnosis given them by previous physicians. Thus the diagnostic effort begins as a problem in differential diagnosis. In the simplest case, some anomaly is apparent from the patient's record or on work up that excludes the prior diagnosis. It will more often be the case that the earlier diagnosis cannot be directly excluded, but must be shown to be an element of the overall condition. This is best done by careful examination and history taking so as to thoughtfully order tests that will identify abnormalities the earlier diagnosis should not cause. The earlier diagnosis in effect becomes the diagnosis of exclusion if mercury intoxication cannot be demonstrated.

Great care must be taken to actually exclude mercury poisoning! In the counting exercise it is best not to include tests done in support of the prior diagnosis, but rather to limit testing and counting to that subset not explored earlier. Alternatively, a large fraction of the suggested tests must be performed, and tabular evaluation used as described in the appendix to perform a differential diagnosis of mercury intoxication versus the prior diagnosis and any other appropriate candidate conditions.

The most likely condition other than mercury poisoning that has similar symptoms and is likely to be missed by large numbers of mainstream physicians is copper poisoning due to problems with copper metabolism. Unlike mercury poisoning this is easy to diagnose with proper tests. Copper will substantially elevated - well above the normal range - in hair, urine and red blood cells. It can be at any level in serum, and may not be significantly elevated in whole blood (if serum is zero and RBC's are twice normal). Copper is often somewhat elevated due to excessive supplementation and this may be due to a supplement another health care practitioner provided and the patient may not be aware it has copper in it. Since the patient's memory is also impaired (a symptom of both copper and mercury poisoning) copper supplementation must be discussed more than once.

Diagnostic checklist for mercury intoxication

In practice, most diagnoses of chronic mercury intoxication will be done by a practitioner not yet experienced or confident enough to do it based on signs and symptoms alone, and will require extensive documentation in your (the patient's) records. A checklist based approach can be used. The rigorous mathematical foundation for this procedure is given in an appendix.

The following is a checklist of test results found to often be abnormal for patients with chronic mercury poisoning, plus signs and symptoms that are uncommon enough among the general population to be useful for

statistical diagnosis. These signs, symptoms, prior diagnoses, and "minichecklists" each count as an "abnormal test result" in the later counting procedure, and in terms of their rarity in the general population.

The intuitively most convincing diagnosis is arrived at by finding distinct abnormalities that are apparently unrelated - unless mercury poisoning is causing them, of course.

Tests which are part of standard screening panels plus those suggested by the patient's signs and symptoms should be performed. If the patient directly suggests tests it is worthwhile discussing these with the patient and ordering them (or tests more appropriate to determine what the patient thinks needs to be measured if the patient does not understand the exact significance of each laboratory test). Patient test requests should be considered because the patients are often unusually sophisticated by the time they discuss amalgam illness with their physician. The likelihood that tests requested by the patient will show abnormalities is much higher than under ordinary circumstances. It can be very helpful for the doctor to talk with the patient about what they are trying to discover with the requested test because ordering a different but related test may be more likely to find it out.

START WITH HISTORY AND DISCUSSION:

1) Anhydrosis (not sweating)

2) Body temperature on awakening averages <97.5°F (2-4 days after end of menstrual period for females)

3) Women, repeated history of amenhorrea

4) Unusually early or late puberty:
Men, signs of puberty before 9th birthday, or no signs of puberty before 15th birthday. Women, first menstruation before 9 or after 15 1/2.

5) Intermittent blurred distance vision

Do you have mercury poisoning?

6) Tiredness after showering

7) Fibromyalgia

8) Chronic Fatigue

9) Any two of: bleeding gums, tender teeth, metallic taste, blisters or sores in the oral cavity.

10) Any three of: sore or irritated throat, loss of appetite, headache, inability to concentrate, dizziness, muscle tremors, chest pains, exactly one item checked in the list above.

11) Any five of: allergy, bad breath, diverticulosis, diarrhoea and constipation, intestinal cramps and pains, fatigue, muscles tire easily, sciatica, leg cramps, joint pains, cold hands and feet, tachycardia (heart racing), one item only checked in the two lists above, or count twice if exactly two items are checked in the two lists above.

12) Any four of: anxiety, tension, depression, forgetfulness, shyness, being easily embarrassed, and count irritability twice.

13) Angina in someone younger than 45

This history taking counts as twelve tests for men, thirteen for women.

PROCEED WITH PHYSICAL EXAMINATION:

7') Perform examination for fibromyalgia[1] if relevant

14) Unusual brunescence of the crystalline lens, or opacities, characteristic of someone 20-30 years older - especially if taking substantial amounts of antioxidant vitamins

15) Findings suggestive of third nerve damage, such as mydriasis, convergence insufficiency, poor accommodation, poor eye mobility, etc.[2]

16) Marked proptosis (bug eyes), or eye changes typical of thyroid disease

17) Crossing changes of the veins and arterioles in the retina characteristic of unexpectedly advanced arteriosclerosis or corneal arcus for age (during optometric exam), or excessively elevated total cholesterol (>270) per blood chemistry lab test

18) Men, arm span / height > 1.00 or height to pubic symphysis / height > 0.500

19) Desquamation on hands, feet or ankles, or notable exfoliative dermatitis or hyperkeratosis on hands, feet or ankles

20) Exceptionally dry skin

21) Markedly poor balance

22) Unusual tics or twitches of the facial muscles

23) Prolonged QT time or T wave flattening on EKG

This examination counts as ten tests for women, eleven tests for men. On items involving a qualitative factor the clinician

---

[1] Pressure applied to 18 tender points on the body (charts available in many publications and on the web) results in pain at 11 or more of them.

[2] Best evaluated by a behavioral optometrist during examination of binocular vision performance. This cannot be evaluated after the pupils have been dilated. Ophthalmologists may not be familiar with this type of examination - it is best to ask optometrists for a referral to a colleague who specializes in behavioral optometry and vision therapy. Symptoms you may experience if you have convergence insufficiency are late day/afternoon headaches, headaches while doing close work, double vision or letters appearing to have shadows or swimming or floating around on the page when you read, eyestrain, blur with reading, loss of place while reading, and reduced comprehension as reading continues. In children, binocular vision defects are often misdiagnosed as attention deficit disorder or dyslexia. Thus if these or related diagnoses of learning disabilities have been suggested for your child binocular vision performance should be examined.

Amalgam Illness: Diagnosis and Treatment

should use best judgment to decide whether the patient's condition is as uncommon as 1 in 40 members of the general population. A more concrete way to put this is that if the doctor didn't see anything quite like this last week, you "pass."

HAVE LAB TESTS DONE IF NEEDED

24)   Hair calcium > 1,150 ppm

25)   Hair lithium < 0.005 ppm

26)   Hair mercury > 3.0 ppm[1]

27)   Urine mercury > 10 mcg/24h or 6 mcg/g creatinine or 6 mcg/liter

28)   Elevated 3-methyl histidine in urine

29)   Elevated sarcosine in urine

30)   Generalized aminoaciduria

31)   Elevated coproporphyrin in urine

32)   Erythrocytes seen on routine urinalysis at any time during period of illness or 1 year prior to perceived onset

33)   IgE > 292 IU

34)   Low total IgG

35)   Low IgG subclass results

36)   Low total T cells

37)   Low CD8 suppressor T cells

38)   Low NK cells

39)   Calculated serum osmolality (the formula is 2XNa + BUN/2.8 + Glucose/18 = osmolality) from blood chem panels average >290 under normal conditions of hydration , or patient produces >3 liters of urine in 24 hours, or abnormal relationship between serum osmolality and urine osmolality, or low ADH for given serum osmolality[2].

40)   Men: ALT elevated more than 4 units above cutoff.
40')   Women: ALT higher than 8 units BELOW upper cutoff.

41)   Elevated AST

42)   Elevated venous CO_2 OR subnormal venous CO_2

43)   Elevated venous O_2

44)   Elevated hematocrit

45)   Elevated MCV (Mean Corpuscular Volume)

46)   Elevated MCH (Mean Corpuscular Hemoglobin)

47)   Serum triglycerides <40 (women) or <50 (men)

48)   Total cholesterol <130

49)   Low HDL cholesterol

50)   Low PRL

51)   Low testosterone (males) or estrogens (females) without elevated LH and FSH (it is preferable to use appropriate age related norms rather than laboratory ranges - see appendix)

52)   Low T3, T4 or TSH; or inappropriate relation (see figure p117 or 185)

53)   Low serum DHEA-S or DHEA or salivary DHEA

---

[1] While some controversy surrounds the hair element test, authoritative sources like *Tietz* accept it as a useful screening test for heavy metal intoxications such as lead and arsenic.

[2] For patients on lithium therapy it must be verified that this is not from the effects of lithium on the kidney, but rather is caused by deficient release of antidiuretic hormone. Approximately one lithium treated patient in 5 has reduced kidney concentrating ability because of lithium.

Do you have mercury poisoning?

(men: serum DHEA-S less than 1.7 - 0.02 * age.

women: serum DHEA-S less than 0.85 - 0.01 * age)

54)   Low serum or 24 hour urine cortisol

55)   Decline in cortisol or ACTH in response to stress (e. g. intense exercise)

56)   Hypoglycemia (fasting or reactive)

57)   Low superoxide dismutase (SOD)

58)   Low serum iron in males

There are a total of 33 relevant laboratory tests that might be ordered for women, or 34 for men.

It is desirable to have either hair or urine toxic and essential elements determined as much for the purpose of screening for other elemental intoxications as for their (limited) utility in diagnosing mercury poisoning. Hair elements, urine essential elements, or red blood cell elements will all identify copper poisoning, which 5-10% of the people believing they may have amalgam illness actually have instead.

There are a total of 56 possible "tests." Those "tests" performed count as m in the tables below. Note that two of the "laboratory tests," hypoglycemia and excessive urine volume, may be determined via history taking instead.

A referral for evaluation under number 14 is suggested if there is a history of dyslexia, reading problems, double vision, or lack of depth perception.

You may be taking large amounts of dietary supplements. These may normalize many of the markers found on a routine blood chemistry panel. If it is important to find abnormalities on the first routine screening, you can abstain from all dietary supplements for several days before having blood drawn. This is very uncomfortable. Do not do it unless necessary.

Test	Affected by
Checklist 9	Vitamin C, co-Q-10
Fibromyalgia	Magnesium, thyroid
19, 20 skin conditions	EFA supplements in large amounts
Balance, twitches	Hydergine, selegiline
EKG changes, angina	Magnesium, co-Q-10, androgens
Hair Ca	Vitamins C and B complex (megadose)
IgE levels	Sulfur food exclusion, accolate, CLA
IgG, T cells	Vitamin A, CLA
NK cells	Echinacea, astragalus, inositol, vit. A
ALT, AST	Silymarin, co-q-10, B vitamins and C
Hematocrit, MCH, MCV	B-12, folate, iron, copper
HDL cholesterol	Silymarin, B-1, B-5, B vitamins and C
Testosterone	Androstenedione, androstanediol, etc.
DHEA	DHEA, pregnenolone
ACTH stress response	Carbamazepine
Hypoglycemia	Glutamine, branched chain aminos
Superoxide dismutase	Copper, manganese, selenium
Iron	Iron supplements

Amalgam Illness: Diagnosis and Treatment

This list is intended to be thought provoking, not complete. If you are taking a lot of supplements and medicines, talk to your doctor about which tests they will make normal, and try to find old tests in your records from before you were taking them to use with this diagnostic checklist.

Standard screening tests that may be informative are: routine urinalysis, complete blood count, and a FASTING blood chemistry panel including glucose Na, Mg, K, BUN, ALT, AST, GGTP, O_2 (venous), CO_2, bilirubin, creatinine, HDL cholesterol, total cholesterol, and triglycerides.

Hair analysis may or may not be an acceptable screening test. It is inexpensive. If it is ordered, ensure that it is sent to a lab that tests for Ag, Sn, Ni, Ca, Li, and S as well as Hg. The ratio of Hg to Ag/Sn/Ni should be very roughly 4 : 3 : 2 : 4 if the major source of mercury is amalgam. It is also an adequate screen for copper poisoning.

IgE is usually an adequate screening test for allergic problems.

Toxic porphyria as demonstrated by fractionated urine porphyrins appears to be the most reliable test but it is not routine, a normal result does not exclude the condition, and laboratory mishandling of samples leading to false normals is distressingly common.

The fall in ACTH on exercise stress must be tested that way. Patients with it usually show normal results on provocative tests using ACTH, CRH and insulin induced hypoglycemia. The proper procedure is to draw blood for ACTH, begin strenuous exercise within 15 minutes, perform exercise for at least 30 minutes, and after exercise is over have a second blood sample drawn for ACTH determination 15 to 30 minutes later.

Counting procedure

Count the number of checklists and tests from this list actually run on the patient, regardless of the result. This is the total number of tests, m. Questions not asked, signs not checked for on examination, and tests not performed do not count in m.

Count the number of positive results as given in the checklist above for these tests. This is n.

Look in the table below to find the correct value of m in the left hand column.

Look across the table. If n is greater than or equal to the first value, then the tests are positive that the patient has mercury poisoning. The greater n is compared to the listed value, the more certain this result is. If n is less than or equal to the second value, then the patient does not have mercury poisoning. They have something else. If n is between these two numbers the test is ambiguous and further work up or thoughtful clinical judgment is required. Careful study of the symptom description earlier in the book and a long talk with the patient about their history and problems is suggested if further testing is not easily arranged.

If some other diagnosis has been suggested that is NOT subject to definitive verification by objective laboratory testing, such as schizophrenia, depression, or most other psychiatric diagnoses, then it is imperative to take a detailed enough history, conduct an adequately thorough examination, and perform tests in a great enough number to definitively EXCLUDE mercury poisoning, rather than simply fail to confirm it. Psychiatric problems do not cause the abnormalities on the diagnostic checklist. If any significant number of abnormalities are seen, something ELSE is causing both the abnormalities and the psychiatric problem. The psychiatric problem must be assumed to be caused by something else unless n is less than or equal to the number in the exclusion column.

Two tables are given. The first is for 97.5% certainty, which is the same certainty that a clinical laboratory test result has when it shows something is "abnormally high" or "abnormally low." The second table is for 99.9% certainty if the physician or patient

Do you have mercury poisoning?

wishes to be extremely conservative due to the poorly understood nature of amalgam illness.

97.5% CERTAINTY, 0.1% INCIDENCE

total tests m	n which confirms mercury poisoning	n which excludes mercury poisoning
1-3	---	---
4-6	4	1
7-11	5	2
12-17	6	3
18-24	7	4
25-30	8	5
31-33	9	6
34-39	10	7
40-44	11	8
45-50	12	9
.	.	.
.	.	.
.	.	.
.	.	.

99.9% CERTAINTY, 0.1% INCIDENCE

total tests m	n which confirms mercury poisoning	n which excludes mercury poisoning
0-6	---	---
7-10	6	1
11-12	6	2
13-16	7	2
17	7	3
18-21	8	3
22-23	8	4
24-27	9	4
28	9	5
29-32	10	5
33-34	10	6
35-38	11	6
39	11	7
40-43	12	7
44-45	12	8
46-49	13	8
50	13	9
51-54	14	9
55-56	14	10
57-60	15	10
.	.	.
.	.	.
.	.	.

Further discussion of diagnosis

Tests directed at alternative diagnoses should be included, such as testing for candida, mycoplasma, Lyme disease, HHV-6, EBV, coxsackie virus, hepatitis, chlamydia and HIV. However, amalgam illness should be EXCLUDED by the standards of this statistical approach even if one of these shows up positive. After all, mercury induced immune suppression may be what is allowing a chronic viral infection to fester. If mercury poisoning cannot be excluded versus the null hypothesis, a statistical procedure for differential diagnosis is given below.

In the not uncommon case where you have a sudden onset of the "mystery syndrome" and have failed to find anything else it could be other than amalgam illness, it is wise to do two things: very definitely confirm that chronic mercury poisoning does exist, and search very hard for the immune system anomaly and infectious agent that caused the sharp onset of symptoms. Understanding WHAT caused the problem to suddenly start may allow it to be just as suddenly reversed - even if the underlying problem is amalgam illness and a year or two of chelation is required to be truly well and not at risk for further "mystery syndromes."

Many other things that appear to occur in amalgam illness were omitted (e. g. assorted autoimmune markers; high normal serum iron in the first few years, low normal (males) or low (females) serum iron later; high hair nickel; leukoplakia; low pitched, poorly enunciated speech; clumsiness; gait disturbances, migraines, non-epileptic seizures, Bell's palsy, bradycardia, fine tremor, withdrawal, impaired interpersonal relationships, particular distribution of dry skin or athlete's foot, night sweats, excessive sweating) because they don't fit into the statistical approach neatly at this very rudimentary level of treatment. Everything given in the symptom description should be checked during history taking and examination to provide a fuller and more convincing context even though much of it is not on the checklist.

Amalgam Illness: Diagnosis and Treatment

All heavy metals cause Mees' lines[1] on the nails. These usually begin a few months after significant exposure starts and may be useful in identifying the source of exposure - dental amalgams or some unrecognized source - if you remember when they started.

In diagnosing children it is helpful to consider the parents histories. If either parent is known to have amalgam illness this suggests that the child is much more likely to be genetically susceptible to the effects of mercury than a randomly selected member of the population. It is also more likely that the child will show up abnormal on tests that came out abnormal for the parent than would an unrelated amalgam illness victim. Another strongly suggestive piece of history for a child is if the mother had fibromyalgia, felt good during pregnancy, and the child had early developmental delays.

Typically mercury toxic children will be weak, uncoordinated, have poor peer acceptance and not fit in very well with other children.

If children have high mercury without elevated silver, nickel and tin, it is very important to figure out what the source of exposure actually IS. Hidden or unrecognized exposure is very common in children and may continue indefinitely if it is not identified.

Several tests can give apparently negative results without excluding chronic mercury intoxication. Urine mercury levels for intoxicated persons may be relatively low (e. g. 3 mcg/d) while those of a healthy person may be quite high (e. g. 80 mcg/d). This is because mercury is metabolized quite differently by different people. The urinary excretion rate is neither a measure of the amount in the body, nor of the person's individual sensitivity to it.

Hair analysis can show both toxic and essential elements low across the board. If anything, this is an indication of intoxication.

For reasons presently unknown some people's hair simply does not incorporate much in the way of trace elements. In many cases, this appears to be from intoxication impairing hair growth and it may go along with thin, fine, slow growing hair.

People who have organomercury poisoning, as from excessive fish mercury, will have low unchelated urine mercury compared to hair mercury, blood mercury, and chelated urine mercury. If it is possible to have serum or plasma analyzed for mercury, those with organic mercury poisoning will have a ratio of serum/plasma mercury to RBC mercury of 1:3 or less, while those with inorganic mercury poisoning will have a ratio of 1:2 or higher. Candida do methylate mercury and it is at least in theory possible for someone with extensive intestinal or perhaps systemic candida problems to convert significant amounts of inorganic mercury to organic mercury.

Perhaps due to the financial pressures of managed care, many large 'chain' clinical laboratories do not employ personnel at every step in their sample handling chain who are aware of the sensitive sample handling requirements of certain tests. The one most relevant to mercury intoxication is fractionated urine porphyrins. False normal results for this test caused by sample mishandling are distressingly common.

Many laboratories pretend that serum cholesterol, triglyceride, and glucose values are not significantly affected by drawing nonfasting samples. They are. Have them drawn 12 hours after food was last eaten.

Given the above considerations in addition to the natural variability in the effects of mercury intoxication on different individuals, one can see why a checklist approach to diagnosis is necessary.

Note that a 25 item check can be run using history, physical examination, chem panel, CBC, and RUA. Essentially all health plans will cover this. Indeed, many patients could be (self) diagnosed from their records

---

[1] White lines that run across them, or along them, or white spots.

Do you have mercury poisoning?

without requiring further testing. An important caveat is that patient use of dietary supplements may normalize some of these values and thus make diagnosis more difficult (e. g. milk thistle would normalize AST and ALT, lecithin would normalize HDL, vitamin C would normalize the "any 2 of" checklist, etc.). In this case diagnosis from old test results in records immediately preceding the beginning of supplementation is most appropriate.

If the number of abnormals in the 25 item checklist is between 4 and 7, or greater certainty is desired, appropriate further tests could be run. Hair elements, fractionated urine porphyrins, urine 3-methylhistidine and other tests appropriately selected based on clinical presentation could then be used. Vitamin C appears to reduce hair calcium levels if taken in adequate quantity. High levels of B-12 and folate should normalize MCH and MCV. Etc. Results which the patient's supplement program would be expected to normalize should be struck from the list of tests to consider in diagnosis and the count of total tests adjusted accordingly.

Excluding the diagnosis of chronic mercury poisoning for a patient whose records support it and who is taking supplements requires the use of the more sophisticated and expensive tests listed above. It cannot properly be done by repeating screening tests and showing that results have now normalized.

The complete list above has more than 45 items. Seventeen abnormals establishes the fact that if there is only one person in the United States with this disease, there is a 97.5 percent chance she is standing in front of you. Eighteen abnormals establishes that if there is only one person on Earth with amalgam illness, there is a 97.5% chance it is this patient.

Note that some patients will have enough abnormalities on history taking and physical examination that the diagnosis can be confidently made without the need for laboratory tests.

Patients who have records containing adequate testing may have the diagnosis strongly suggested if serial measurements of the parameters listed above trend in the expected direction. If a reasonable number of apparently unrelated physiological parameters are marching in lockstep towards the goal of definitive abnormality and overt illness, it is not necessary to wait for them to get there to make a well founded diagnosis and stop the disease process early.

Many people have an unusually high daily urine production[1] and are unaware of this. Serum osmolality calculated by formula $(2 \times Na + Glucose/18 + BUN/2.8$: which gives a slightly different numerical value than a measured osmolality) for tests drawn under conditions of free access to water - most routine blood chemistries - can be informative. People with proper water regulation have an average osmolality of 287. People with partial diabetes insipidus will usually have an osmolality over 290 - and such a result should motivate appropriate inquiry. People who have primary polydypsia (they want to drink a lot in the absence of a physiological need) will have a result <285. People with primary polydypsia do not usually have to get up at night to urinate. Primary polydypsia is a sign of some psychiatric disorders - which may in theory be due to mercury poisoning and hence curable by mercury detox - but a low calculated osmolality should direct inquiry into defining what is causing the polydypsia as well as identifying or excluding independent abnormalities that will allow the diagnosis of chronic mercury intoxication to be confirmed or excluded. Partial diabetes insipidus suggests further endocrine testing will find further abnormalities. Primary polydypsia alone does not.

Chronic mercury intoxication without ongoing high levels of mercury exposure does not typically involve the kidneys. Generalized aminoaciduria, elevated serum creatinine, impaired creatinine clearance, or elevated urine protein suggest recent or ongoing high levels of exposure, or

---

[1] More than 2.5 liters in 24 hours.

63

autoimmune processes involving the kidneys, or the aftermath of iv DMPS "therapy." In this case magnesium wasting is likely and some care must be taken not to exacerbate kidney problems through chelation - low, constant doses must be used. The most important consideration is identifying the source of exposure and removing it.

Old (possibly unrecognized) exposure

Patients who had an exposure much earlier which is no longer present, or which they are currently controlling the effects of through diet and supplements, may not at present show abnormalities on some of the more common tests. If an adequate number of abnormalities are present in records to diagnose chronic mercury intoxication for a past health event which was never satisfactorily explained, the patient has mercury intoxication at present unless appropriate chelation was performed to clear all internal organs, including the brain, of their mercury burden. A very carefully constructed history, verified and reverified, which the patient has spent many hours poring over to ensure accuracy is essential for such a retrospective diagnostic effort. For a patient without ongoing exposure retrospective diagnosis may be the only way to establish a definitive diagnosis short of a prolonged therapeutic trial.

The most difficult diagnostic problem is presented by someone who had a high level of mercury exposure that ended several years ago - e. g. an optometrist exposed to thimerosal containing contact lens solutions that are no longer on the market, or an adult who played extensively with mercury during childhood, or a former dental assistant. Such a person may have cleared her body of mercury, with the only remaining deposits being in the brain. Thus symptoms are likely to be entirely of central origin - psychiatric problems or centrally mediated endocrine dysfunction. In women endocrine dysfunction may take the form of inability to conceive despite otherwise apparently normal cycles. In this case a very thorough reconstruction of medical history by repeatedly going over it is extremely helpful in deciding whether you are mercury poisoned or not.

In this case the only potential abnormalities that can be verified through clinical laboratory tests are endocrine problems due to central or pituitary defects. Not everyone will have those - some will have "psychiatric" problems without any endocrine component. If adequate history and medical records do not exist to make a retrospective diagnosis possible, careful consideration of the person in relationship to the description of chronic mercury intoxication, possibly coupled with testing of the kinds of neurological problems seen to persist in former mercury miners (as described by Kishi *et al.*) may be necessary. In addition, a mobilization test using DMSA plus lipoic acid may be informative. It is recommended that standard therapeutic amounts - 100 mg DMSA + 100 mg LA every 3-4h - be administered for several days and serial urine mercury determinations (preferably 24 hour) be made. Unfortunately there are no standards to compare the results to so, at present, it is difficult to say what number corresponds to a "large increase" in mercury excretion. However, the side effects experienced during this test may be diagnostic. A person who does not have significant problems due to the mercury in their brain would not have their troublesome symptoms exacerbated by this test. One whose problems do derive from brain mercury would experience a growing exacerbation of symptoms as therapy continued over several days. Indeed, a dramatic aggravation of behavioral symptoms is possible during this test. NB: lipoic acid will mobilize many things in addition to mercury, e. g. arsenic, and will access most body tissues, not just the brain. Thoughtful interpretation is required.

Due to the great number of potential sources of occult mercury exposure, anyone with psychiatric or neurological problems which are not responding to treatment, or which are generally considered to have a poor

Do you have mercury poisoning?

outcome[1] (prognosis) is a legitimate candidate for a lipoic acid/DMSA therapeutic trial. People who are mercury toxic ought to respond positively to antioxidants (minimally, vitamins C, E, selenium and hydergine), ought to have some symptom exacerbation during LA + DMSA therapy followed by temporary improvement about 1 week afterwards, and ought to show an unexpected increase in urinary mercury excretion during chelation. In addition, urine volume may increase and pituitary factors fall during and shortly after chelation even if they are normal otherwise. All of these should be reproducible. At least one urine sample taken during chelation should be analyzed for lead and arsenic as well as mercury.

Arsenic, cadmium, lead and copper

Arsenic and lead are synergistic poisons with mercury. They may complicate mercury poisoning, and may lead to serious intoxications when none of the individual toxins are present at levels where they would individually cause overt illness.

Symptoms or history may suggest any of these toxins be considered.

There are a variety of laboratory tests for the metabolic effects of lead. In addition, certain changes observed in a blood count are typical of lead and not of the other toxins. Lead levels in hair, urine and blood are representative of body burden. Free erythrocyte protoporphyrin, zinc protoporphyrin and urinary aminolevulinic acid are specific tests for lead intoxication.

Coexistence of gout is diagnostic for lead.

Wrist or ankle drop is diagnostic for lead.

Chronic mercury intoxication can be difficult to diagnose because large quantities of mercury can be sequestered in the internal organs yet most of the mercury in the extracellular compartment may have been excreted long ago. Thus a "low" mercury excretion may mean someone is fine, or it may mean someone was poisoned to the gills so long ago it is no longer apparent by measuring excretion. Unlike mercury, lead has a long excretion half life, so lead excretion will be indefinitely elevated if lead poisoning has occurred and no chelation treatment has been given in the meantime.

Cadmium concentrates in the kidneys and the most sensitive test for it is ß-2 microglobulin in urine. Like lead and mercury, cadmium is ubiquitous and may be encountered from rechargeable batteries, artists' paints, the pink pigment in denture plates, etc. as well as from industrial sources.

Arsenic is the most difficult to test for since hair, blood and urine levels are NOT representative of body burden. Arsenic is the only case where a provocative test is necessary. Exclude seafood from the diet for a week, and perform a 24 hour urine collection to analyze for arsenic while administering 50-100 mg of lipoic acid ever 3 hours during the waking period (administering 50-100 mg of DMSA with the lipoic acid will reduce side effects and protect the patient somewhat from mercury entry into the CNS if this is a concern). A substantial rise in arsenic concentration when compared to a prior collection is diagnostic of an elevated body burden. This test should not be performed simply for informational purposes if the patient is to be treated for mercury poisoning anyway, since the treatment is the same and will cure both conditions at the same time. If mercury detox is performed this test can be combined with it at an appropriate phase of treatment if curiosity gets the best of everyone involved.

Extracellular chelators like DMPS and DMSA do not mobilize arsenic from its stores without the aid of lipoic acid.

Behavioral changes as described above under symptoms may be diagnostic for arsenic to an experienced practitioner.

---

[1] such as Parkinson's disease, Alzheimer's disease, schizophrenia, borderline personality disorder, or bipolar disorder.

Amalgam Illness: Diagnosis and Treatment

If mercury poisoning is apparent, the mobilization test for arsenic can be deferred until chelation with lipoic acid is appropriate therapy for mercury removal since the order of therapeutic interventions will not be altered by the presence or absence of arsenic.

Copper versus mercury poisoning

The symptoms of copper poisoning are very similar to the symptoms of mercury poisoning (amalgam illness) and a significant number of people who believe they have amalgam illness turn out to actually be copper poisoned and have no problem with mercury.

There are a wide variety of abnormalities in copper metabolism, one of which is the rare textbook condition Wilson's Disease. There are many more less rare problems with copper metabolism that haven't made it into standard texts yet. It is well worth checking RBC copper, hair copper and urine copper if corresponding tests for other elements are to be performed. Serum copper and ceruloplasmin are not informative tests as they are normal in many of the more common forms of copper poisoning even though they are low in Wilson's disease. As copper is an essential element, LOW copper can also cause problems.

Typically hair analysis for a copper toxic person will show everything fairly normal except that copper will be vastly elevated. This is in contrast to a mercury poisoned person where calcium will be vastly elevated and the essential elements will vary widely from the norm. Urinary copper excretion will also be vastly elevated.

In copper intoxication it is important to perform a stool analysis for toxic and essential elements. In normal individuals, 96% of copper is excreted in the feces. If no copper is excreted in the feces then lipoic acid can be used therapeutically since it increases urinary copper excretion. However LA decreases fecal copper excretion and will make matters worse if it is given to someone who is excreting significant amounts of copper in the feces.

The traditional treatment for copper poisoning is penicillamine, which many people do not tolerate well. DMPS does increase urinary copper excretion significantly. DMSA does not. LA increases urinary copper excretion and decreases biliary copper excretion.

Copper absorption can be reduced by excluding high copper foods, scrupulously avoiding copper in supplements, and taking 10-30 mg of zinc and 250-1000 mcg of molybdenum with each meal. Vitamin D supplements may increase metallothionein formation and thus copper excretion. Selenium supplements may increase the binding of copper to metallothionein which sequesters it safely inside the cells.

The antioxidant, liver support and brain support medications given in the treatment section will be helpful for copper toxic individuals and they will also have imbalanced fatty acids and need to take flax oil. Other sections, e. g. on allergy, will also be helpful if relevant. Copper poisoning acts similarly to mercury poisoning in that both metals are oxidation catalysts.

The Carl Pfeiffer Center has extensive experience in treating copper toxic individuals and may be willing to cooperate with your doctor to help him know how to treat you best. They also accept patients who go there in person for a few days and can usually be managed by telephone thereafter. The Pfeiffer center can be reached at:

Pfeiffer Center
1804 Diehl Road
Naperville, IL

(630) 505-0300.

Before the initial visit it is helpful if you can have the following tests available so they can determine whether they can get insurance to cover your treatment, and get some idea of what you have: Zinc, copper, lead and manganese in blood and a hair analysis heavy metal screen, kryptopyrrole urine analysis, blood histamine, thyroid panel, ABO blood type and an extensive blood chemistry panel equivalent to Chemzyme® Plus.

What to do about mercury poisoning

What if you can't get medical help

If you feel terrible and don't know where to start: get the following vitamins and take the suggested amounts: "B50" or "B100" once or twice per day[1]. Buffered vitamin C, 4 grams per day, 1 gram with each meal and one at bedtime. Magnesium, any form, 100 mg magnesium equivalent with each meal and 100 at bedtime to start, and increase this to 200 in a few weeks. Vitamin E, 400-1000 IU per day. Coenzyme Q-10, 75-200 mg per day. Zinc, 50 mg per day. Flax oil, 10+ grams per day. Borage oil, 1+ gram per day. Milk thistle, 1-2 capsules with each meal. Folic acid, 2-6 tablets (400 or 800 mcg) each day. Get a "weekly pill minder" box to count these out into each weekend.

See the "therapeutic agents" section for details on dosage. When dosages are not listed here they need to be individualized using the information there, and by experiment.

Read the diet section and control your diet strictly. Dramatic symptom relief is often possible.

Try lecithin, choline, and B-12 and see how you respond to them.

For dry skin, take lots of flax oil (30-100 gms - 1 to 3 oz) and some borage oil (2-10 gms). Try extra vitamin E and beta carotene.

For anxiety, take gotu kola + niacinamide + vitamin B-6 + GABA. If you are thin or have poor digestion, add taurine and go very lightly on the GABA. If you have trouble with codeine, go lightly on the GABA.

If stress bothers you, take DHEA and pregnenolone.

For depression, take 100 mg a day of zinc plus 2-3 mg (2,000-3,000 mcg) a day of folic acid as these may work quickly. Also take St. John's Wort + niacinamide 500-1000 mg + acetyl-l-carnitine 500 mg with each meal and at bedtime, + pregnenolone with breakfast and lunch. If you are not anxious, add phenylalanine or tyrosine or pseudoephedrine (sudafed®) with breakfast and lunch.

If your depression, inability to concentrate, etc. is NOT RESPONDING to other supplements, medicines, etc.: take phosphatidylserine 300 mg each day, start with 600 mg a day the first two weeks.

If you have no energy, motivation, and can't get anything done: take ephedrine 12.5 mg in AM + 6.25 mg every 4-6 hours until 6 PM. Various people respond to ginseng, gotu kola, ginkgo biloba, licorice, ginger and astragalus, which you can try if the ephedrine doesn't do what you want. You can also try pseudoephedrine or tyrosine if the ephedrine did something helpful but it wasn't quite what you needed.

If you have autoimmune problems, take niacinamide 500-1000 mg with each meal and at bedtime, + DHEA + borage oil + forskolin.

If you have rheumatoid arthritis or fibromyalgia, take ginger. For fibromyalgia, also take 1-3 ounces per day of flax oil, plus 4-8 grams per day of fish oil in divided doses the first month, plus religiously avoid partially hydrogenated oils, and take as much magnesium as you can tolerate.

If you have hypoglycemia, take 200 mcg chromium picolinate with every meal, eat a high protein diet, take 1-2 grams branched chain amino acids with meals and at bedtime unless you are very thin and can't gain weight, eat frequent meals, and learn about ADRENAL FUNCTION in the treatment section.

---

[1] It is even better to break them in half and take them twice as often, or to take "B-50's" 3 or 4 times per day.

67

If you have migraines, take ginger and limit the amount of arginine you take to a level that doesn't bother you.

If you have heart pain (angina), take as much magnesium as you can tolerate, take lots of arginine, take acetyl-l-carnitine 1/2 - 1 gram 4 times per day, take 200-400 mg per day of coenzyme Q-10, take 200 mcg of chromium every time you eat and don't eat sweets or high carbohydrate meals.

If you have difficulty paying attention or concentrating, take DMAE + lecithin + choline. Consider nicotine patches. If you are chemically sensitive (have MCS), start with low doses of DMAE only.

If you are upset or emotionally disturbed, or have "crazy thoughts" that bother you, take glutamine. If you are not subject to runny nose, skin rashes, etc. AT ALL, also try histidine and niacin.

Also try glutamine if you are thin, weak, fatigued, have periodic depression, or are hypoglycemic.

If you have allergies or asthma, take 2 grams vitamin C 4 times per day + more magnesium + borage oil + DHEA + forskolin + selenium + drink a lot of strong black tea.

If you have allergies, take short showers and rinse your hair whenever you are having trouble.

If you have trouble with viruses (e. g. herpes of any form, long colds) take 1/2 gram of lysine with each meal and also take inositol routinely.

When you come down with a virus, take elderberry or grapefruit seed extract + echinacea or astragalus for the duration.

If you have trouble with bacteria, take 1-2 grams of arginine with each meal.

For either kind of infection take grapefruit seed extract.

If you have poor digestion and you don't think your guts can handle all this stuff, start off with E, C, magnesium and B-25 while you prepare your digestion for additional supplements by taking bifidobacteria and lactobacillus acidophilus, starting at recommended doses on the bottles and working up to 10 or 15 times that over a few weeks. Take with a very small amount of liquid iron supplement, a lactose food, or fructooligosaccarides (FOS) 5-10 grams per day. Then try glucosamine (2 grams), glycine (2-10 grams), ginger, digestive enzymes (animal derived, as directed on bottle) to see what helps, and try to eat as little processed and packaged food as you can. Eating a raw fruit or vegetable daily is helpful, as is anything to increase fiber. Psyllium husks cause less gas than bran. If dairy products are OK with you, eat lots of yogurt. Take ginger if taking all this stuff makes you nauseous, or you need to improve your appetite.

Sublingual coenzymated B complex vitamins can be found for those with the most serious digestive problems.

If you are trying to take as much magnesium as you can and it seems to be helping some but is giving you diarrhoea, take epsom salt baths by dissolving a carton (3-4#) of epsom salts in the hottest bath you can stand and soaking in it until the tub is cool. Do this several times per week.

If you can't control your diet tightly, try not to get any of the food preservatives BHT, BHA, TBHQ, or sodium sulfite or sodium metabiulfite (or similar names) in your food, no partially hydrogenated oils, and no FD&C yellow #5 (tartrazine).

Find other people with similar problems. Talk to them. Find out what helped them. Try it if it sounds good for you. The internet can be good for this.

Try to be happy, trusting, optimistic, exercise regularly and get enough sleep. It boosts your immune system as well as being fun.

What to do about mercury poisoning

Keep poring over this book, and any other source that seems to be helping you to find more things to try.

Diet

Since mercury poisons the enzymes in the liver and elsewhere in the body that metabolize food, control of diet is essential to feeling good. Unfortunately, the proper diet for a mercury poisoned person does not follow any of the other diets that are easy to find. Diets are also surprisingly difficult to follow strictly.

Many of the problems you can have from things in your diet do not cause you to have indigestion. Your digestive system may feel fine. The rest of your body can feel terrible from things in your food that got digested and distributed to your body but were not properly processed by your liver.

The only way to find out what kind of diet you need to follow is to start with an extremely simple diet of only a few components you prepare yourself and eat only that for several days, then try adding one thing at a time and paying attention to how it makes you feel. If other people make food for you they will not be careful enough about reading ingredient lists and using only certain specific ingredients unless you watch closely and are involved in food preparation. They will tell you what you want to hear and keep doing what they are doing. They simply can't believe you could be so sensitive to things and the effects could be so subtle unless they have been through it themselves. They will think you are upset over nothing and will humor you to keep you from making their life difficult by actually requiring them to follow your diet rules. If you want to feel good - or to even find out how much better you can feel - you will have to be involved in food selection and preparation.

Each person has to find which diet works for her. For practical purposes, most people will have to restrict their food selection very sharply to those things known to be safe for them. They will have to pay careful attention to what they respond poorly to and exclude everything with those components from their diet. This leads to a very boring diet!

Different classes of things you might benefit from excluding are:

- Partially hydrogenated fats and oils[1].

- Foods cooked in polyunsaturated oils[2].

- Spices and seasonings.

- Sulfur foods.

- Tyramine containing foods.

- Sulfite containing foods.

- Foods high in materials that are metabolized by MAO.

- Preservatives and colorings, especially BHT, BHA, TBHQ and FD&C yellow #5 (tartrazine).

- Pesticides.

- The antibiotics fed to animals to make them grow fast (a lot of "hormone free" meat is full of antibiotics).

Not everyone will have trouble with all of these materials. Other things might bother some people. Tyramine containing foods, "sulfur foods," and foods containing sulfites, MAO metabolized foods, plus some other types of foods are listed in an appendix.

---

[1] It takes a month or two for your body to clear these out. This is the only exception to the rule that excluding it for a few days and reintroducing it is a good test of how you react to it. You have to diligently exclude these for a month or two before you know if they affect you. They are in pretty much everything fried or baked you find at restaurants and in almost everything in the bakery department or baked goods aisle at the supermarket.

[2] The oils form peroxides on cooking. These peroxides oxidize more things in your body and also activate your immune system when there is nothing to fight but you. They are actually LESS healthy for you than foods cooked in butter or lard.

Amalgam Illness: Diagnosis and Treatment

There is a lot of difference between "healthy," "natural," and "organic." If in doubt, assume that if it is not certified organic it has stuff in it you don't want to eat. The staff at grocery stores is not always knowledgeable about what is in their stock and may tell you what you want to hear instead of what you need to know. Also be aware that labels are not always completely accurate.

Certain dietary manipulations can also be used to help with other problems. People with low blood sugar problems (hypogycemia) should avoid sweet things, and if possible eat a diet high in fiber and protein but low in carbohydrates.

People with lots of problems related to inflammation can reduce the amount of the inflammation precursor arachidonic acid in their diets by excluding meat, dairy products, and shellfish. Taking a lot of flax oil and some fish oil helps replace AA with antiinflammatory materials.

People whose bodies seem to have trouble making energy should exclude partially hydrogenated fats and oils and eat a low carbohydrate diet which increases pyruvate and pushes energy making substrate through the Krebs cycle - the basic biochemical process that produces energy in the cells. If you are cold, achey, and have a high pulse and respiration rate you should try this for a month or two.

If you crave protein, try taking branched chain amino acids.

A lot of people have trouble digesting what they eat. They will benefit from taking betaine hydrochloride (extra stomach acid) or taking their vitamin C in acid form with meals, plus digestive enzymes. Animal derived digestive enzymes are far superior to plant derived ones for this purpose. Not digesting food properly leads to two different kinds of problems - not getting the benefit of the nutrients in it, and having the undigested food cause trouble in your intestines. Not digesting food properly leads to a feeling of indigestion which is relieved by taking digestive enzymes with meals.

If you do find some class of food you have to exclude from your diet in order to feel good, you can quickly break your subconscious of craving it (e. g. sweets) by remembering eating it when you are having your reaction and feel terrible, and focussing on how eating it felt and tasted while also trying to wallow in how miserable you are feeling from it. Your subconscious learned to associate the food with how good it tasted and how great you felt just after you ate it. Put together the good feelings of the food with the miserable feelings of the problem it causes and you will quickly learn to avoid it. If you try to do this all intellectually by "knowing" what is bad for you, adequate self control will be lacking.

Food components people may be sensitive to follow. You don't need to exclude ALL of these things from your diet! You need to figure out what is giving you trouble and limit or exclude the relevant foods. Lists of the foods containing each material are in an appendix.

- "Sulfur foods."

- Tyramine.

- Sulfites.

- Melatonin.

- Tryptophan.

- Phenylalanine.

- Aspartame (Nutrasweet®).

- Salycilates and other things that require sulfation.

Rotation diets are described in many places. They are beneficial to people whose immune system is in a "universal reactor" state where they sensitize to antigens very easily. Rotation diets are not helpful for most people. They are also difficult to follow and

What to do about mercury poisoning

should not be used unless necessary since they are very time consuming.

Day to day practicality

Organizing the treatment program so it is straightforward and simple increases the likelihood you will be able to comply with it and gives you more time to get on with the rest of your life. Prescribing treatment programs of byzantine complexity is the most common error alternative physicians make in managing their mercury intoxication cases. If the treatment program becomes too burdensome for you to comply with, symptoms previously suppressed reappear and further reduce your ability to follow the program.

The most important thing to do is to get your day to day life really organized so you can focus on treatment - taking those vitamins, chelating, etc., and do it every day. Get vitamin minder boxes. Keep calendars. Do what it takes. When you miss some supplements, put off chelation, or what have you there is a big risk you will start feeling really terrible, get your brain all fogged in, and not be able to pick up the pieces and get on with your life for weeks on end.

Your most important priority is to take your supplements and medicines on your regular schedule. This is what makes it possible to get anything else done. If you skip this to do something else, you soon won't be doing ANYTHING.

You also need to make a written "punch list" of all the things that work to rescue you from a funk when you eat the wrong thing, forget your vitamins, etc. Put copies all over the place. Give them to your friends. You won't think to do the right thing when problems happen, so make it easy to find a piece of paper that reminds you what it is!

Mercury poisoned people are also prone to depression, which makes it very difficult to comply with complex treatment programs.

Mercury poisoned people also do not have as many hours in the day that they are able to concentrate, pay attention and be active as other people do. Thus a few minutes of unnecessary work on their health care is a greater burden on them than it is on other patients.

You have to develop a clear understanding of priorities and of what is important. Your physician may not know. Everything is not equally important. If you view everything as equally important you will make potentially dangerous decisions during treatment (e. g. to stop a prednisolone taper during the high dose portion after a few days in order to keep taking your B vitamins and selenium supplement).

You must organize your life and home in such a way that treatment becomes routine. Buy weekly vitamin minder boxes and pack them on the weekends. Find inexpensive supplement stores and mail order catalogs that carry the materials the patient needs. Find nearby sources of safe foods. If attempting to keep a rotation diet (which should not be prescribed unless NECESSARY to control serious food allergy problems) a large wall calendar should be annotated to keep track of it. A calendar should also be used to note when to refill prescriptions and order more supplements, as well as to keep a record of chelation, medications, supplements actually taken or omitted, medical tests, and symptoms.

Procrastination is a symptom of mercury poisoning. You will do it a lot. Learn all of the ways you can to defeat it and use them. Have your friends and family help with this too.

The physician should assist you in convincing your family, friends, and co-workers of how important their help will be if this is necessary to enlist their support.

71

Amalgam Illness: Diagnosis and Treatment

How to keep your life together during treatment

Be realistic. There will be a long period of time during which you just won't be able to get as much done as you would like. You are probably already behind in life because of this. Focus on catching up and keeping up! Don't take any new things on! Do essential things and ignore the rest!

For practical purposes you don't have as much time in the day as other people. So don't take stuff on that 'just takes a minute.' You don't have as many minutes to spare as other people do!

- Keep to do lists (including daily stuff like tooth brushing and taking pills).

- Keep logs and diaries so as to be able to figure out what helps you and what hurts you.

- Keep a calendar - desk blotter calendars work well.

- Make a list, pick the most important thing on it, do that, cross it off.

- Enlist the support of friends and family on deadlines and tasks.

- Simplify life, avoid stress.

- Read appropriate parts of this book repeatedly.

- Have your friends and family read the description of symptoms repeatedly.

- Get a good time management book and read it.

- If you aren't sure whether you need to do something, don't do it.

- If you are having a hard time making a decision, flip a coin.

- Every time you get something important done, do something nice for yourself.

- Arrange your finances as conservatively as possible.

- Be aware of emotional symptoms in order to intellectually circumvent them when they are out of control.

- Get a new attitude towards physicians - they are body mechanics, not godlike beings. You will see a lot of them. No single one knows enough to get you well.

- Do not experiment excessively with your diet, supplements, and medicines, and don't let your physician do so[1].

- Plan and expect this to be a long, drawn out process with lots and lots of frustration and delays.

- Stick to the diet, supplements and medicines longer than you think you need to. Be SURE you are well before discontinuing them.

The physical symptoms resolve before the emotional ones. Shyness and withdrawal are among the last symptoms to go.

You are poisoned. You are not CRAZY. Sometimes you might ACT crazy until the mercury is gone. You might even FEEL crazy while there is a bunch of mercury banging around in your head. When it is gone you might need some time to cope with all the emotional baggage it left behind.

---

[1] If they do testing and dosage adjustment on one thing more than 3 times and there is other stuff you want to get on with, just tell them what the dose is going to be and refuse to let them do anything about it until the rest of your issues are addressed. If they insist, see another doctor for a while. You are trying to find something that works so you can move ahead. Your body will change as you detox and you can't get everything perfectly adjusted - nor is it really important.

What to do about mercury poisoning

The baggage isn't only emotional. Chronic illness is like a war being fought inside your body. After the soldiers are gone, it takes a lifetime to clean things up and they may never be perfectly right again.

WHAT IS IMPORTANT:

- Take your DMSA/LA or DMPS/LA like clockwork

- Take water + lipid soluble antioxidants

- Take everything on your program every day

- Find doctors who will help

- Do tests, exams, try things

- Try new doctors, labs, etc. to find out what helps

- Do things now

WHAT IS NOT IMPORTANT:

- Exactly how much DMSA, DMPS, LA, vitamins, etc you take

- Exactly which medicines and supplements you take

- Taking exactly the right things in the perfect proportions

- Finding exactly the right doctor, therapy, lab test

- Doing things perfectly

- Having a doctor who thinks he knows exactly what to do

- Forcing a doctor to help who doesn't want to, even if it really is his job

Short instructions to the doctor when amalgam illness is suspected

Prescribe the following program of supplements and medications:

MEDICATIONS

- Rx Hydergine 3-5 mg 3-4 times per day - increase over 1-2 weeks to avoid nausea, or use Hydergine-LC

- If the patient is thin and either allergic or weak or depressed or anxious, Rx hydrocortisone 5 mg 2-4 times per day

- If allergic, Rx accolate 20 mg bid + antihistamine as appropriate + inhaled steroids.

- If fibromyalgic, Rx celebrex 1-2 caps bid + NSAID.

NUTRITIONAL SUPPLEMENTS

- 2 grams buffered vitamin C 3-4 times per day

- B-50 or similar multi B vitamin 2-3 times per day

- Vitamin E 1000 IU per day

- Flax seed oil 10-30 grams per day

- 200 mcg chromium picolinate with each meal

- Magnesium (any form) 500-750 mg elemental equivalent per day in divided doses

- Milk thistle extract 3-4 times per day

PATIENT MANAGMENT

Instruct the patient that dental work will begin in 4-6 weeks if testing confirms that they have amalgam illness, and that the dosages of supplements, medicines, etc. will be optimized later.

Work through the diagnostic checklist earlier in the book, and order other tests as appropriate to understand the disease process or exclude alternative diagnoses.

Schedule 3-4 appointments in the next 3-6 weeks to review test results, review history, and order further tests as appropriate.

Assign the patient their homework of making their life as routine and organized as possible so they can prepare to "hunker down" for about 1 year if they do have amalgam illness.

Instruct the patient to eat 3 meals per day, and snacks, even if they are very simple. Instruct them to eat protein and fiber but avoid sweets and limit caffeine.

If the patient is anxious or depressed, wait one appointment to see if the medications, supplements and regular meals help unless their suffering is great. It is difficult to find anxiolytics and especially antidepressants these patients respond well to.

If the diagnosis is confirmed, schedule the dentistry as soon as possible and read the treatment section.

Modify therapy as test results come in.

After amalgam removal, use 50-100 mg DMSA every 4 hours on alternate weeks for 3 months, then 50-100 mg DMSA + 25-200 mg LA every 3-4 hours for 3-4 days per week.

Tutor the patient on the natural progression of treatment at every appointment (initial remission in the first few months, followed by exacerbation of symptoms from 4-9 months post removal which will be severe if appropriate medication and supplementation is not continued. See figure 15).

Outline: treatment for mercury tox

The proper protocol first addresses the need for correct diagnosis, then gives a high priority to removing exposure and clearing the body of toxins, and finally provides ongoing support in all ways necessary to keep you, the patient, comfortable and healthy during the prolonged detoxification process.

#1, Ensure correct diagnosis by considering and excluding other (real, not latinized symptoms or "garbage pail diagnosis") conditions. Patients with otherwise intractable conditions (parkinsonism, lupus, schizophrenia, anything with long term disability and poor prognosis) should be worked up extensively to definitively exclude amalgam illness as the root cause of their condition since it is readily curable. A therapeutic trial as described in the appendix should be used if definitive exclusion of the diagnosis is not practical for economic or other reasons. Amalgam illness should not be considered excluded just because there is a name in the medical textbooks that sounds a lot like their problem.

Do not perform challenge tests - they are not useful and can be quite harmful. The only exception is when a challenge test is needed to get insurance coverage, to protect the physician from overzealous licensing authorities, etc. Challenge test protocols are described in an appendix.

A summary of laboratory abnormalities which are described below in greater detail: the patients will often have toxic porphyria per fractionated urine pophyrin test, relatively low or abnormally low hormone levels AND stimulating factor levels, elevated ALT and sometimes AST, either malabsorption leading to low cholesterol and low triglycerides, OR high LDL cholesterol with relatively low HDL cholesterol, etc. Many patients have nocturia and will show an abnormal relationship of urine and serum osmolality on dehydration. Urinary excretion of 3 and sometimes 1 methylhistidine is usually quite elevated. If the patient is not yet taking much in the way of supplements, hair calcium is also quite elevated and lithium reduced.

NB: I believe an experienced practitioner can make the diagnosis with perfect certainty by physical examination and history taking alone, but testing both allows exactly what problems are secondary to mercurialism to be identified and also provides defensive documentation to convince insurance companies, patients and their families, and, if need be, licensing authorities that a reasonable diagnosis has been made.

#2, Appropriate nutritional and pharmacologic supportive treatment includes: "B100" vitamins - preferably time release; 8 gms buffered vitamin C, 1000 IU E, 500 mg B6; 10,000 mcg+ sublingual B-12 or B-12 injections, milk thistle extract 300+ mg, omega 3 (flax, 10+ gms) and 6 (borage, 1+gm) oils, 10+ grams lecitin, 100+ mg co-q-10, 50 mg DHEA, echinacea 5 days per month, and other supplements depending on symptoms and budget. If there is any evidence of autoimmunity 2-3 g of niacinamide should be included unless phase 1 metabolism is slow. NB: thiol containing foods and supplements are harmful to many patients and must be excluded from their diets. This can be determined by proper standard laboratory testing, perhaps by other testing, and by patient experiments. People who are chemically sensitive or who have reacted badly to supplements before should start at very low doses and ramp up slowly, adding a few at a time. People who have never tried supplements should introduce a few every week at a half or quarter dose and increase them the next week. Most people will find they need high dosages of many supplements to really help them. A few will be brand sensitive, need to get the dose just right, etc.

If prescription drugs are available (e. g. by overseas mail order) therapy should include 20 mg ergoloid mesylates plus hormone supplements (unless contraindicated) like armour thyroid and testosterone/bi-est or tri-est creams and hydrocortisone 5 mg four times a day, plus inhaled glucocorticoids unless contraindicated or clearly unnecessary. Candida problems sometimes contraindicate hydrocortisone and inhaled steroids. Many patients also require antidepressants (selegiline being a good choice) or anxiolytics.

The purpose of this is to ameliorate symptoms during the prolonged detoxification process, not to distract attention from detoxification or delay it. Excessive experimentation with diet, supplements and medications causes unnecessary patient discomfort and wastes time.

#3, Remove amalgams and other sources of exposure using any reasonable protocol (e. g. dam and independent breathing air). Expect symptom exacerbation regardless of the care taken during removal. Symptoms can be relieved for a few days by intravenous vitamin C. SMALL doses of DMPS given intravenously (e. g. 25-50 mg) will also relieve symptoms with modest risk of side effects.

#4, Use oral DMPS by mouth every 8 hours on a week on-week off or 10 day on 4 day off schedule starting no earlier than 4 days after the last amalgam removal, and/or DMSA by mouth every 3-4 hours on the same schedule to suppress urine mercury by 80%. Select dosage on an economic basis. DMSA is more economical per unit mercury removed than DMPS, but DMPS suppresses symptoms more effectively. Reasonable dosages are 50-300 mg. Always test the chelators for side effects by ramping up dosage from 25 or 50 mg the first time. Penicillamine and dimercaprol are always contraindicated.

#5, Use lipoic acid every 3-4 hours starting at 25-50 mg and working up to 100-200 mg per dose as side effects are tolerated, plus at the same time use DMPS or DMSA per the above schedule. Do this in campaigns of a few days to a few weeks, with rests in between. Continue for 6 months to 2 years until chelation at high levels is not causing much side effects, urine mercury is low during chelation, and other symptoms are gone and do not recur after several months without chelation.

#6, Allergies and fatigue may be controlled with 5-8 day prednisolone tapers (at fairly high doses) every 2 months during therapy if needed. Note that DMPS and DMSA affect the immune system, often by stimulating it. Thus there is a tradeoff between more rapid removal of mercury and hence amelioration of CNS and endocrine symptoms, and more effective allergy suppression.

#7, Appropriate testing includes fasting plasma amino acids to determine which to supplement and which to exclude (remember that you don't have to treat it if it doesn't correspond to a symptom or problem), ACTH response to exercise stress to determine whether exercise restriction or therapy (e. g. Tegretol), is appropriate, for phase 1 and 2 liver metabolism to determine which therapeutic approaches (e. g. Tegretol) are indicated or contraindicated as well as to determine diet, and T, B and NK cells to determine immune status and whether certain therapies are indicated or contraindicated (e. g. ginseng, echinacea and inositol for low NK cell number, which also contraindicates prednisolone tapers). Further appropriate testing (e. g. to identify endocrine or gastrointestinal abnormalities) should be guided by signs and symptoms. PDR discussion of DMSA indicates frequent CBC's to check for white blood cell suppression. Under ideal circumstances, occasional CBC's should be ordered when other tests are being drawn anyway, since these patients are on (usually low doses) of medications known to affect the immune system and often have immune abnormalities to start with. Under less than ideal circumstances the patient does not assume a large risk if he refuses the CBC's, since the risks the CBC's are meant to catch are small to start with, the doses of the immune suppressing agents are low, and symptoms are likely to occur if problems get out of hand.

#8, Pay attention to the fact that there are usually psychiatric disturbances secondary to mercurialism - and exacerbated by therapy - which may require intervening in the patient's social or legal context and which may influence the choice of medications in some instances. Mercury poisoning can cause schizophrenia spectrum disorders, anxiety with agitation and panic, and depression with suicidal ideation. Patients may be more compliant and behave more appropriately if they are well informed of these possibilities beforehand. Some patients experience these at clinically significant levels, others do not.

Less dramatic difficulties include confusion, difficulty concentrating, indecisiveness, feelings of hopelessness, lethargy and fatigue. These may interfere with the patient's ability to comply with therapy, file and appeal insurance claims, pay bills, maintain employment, etc. Compassion, reminders, checklists, and encouraging the patient to enlist the help of his social network for the next 6 months to one year are appropriate means of addressing these very real problems.

If you don't bother with #1 you might end up treating a problem you don't have and not get well!

If you don't bother with #2 you will suffer a lot more than you have to for the next year or two.

If you don't bother with #3 you won't ever get well.

If you don't bother with #4, you won't feel as good the first few months but things aren't slowed down.

If you don't bother with #5, you will experience a great exacerbation of symptoms during months 3-9 that can be minimized, and in addition mercury will never be removed from your brain. If the DMPS or DMSA is not used with the LA the treatment is not as comfortable and takes longer, but still works.

If you don't bother with #6, you will be more allergic and a LOT more tired and lethargic for a couple of years.

If you don't bother with #7, you have to guess what to do if you want to use supportive therapies. Sometimes you will guess wrong and suffer a lot.

If you don't bother with #8, the next year of your life will be a much bigger mess than it has to be.

What to do in case of an adverse reaction to improper chelation protocol

Some physicians or patients may not realize that monthly DMPS injections, DMPS challenge tests, or DMSA therapy every other day are dangerous until an adverse reaction occurs. If at that point they happen upon this book, the following are some things that have helped people control and end such adverse reactions.

These adverse reactions can be life threatening in two ways, one is directly, and the other is through inducing suicidal depression - even in patients with no personal or family history of depression or suicide. Do not permit a suicidally depressed patient to be confined in a psychiatric hospital, since the hospital will not do any of the things that might help, and is likely to do some things that will worsen the depression and the patient's long term prognosis.

Dementia and psychosis may also be induced by inappropriate chelation. Hospitalization is again harmful. The major difficulty is getting the patient to accept and comply with helpful therapy at that point.

In all cases of adverse reactions, immediately ensure the patient continues to take appropriate nutritional supplements.

Many adverse reactions can be put on hold for a few days with 20+ grams of vitamin C (sodium ascorbate, not acid form) administered intravenously which is easy to do by putting commercially available sodium ascorbate for injection into standard iv bags and setting up an iv drip to run it in over an hour or two. Even made in distilled water, the solution is hypertonic (more concentrated than blood). Other vitamins and minerals can be included as appropriate. This does not end the adverse reaction - it will reappear - but it buys time to figure out what to do.

The adverse reactions are caused by redistribution of mercury caused by rapidly rising and falling blood levels of the chelating agent. PROPER chelation can clear out this freshly redistributed mercury and cure the adverse reaction. DMPS is much more effective at this than DMSA. If DMPS is available, 100 mg by mouth every 8 hours for a week is very helpful. It may be necessary to repeat this a few times. Since DMPS is investigational it may be necessary

to use DMSA, which must be given every 4 hours (even at night) and should be used in larger doses up to the dosage limit of 5 mg/kg.

Further mercury redistribution can be lessened by immediately excluding "sulfur foods" from your diet, and stopping any supplements containing garlic, cysteine, or glutathione. NAC should not be discontinued unless you are believed to have adequate liver phase 2 glutathione conjugation, but it should be used at the lowest appropriate level. The "sulfur foods" are: eggs, dairy products, bakery products containing whey, cysteine, eggs, or "enzymes," cabbage, bok choy, cauliflower, broccoli, broccoflower, brussels sprouts, kale, turnips, rutabagas, asparagus, onions, shallots, leeks, garlic, and coffee. If you think it is related to one of these, don't eat it.

The prescription drug hydergine, in divided doses totalling 20 mg per day, is very helpful at protecting the brain from oxidative damage and at elevating mood. Dosage must be worked upward from 1 mg per time to avoid nausea. It can be increased every few days. Hydergine LC is less likely to induce nausea.

Always consider anxious, agitated, nervous depression to be due to reactive hypoglycemia and treat it with a high protein diet of frequent, small meals, each with 200 mg chromium picolinate, plus supplementary branched chain amino acids and glutamine, and also give cortisol 5 mg 2-4 times a day if possible.

The supplementary amino acid glutamine will often elevate mood and reduce "crazy thinking." A plasma amino acid analysis with proper supplementation or dietary exclusion can be quite helpful.

If there is any tension, anxiety, or signs of low bile flow, use supplementary taurine.

If there is depression use fast acting antidepressants other than of the SSRI class.

Amalgam Illness: Diagnosis and Treatment

Cortisol elevates mood and reduces anxiety and relieves tension by direct action on the brain. 5 mg 2-4 times per day is enough to have some of this effect, it happens quickly, and this is not enough to lead to the negative side effects of glucocorticoid use like HPA suppression or excessive weight gain.

If you are depressed and have responded well to SSRI antidepressants before, also use these after a quick trial of 5 hydroxytryptophan. Also consider tryptophan by prescription from a compounding pharmacy.

Rapid flareup and dissapearance of autoimmune disease attacking first one organ, then another, may occur. This may lead to fluctuations in hormone levels if the targets are in the endocrine system. Appropriate use of glucocorticoids or other methods to handle autoimmune disease should be considered.

If reduced kidney function is seen, it is often caused by deposition of immune complexes on the glomerular membranes and can usually be cleared temporarily by administering intravenous immune globulin.

Whatever medical problems characterize the adverse reaction are likely to be either centrally mediated, due to liver and pancreatic damage, or of autoimmune origin.

The doctor's approach to the patient with chronic mercury poisoning

The most fundamental question is "how poisoned is this patient?" The answer is not immediately apparent. Extremely poisoned patients do not look as sick as they are. In addition they usually have an impaired adrenal response so they are unable to make adequate cortisol after stress (such as their doctor's appointment) but do make adequate adrenaline during the stressful time and perform. Then they collapse for a long time while nobody is around.

Under ideal circumstances, a patient should be subjected to reasonably thorough laboratory work up as soon as she is willing to undergo it in order to determine how sick she is and what particular parts of her physiology are compromised. Some patients will refuse a lot of laboratory tests and need to be handled using a more clinical approach. This approach will involve a fair amount of experimentation and ambiguity. It is especially important that detailed notes be kept in the file and reviewed shortly before each appointment when a more clinical approach is being taken. It is important for ALL patients that at least a summary page be kept in their file and reviewed shortly before each appointment.

It is appropriate to schedule several appointments at short intervals during the initial work up period so as to not inordinately delay therapeutic measures which can ameliorate the patient's symptoms. If certain laboratory test results must be received before the next appointment, the patient can be given the responsibility to check with the lab and make the appointment as soon as the results are available.

If a fair number of therapeutic trials are needed to identify agents which ameliorate symptoms, these should be conducted rapidly (e. g. by having the patient spend several days in the physician's waiting room and trying the agents one at a time until an effective medication has been found).

It is important to go over and retake history several times at different appointments. Further useful information will be gleaned each time. The patients usually have memory and concentration difficulties which make it difficult for them to offer all relevant information at one sitting.

The patients have subtle emotional changes and impaired interpersonal relationships. It is best to be simple and direct with them, not to infer their attitudes and opinions from tone of voice or behavior and not to agree to procedural things unless you will actually do them exactly as stated. Example: the patient may interpret the question "how are you?" socially rather than

What to do about mercury poisoning

as an attempt to elicit symptoms or a complaint and politely answer "fine."

The patient's experience with nutritional supplements and OTC drugs is quite useful as most patients have experimented extensively. The information gleaned may suggest prescription drugs which will be more effective, or which are likely to lead to adverse reactions.

How sick is the patient? Choices are:

1) Seriously chronically poisoned

2) Seriously acutely poisoned

3) Moderately chronically poisoned

4) Has some other problem

APPROPRIATE ACTION: 1) the patient is seriously chronically poisoned: the patient will be very sick for at least a year and will need extensive testing and ongoing medical assistance during this time. Amalgam removal, creative use of supplements and medications, and a well thought out chelation regimen are required. Complications are expected. The patient is most likely already using most of the supplements and medicines that can improve their condition. The patient's life will be seriously interfered with for a year or more.

2) the patient is seriously acutely poisoned: The patient probably has a sudden large exposure to mercury from, for example, dissimilar metals touching in the oral cavity. The most important thing to do is immediately resolve this situation by appropriate dental work to reduce exposure. Immediate improvement is often experienced. The major symptoms will resolve in 3-6 months. Simple testing will usually eliminate most of the major problems of long term exposure and amalgam removal, a simple supplement program, and a modest chelation program will resolve all problems within a year. Complications are not expected.

3) the patient is moderately chronically poisoned: the patient will be sick for at least a year and will need proper initial testing to identify the areas which require routine therapy during this time. Amalgam removal, standard supplements and a proper chelation regimen are required. Complications are not expected. The patient will experience prompt relief from the prescription of standard supplements and medications to start with, and their life need not be greatly interfered with.

4) the patient has a problem other than amalgam illness: much discomfort, expense and delay can be avoided by diagnosing the underlying problem before a large investment of time, effort, and money is made in amalgam removal, chelation, etc.

In the rare instances where a patient is found to have amalgam illness before it is very bad or the more common one of a patient deciding to remove her amalgams despite a lack of serious symptoms the need is for modest medical monitoring with one or two follow up appointments to ensure that no problems develop. It is generally appropriate to suggest that the patient have the fillings removed one tooth at a time with several weeks between removals. If the patient has CNS related symptoms that do not resolve, a therapeutic trial of chelation with DMSA and lipoic acid is appropriate some time after amalgam removal. If these do not improve after 3-6 months of therapy another cause should be sought.

A patient with a serious chronic condition (schizophrenia, multiple sclerosis) who chooses to have his amalgams removed or wishes to consider it should be worked up like a patient considered likely to have serious chronic mercury poisoning. Amalgam illness and other organic causes should be definitively excluded and some creative energy should go into this. Failure to do so ensures that the patient will not accept the physician's advice - especially if the problem is psychiatric - and will not seek the recommended help. It is entirely possible that the root of the patient's problem IS mercury intoxication or a related condition, which is curable. Even in this case, counseling may be an appropriate adjunct or follow up to treatment, and the patient is unlikely to heed advice to seek it unless the physician has been diligent in diagnosing and treating the physical aspects of the disease.

It is common for a patient to have never had a thorough work up and to desire to avoid blood draws or other unpleasant tests at first. After all, they may be difficult to draw blood from, bruise easily, be unusually sensitive to pain, and not have had any prior physician put earlier test results to productive use. This disbelief that testing will help is best handled by explaining what the value of each test is, ordering noninvasive tests at the first appointment or two, and taking a clinical approach so the patient can honestly be told - and convinced - that information from specific blood tests is necessary to make further progress. Patient response to the "doctor knows best" approach to justifying the need for tests is likely to be poor since most of these patients have had prior doctors take this approach and then fail to resolve their problem.

Common problems and treatments are tabulated below:

Hypothyroid symptoms	Desiccated thyroid or equivalent, 1-5 grains
Adrenal hypofunction symptoms	5 mg hydrocortisone 2-4 times a day, 1-3 grams per day borage oil, B vitamin supplementation
ACTH fall on stress	Carbamazepine
Male hypogonadism	Testosterone transdermal gel
Female hypogonadism	Birth control pills if desired
Hyperinsulinism	Chromium picolinate with meals, avoid sweets
Low magnesium (causing fibromyalgia, anxiety and cardiac problems)	500+ mg magnesium supplementation by mouth, 2 grams per day taurine, DDAVP if excessive urine volume, alkalinize urine, no caffeine, maximum tolerable thyroid supplementation, weekly injections iv (preferable) or im if needed.
Yeast (candidiasis)	Correct cortisol defect, assorted literature approaches, lamisil, diflucan, etc.
Allergy	Flax oil, Accolate, H1 blocker + histidine, exclude H2 blockers, inhaled steroids, 5 mg cortisol 2-4 times per day, NAET or other alternative treatments.
Malabsorption	Animal derived digestive enzymes, arginine + glutamine, 5 mg cortisol 2-4 times per day, DHEA
Partial diabetes insipidus	Carbamazepine, DDAVP if needed, wait for chelation to take effect.
Autoimmunity	Standard therapy + DHEA in large amounts + NAET + androgens if possible
Low immune fctn, susceptibility to infection	Echinacea + astragalus 1 wk/month, inositol, arginine + lysine, vitamin C
Concentration difficulty or brain fog	Hydergine 3-5 mg 3-4 times per day
Anxiety on hydrocarbon (exhaust) exposure	Niacinamide
Anxiety, general	Treat first as hypoglycemia, low cortisol. If ineffective try taurine + pregnenolone + DHEA + Gotu Kola, then GABA, then Rx drugs

What to do about mercury poisoning

Depression	Tyrosine or tryptophan (5HT) per amino acid test, B12 + folate at high levels + trimethylglycine, niacinamide, Rx antidepressants of different types to find the class that works, start with selegiline.
Schizophrenia spectrum disorder	Histidine (exclude if histadelic) + niacin + vinpocetine + borage oil. Limit copper absorption with 100 mg zinc + 1 mg Mo each day. Neuroleptics only if unavoidable.
Poorly regulated emotions	Carbamazepine
Bipolar disorder	Carbamazepine or lithium, phosphatidylcholine, choline, exclusion of histidine
Mania	Choline + phosphatidylcholine
Attention deficit	DMAE

Dental treatment

Unlike physicians, many dentists believe in amalgam illness. Unlike the medical treatment of amalgam illness, many dentists do know how to handle its dental treatment. Unfortunately mercury toxicity is such a hot political issue in the dental profession that most state licensing boards will revoke the license of a dentist who advertises too openly that s/he is "mercury free." So you have to ask around. There are several books discussing how to find a mercury free dentist and how they should remove your fillings safely.

You can get books from:

Bio-Probe, Inc.
PO Box 608010
Orlando, FL 32860-8010

as well as finding many in public libraries or through bookstores.

Referrals to mercury free dentists can be had from:

DAMS
PO Box 64397
Virginia Beach, VA 23467
(800) 311-6265
NatlDAMS@aol.com

www.amalgam.org

or from friends - ask around! You would be surprised how common this is, despite its lack of publicity.

The things you want to know about the dentist are: is the practice mercury free? If not, does he only place amalgams if a patient really, really, really, really insists so that he doesn't get in trouble with the state licensing board? Does he have experience removing people's amalgam fillings? Does he have lots of experience placing composite fillings? Experience with composites is very important as these are much harder to place properly than amalgams. Does he guarantee the work once you pay for it? Will they fix it for free if there is a problem? Do you know any satisfied customers? Does he take precautions to keep you from inhaling dust and vapors, swallowing amalgam chips during removal, or generally being exposed to mercury? You can find out if he really believes mercury is a toxic hazard by finding out: how does he protect himself while he is working on you?

Do be aware that in most states if a dentist says "mercury is toxic," or "amalgam is not good for you," the licensing board will take their license for saying that. Thus most of them will not respond directly to questions such as "Can I get mercury poisoning from my amalgam fillings?"

Amalgam Illness: Diagnosis and Treatment

If dissimilar metals touch in your mouth they make a battery and one of them dissolves. If amalgam touches another metal it is the amalgam that dissolves. Very rapidly. This releases vast quantities of highly toxic mercury ions. This may occur if a crown touches an adjacent filling, if a crown is places OVER a filling (which is hard to tell, though an amalgam tattoo around the base of the tooth is a giveaway), if a root canal is done through a crown and an amalgam filling is used to close it, if a bridge is placed over or next to amalgam fillings, etc. If health problems start to happen rapidly after a crown, bridge, etc. is placed this is most likely the problem. The work has to be re-done IMMEDIATELY, removing all amalgam from contact with a dissimilar metal. This is a very dangerous situation if you let it go! On the other hand, you will get well pretty quickly if you do correct this problem right away.

When the dentist is working on you he has to use an anesthetic. Most of the choices he has don't just contain one drug. They contain several plus half a dozen other things to preserve those. It is pretty common for mercury toxic people to be sensitive to at least one of these materials and feel pretty terrible after they had some "Novocaine®" in their mouth. There are some anesthetics that contain only water and one anesthetic medication. One of the more common of these is Carbocaine®. Ask the dentist to talk to you about what is in the anesthetics and to select one that has only a single ingredient - the anesthetic.

There is much discussion in the alternative medical community of administering vitamin C intravenously for amalgam illness. There is some merit in using it during or shortly after amalgam removal though it is certainly not essential. Vitamin C IV's should not be given before dental procedures since they can interfere with local anesthetic action. A vitamin C IV given shortly after or during amalgam removal will eliminate the symptoms of increased mercury exposure that would otherwise occur regardless of how careful the dentist is. If you and your doctor are comfortable with intravenous vitamin C you should use it, but if you are not there is no need to worry that you will suffer irreparable harm if you skip it.

There is a condition variously referred to as a "cavitation" or as "NICO" (neuralgia inducing cavitational osteonecrosis) that sometimes occurs in seriously amalgam ill people. In this condition some portions of the jawbone die and store toxins. These toxins are then continuously released and amalgam removal alone does not cure the patient. There is much debate among mercury free dentists as to the prevalence of this condition, but a patient who stops getting well after a few months should look into it. In these cases removal of the dead tissue by an oral surgeon experienced in this procedure leads to resumption of healing.

If cavitations are apparent at the initial exam or during the amalgam work, they should be treated at that time if they are real. The key question for the dentist is what fraction of his patients appear to have cavitations. If it is a small fraction the dentist is conservative in diagnosing them and a second opinion may be sought depending on cost and patient interest. If a large fraction of patients have cavitations (<25%) a second opinion is a very good idea. If a cavitation clearly exists there is no point delaying its treatment.

Any tooth which has had a retrograde amalgam filling of a root canal (amalgam surgically placed in the bottom tip of the tooth to seal it) has a reasonable likelihood of requiring cavitational surgery to remove the mercury impregnated tissue around it.

DENTAL WORK DETAILS

Do not take any chelating agents by mouth one day before or for 4 days after having amalgams removed. They may increase mercury absorption from the amalgam chips the dentist turned your old fillings into that will inevitably find their way into your gut.

What to do about mercury poisoning

There are many protocols for amalgam removal. Any involving a dam and independent breathing air or equivalent protection for you is suitable. For those who wish to be patient, removing one amalgam every 4-6 weeks will eventually do it and makes protection less of an issue. No matter how you do it, expect some exacerbation of symptoms and extra exposure from the procedure.

Think long and hard about whether you may have amalgam sealing a root tip or under a bridge or crown before doing all of this. If so, fix it early. Root tip amalgam shows up on x-rays. Amalgam under crowns does not.

Patients experience far fewer negative effects and symptom exacerbations from amalgam removal if they receive IV vitamin C shortly after dental work is completed. Small doses of DMPS administered intravenously at this time (e. g. 25-50 mg) may also be helpful, though the author recommends vitamin C alone. The few days following amalgam removal are the only time DMPS and DMSA should not be taken orally. Thus iv administration is required if they are to be used. Only DMPS is available for injection, and it is investigational[1] in the United States.

Some dentists administer vitamin C intravenously at the time of amalgam removal. If this is done competently (e. g. the IV solution is properly neutralized and buffered to pH 7.2 so it doesn't sting) it is fine and saves a later trip to the doctor's office if one wishes to have IV-C.

Some people (1 in 10?) need further attention to amalgam tattoos, amalgam chips, NICO, etc. The basic rule is to look for this stuff if you stop getting better and don't make the level of progress expected. It is normal to have progress slow down or even stop getting better for a few months starting about 3 or 4 months after amalgam removal. Some people have serious brain or liver intoxication and have to treat it properly to fix it - they

won't get better if they treat a "cavitation" instead. People who clearly have an unresolved problem should look into cavitations and have them surgically cleaned out if one is actually present.

When having dental work done, remember that there are risks and even the best dentist isn't perfect. Not all dentists are the best, either. Having a lot of fillings replaced when you are not in the best of health can result in one or more tooth roots becoming infected, which is exceptionally painful and requires a root canal or having the tooth pulled. If this kind of thing happens you are in for at least several days of really intense pain plus quite a bit of additional expense. Consider these risks and make sure you select a dentist who has a lot of experience with the materials that will be used, has found them satisfactory in many prior patients, and will be there and take care of you if there are problems.

Medical Treatment

INTRODUCTION

Amalgam illness is analogous to a war. Your enemy, mercury, captured a beachhead in your teeth and fortified it with amalgam. Then it launched an attack. House to house. Organ to organ. Cell to cell. Slowly capturing your body. You win the war with a surgical strike. Dental surgery. Drill out those fillings. Removing your amalgam declares an armistice. Fighting stops, but the mercury atoms are still dug in wherever they reached. Chelation sends clean up squads off to round up the enemy and escort them out. Meanwhile the surviving cells in your body get to work and to repair the war damage. Supplementation is like disaster relief - it makes the process go a lot faster.

There are two goals to treatment. First, get rid of the mercury. Second, control symptoms so you can be comfortable and productive during the prolonged period when mercury is removed and healing takes place. In order to control your symptoms it is

---

[1] not yet fully FDA approved.

83

necessary to identify the metabolic defects mercury is causing for you.

In your ongoing battle to control symptoms while the mercury comes out and your body repairs all the damage, you need to take a straightforward, common sense approach.

- Know yourself. If you react to everything, go slow, start with small doses of things, be patient. Don't be any more aggressive than your body and your psyche can tolerate.

- Start with the problems that are causing other problems.

- If your digestion is not working, get your guts fixed up since this will take a load off your liver and let you get helpful supplements and medicines into you.

- Make sure your hormones are working right. Treat your body, not numbers on a lab report.

- Solve the other troublesome problems, and find solutions that work for you.

It is very common for mercury poisoned people to have been treated for depression, and for most MD's to diagnose them as "just depressed." While depression is often present it is not the cause of the problem. It should be treated to reduce suffering. The underlying problems causing it must be identified and treated too - just treating depression is like continuing to give painkillers day after day for a broken arm instead of setting it and putting it in a cast.

People who became seriously chronically poisoned before anyone figured out what is going on need to pay diligent attention to this section as they will be very sick for a very long time if they do not take active medical measures to support their ailing physiology for a year or two while they detox. These people are pretty much holding their metabolism together with baling wire and duct tape until they get enough mercury

chelated out for their body to start working like it is supposed to again.

People who are not too seriously chronically poisoned, or who are acutely poisoned, can feel a lot better very quickly if they take appropriate supplements and use this section to identify and correct their one or two big problems. This way they can get well immediately and get the mercury out later.

SYMPTOM CONTROL IS NO SUBSTITUTE FOR AMALGAM REMOVAL AND MERCURY CHELATION. GET THE MERCURY OUT!

The most important part of treatment is to engage in regular chelation using appropriate chelating agents given in proper dosages on a safe administration schedule. It is especially important to realize that stretching the interval between doses does NOT make chelating agents more safe, it makes them more dangerous! Proper chelation is described in a separate section. As a rule, you will take one or two chelating agents during a "chelation campaign" and then take a break. You have to keep repeating this every 1-3 weeks for many, many months if you want to get well. You have to keep repeating this even after you start feeling well - there is a long period where it is KEEPING you well by removing the mercury that is leaking out of your tissues before it can build back up to harmful levels.

People who are not too toxic may not need much of the testing and intervention described below. However, even in the mildest case, amalgam removal is only half the cure. *Mercury in the brain does not come out at a reasonable rate and chelation with lipoic acid is necessary if it is to be removed.*

There is some evidence from animal studies (Zorn and Smith) and from people's experience that proper vitamin supplementation reduces the amount of new mercury that accumulates in your system. However it does not appear that vitamins or other nutritional supplements remove mercury that is already there unless they are monothiols that mobilize it or dithiols that chelate it. You can slow down the rate at which you accumulate new mercury with the right vitamins, but you have to take chelating agents if you want to get rid of the mercury already in you.

Taking appropriate nutritional supplements can make you feel MUCH better by interfering with the basic chemistry of how mercury messes up your body. Supplements can disagree with a person just like some foods do. It is often herbal supplements that cause trouble. Pay attention to your supplements and stop taking ones that bother you. I have included long lists of supplements and medicines in the therapeutic agents section so you can find ones that agree with you.

The most important supplements are: antioxidants such as vitamins C and E, essential fatty acids to repair cell membranes, things like forskolin to directly counteract the effects of mercury, and things like B-6, B-12, DHEA, thyroid and other hormones to replace the things which mercury interferes with the production or use of. It is generally a good idea to keep supplementary manganese (Mn) copper (Cu) to a minimum, and take supplementary zinc (Zn), magnesium (Mg) and molybdenum (Mo) regardless of how tests come out. Potassium (K) supplements should only be taken if serum or red blood cell potassium is notably low.

Some people are "universal reactors" and their immune system quickly sensitizes to new materials. These are the people who will benefit from a rotation diet. In addition, these people may also become sensitive to their supplements. Since these supplements are very beneficial, it is important to desensitize the patient to them. This may most conveniently be done using acupuncture and acupressure related techniques such as NAET. *Cutler* describes NAET, and information can be found on the web at www.naet.com or www.allergy2000.com. Practitioners who insist "the body knows what order to do things in" and will not flex what order they do some crucial items in for patient convenience are not adequately skilled

and another practitioner should be sought. Also, if treatments do not "take" or do not last and you start to become resensitized to previously treated materials, find another practitioner. Patients with a lot of sensitivities can have family members or friends taught how to treat them for each allergen.

Traditional allopathic approaches to allergy desensitization are too time consuming to be of practical utility.

Close attention to diet is crucial. Mercury stops some parts of your metabolism from working, so each and every chemical compound in the food you eat might be as foreign and indigestible to your body as kerosine is to most people. There is much superstition about such things as rotation diets. These are only helpful for people with problems directly caused by allergic reactions to foods they eat who sensitize easily. What seems to work best for most people is to eat a very limited number of things that they are absolutely sure are safe for them. Immediately removing spices and coloring agents and partially hydrogenated fats and oils (margarine, shortening) will be quite helpful. Most commercial baked goods are full of these "no-no's." Learn to religiously read lists of ingredients. Many stores claim their stock is "all natural." Sometimes it is. Ask around. Many people have trouble with, for example the antibiotics in meat. It is impractical in most cases to figure out exactly what you are having problems with. Find stuff you can eat and stick to it.

When you have gotten sick but don't yet know what to do about it or are in the process of learning, you may unintentionally eat the wrong things and fill your body up with toxic nasties that make you feel horrible. You can clear these out quickly if you either fast (which guarantees you don't get any more nasties accidentally) or stick to a diet of one or two things that are very simple and safe (like corn or potatoes) for a few days. It is a good idea to take your basic water soluble antioxidant supplements during this time. People who have low adrenal function will not tolerate a fast well - they will have hypoglycemia with associated fatigue and anxiety. People who may be reacting to antibiotics in their meat can get protein (also important in low adrenal function) from peas or beans[1] or from fish caught at sea instead of farmed (e. g. halibut, flounder, sea bass, snapper, etc. but not salmon, trout or catfish) if organic meat is not available[2].

The amount of mercury in fish is not so large that eating it a few times makes a significant difference. Fish that feed on the bottom (especially shellfish) and large fish that eat smaller fish like swordfish, tuna and sharks contain more mercury than other fish. Daily consumption of high mercury fish can make a significant difference, or even lead to mercury intoxication in especially sensitive people. Those who have liver problems leading to low bile secretion, and who have an especially high sensitivity to mercury intoxication are at risk. People who showed up toxic with perhaps 10-20 mcg/day of urinary mercury excretion and who have adequate bile secretion are not at significant risk if they consume fish during detox. People with low bile secretion will often be constipated, will have difficulty digesting fat, will often have light colored stools, and will have occasional jaundice.

Many people believe they are very brand sensitive in all their supplements. This usually turns out not to be true if they stop the rotation diet, other superstitious rituals, and instead eat only those few foods known to be safe for them. There will be occasional brands of this or that people don't tolerate, but it is not a widespread problem - most brands are fine for most people.

The most common physiological problems mercury toxic people have are with the adrenal and thyroid glands. Some have

overall low hormone production. Others have apparently adequate cortisol production that is not properly regulated to respond to the body's needs. In most cases the patient has strong symptoms of adrenal insufficiency and hypothyroidism, but blood test results are low-normal. The patients usually improve A LOT if modest amounts of supplemental hormones are given. Seriously toxic patients will need more than modest amounts of supplementary hormones. It is usually difficult to establish the proper dose.

Some people have the usual endocrine related antibodies which indicate they need hormone supplementation. Many people do not have these antibodies. Most of them still needs supplementation, even though their blood tests appear normal.

Exercise mobilizes mercury and needs to be done in MODERATION. It is NOT always good for you. Exercise is STRESS, and there is a particular physiological response to stress that is messed up in most mercury toxic people - cortisol goes DOWN instead of UP like it is supposed to. So you can release adrenaline and feel really good WHILE you are active, but then crash afterwards and take a long time to recover. Depending on how sick you are this can be from hours to days. Moderation is doing exercise in small enough bits that you don't get this "crash" after it. No hours of sitting and doing nothing. No inability to think. No being woozy with allergy symptoms.

If you have a paradoxical cortisol (or ACTH) response to stress, getting small amounts of exercise a few minutes at a time during the day will help you feel better, but be CAREFUL not to overdo it! Everyone has to learn their own limits by paying attention to their body and remembering how they reacted to exercise in the past. You will always feel good DURING exercise - that is the danger. The question is how you will feel an hour or two after you stop.

Controlling this aberrant stress response with medications such as cortisol and carbamazepine is described later.

---

[1]High in sulfur and copper - some people must limit these elements.

[2] "Natural" does NOT mean organic! Organic is the identifying mark that means no hormones, antibiotics or feed additives were used. Natural means pretty much whatever the producer feels like it means that day - which is usually not much.

What to do about mercury poisoning

Once amalgams have been removed, symptoms can be directly controlled by taking small amounts of oral DMPS or DMSA on a rational administration schedule. DMPS 50-100 mg every 8 hours. DMSA 50-300 mg every 4 hours. A few people who have fast liver "phase 1" metabolism may need to take DMPS and DMSA more frequently than this to maintain even blood levels and suppress symptoms effectively. Do this for 4-10 days, then skip 3 or 4 days. This does not reduce the total amount of mercury in your body significantly and is not intended to do so. The purpose of this is to passivate the free mercury in your blood so as to suppress symptoms somewhat.

Citrate, as in supplements like magnesium citrate is a very mild chelating agent. Barely a chelating agent. But it is one. It does have some ability to reduce symptoms like "brain fog" in many people.

If you find yourself and your doctor spending a lot of time adjusting a particular medication or protocol up and down and back again, and doing a lot of testing relating to it, most likely it isn't the real problem. You have to convince the doctor to stop thrashing and get a correct diagnosis instead of the one you are working from. You and your doctor have to "think outside the box." Talk to other people. Do different tests. Once you identify the real problem you will be able to get all of your dosages and treatments adjusted properly and have them stay that way indefinitely.

CHILDREN

Many children are poisoned by mercury or other environmental toxins. These often cause developmental delays, learning disabilities, autism, hyperactivity, allergies and asthma. These can all be cured by appropriate detoxification, and if this is performed in childhood, most or all of the deficits in intellectual, emotional and physical development can be made up for during the ongoing process of growth which naturally changes and improves things.

Unfortunately many physicians are afraid to try to do anything to help children for fear of liability, because children's metabolisms are less well understood than adults, and because test results have to all be looked up to see which ones are naturally different in childhood. In addition, drug dosages have to be routinely weight adjusted which requires calculation for every prescription instead of just writing down the same thing for everyone as is done with adults.

It is important to treat children early so as to not miss the opportunity for complete healing that growth represents. Children recover faster and more fully from many things than adults. Children also have the great advantage that they actually are being taken care of all the time. Adults have to devote much energy to taking care of themselves, making a living, and staying organized. Children do not have these burdens. It is best to detoxify them early while they still have the advantage of a supportive environment.

There is one very good pragmatic reason to detox children early. During the process of growing up, becoming sexually mature and experiencing puberty large amounts of new hormones surge through their bodies and cause tremendous growth and changes. In particular, their brains grow and change a lot. During this time it is well known that many earlier learning or behavioral problems disappear. If you detox your children BEFORE this is complete, there is a much better chance they will become a reasonably normal well behaved adolescent. If you do NOT detox them they may develop NEW behavior problems in adolescence, and it is much more difficult to care for and control adolescents than small children. Don't lose your golden opportunity by waiting!

The most obvious difference in the biochemistry of children and adults is that children do not make and use the steroid hormones (adrenal hormones and sex hormones) during the earlier parts of their lives. These are also hormones that can interfere with and affect growth until full adult height is achieved. Thus in treating children it is best to avoid using any steroid hormones if possible. These include pregnenolone, DHEA, cortisol, glucocorticoids, estrogens, androgens, androstenedione, testosterone, etc. Do not use these unless absolutely necessary.

The major hormone problem to be concerned about in children is thyroid deficiency. Quiet , sedate, weak children with slow growth should be suspected of having low thyroid if there are other reasons to believe they are mercury toxic. If they also have a history of bed wetting or wetting their pants to an unusually late age you should assume that their pituitary is not functioning well and that they need to be treated but that the TSH test is useless for tracking and controlling treatment.

Other differences include: children use more food per weight and thus can use more of supplements like flax or borage oil than their weight would suggest; iron is more toxic to children than to adults and should not be used unless clearly indicated; children's metabolism is faster so things given in small frequent doses should be given somewhat more frequently than for adults if the child appears to be having trouble with it; children's immune systems are much more active than in adults; and the amino acid arginine actually is essential for children.

The prescription drug DMSA is specifically approved for use in treating lead poisoning in children. It is safe for children. In a technical sense DMSA has only been proven to be safe in children - it's use in adults is "speculative." It is appropriate to use DMSA to treat children who have heavy metal poisoning. That is what it was made for.

If you have a child you want to detox, find a doctor who wants to help sick children get well and who is open minded, instead of one who went into pediatrics because they enjoy seeing a lot of kids who are basically fine and not having to worry about them too much. The doctor you need may or may not be a pediatrician. It is a very rare family practice physician who will stick with you

through a difficult project like this without wanting to refer you somewhere - anywhere - because it is hard to figure out what to do next.

Mercury and other heavy metal intoxications affect the emotions. Marlowe has shown that emotionally disturbed children have elevated levels of lead and mercury. Pay attention to how your child feels. Most adults have difficulty believing that a child is seriously emotionally distraught and won't come out of it on their own. Yet this happens frequently in mercury poisoning. Children don't have the maturity to handle themselves when their emotions are bouncing around like a ball in a pinball machine. You have to help them do that. Learn to talk to your child about their emotions, be very open and accepting so they don't learn to tell you what you want to hear, and believe what they are telling you.

Mercury affects the third cranial nerve and can cause a variety of binocular vision defects. Since ophthalmologists (MD's who are trained to perform surgery on the eye) don't know how to look for these or indeed what they are, these are usually missed and diagnoses of attention deficit disorder or dyslexia are made instead. The problem can be cured[1] with active vision therapy after detoxification[2]. This vision therapy should be performed by a behavioral optometrist rather than an ophthalmologist as the

---

[1] which has a large positive effect on behavior, school performance and sports ability. It is often covered by health plans as a medical benefit.

[2] Unlike adults who develop visual problems due to mercury poisoning, children who develop these problems often do so before they have learned to use their visual system properly. There is an age at which learning how to use binocular vision to see in depth, with perspective, and learning to use the eyes together comes naturally. If these skills are not learned at that time then they must be actively taught. Adults with toxin induced visual defects will usually have learned these skills at some point in childhood - and like learning to ride a bicycle, once you know how you don't forget even if it is years since you did it last. Adults with a childhood history of unresolved learning disabilities may require active vision therapy.

What to do about mercury poisoning

likelihood of a favorable outcome is much higher. If there is regression after vision therapy it is usually a sign that further detoxification is necessary.

Increasing mercury correlates with childhood intelligence (Marlowe *et al.* 1986). Since intelligence correlates with success at school, in social circles, at work, and ultimately at life, it makes sense to detox children as early as possible so they don't have a lot of catching up to do once they have full use of their brain back. It is not known whether artificially induced intelligence deficits during the formative years lead to permanent deficits that cannot be caught up on later.

The opportunity to make your child smarter, healthier, more emotionally stable and give them the opportunity to catch up on past problems through natural growth and development it is well worth taking.

It is common for more than one family member to be mercury poisoned. In this case it is best not to delay detoxing everyone. If both adults are poisoned, it is best for the healthier of the two to delay detox, or begin it very slowly, while the other adult and the children detox aggressively.

CHELATION

Chelation takes the mercury out of you and makes you healthier. Everything else in this chapter corrects the problems mercury causes and makes you feel better while you are detoxing, but it does not cure you. Chelation is what cures you. Chelation is the most important part of your treatment.

In the few months post amalgam removal, you may patiently wait for your fast body pool to drain while taking minimal chelating agent to suppress symptoms, or you may take large amounts of oral DMPS or DMSA to reduce it faster. DMPS is MUCH more effective for this purpose. Symptoms relieved by chelation are brain fog, attention deficit, inability to concentrate, anxiety, and other emotional disturbances. Allergies may or may not be suppressed.

Distributing the chelating agent over a couple of months (with breaks) is more effective at removing mercury than is taking a bunch over a short period. Under ideal circumstances the total amount of chelating agent used would not be limited and high doses would be used to cure the patient quickly. A typical dose would be 200-400 mg DMSA every 4 hours, or 400-800 mg DMPS every 8 hours. The dosage used in high dose regimens is 10 mg/kg of body weight (DMPS) or 5 mg/kg (DMSA).

Some highly poisoned patients may want to get well quickly through aggressive chelation. Even the most well optimized protocol will cause side effects as the dose is increased. Thus high dose chelation followed by intravenous vitamin C (a vitamin/mineral drip) to cut short the prolonged recovery from side effects may be appropriate early in therapy.

If chelating at high dosages it is wise to get a routine urinalysis every few weeks and to stop if red blood cells start to show up. At high doses, occasional blood counts are more important than otherwise.

Several months after amalgam removal, the 'fast' body pools of mercury should be much reduced and it is time to mobilize the 'slow' body pools. This can be done with lipoic acid, 30-200 mg every 3-4 hours (0.18-1.2 grams per day). Unlike the other chelating agents lipoic acid will not suppress symptoms. DMPS or DMSA in the low doses mentioned above should be taken with the lipoic acid to suppress symptoms. This regimen must be pursued continuously for 6 months to 2 years to rid the body of mercury.

Therapeutic approaches currently offered by some practitioners but which should never be used include: DMPS by injection except when oral administration is contraindicated and dosage is low, DMPS or DMSA on any schedule not involving frequent administration of equal doses for at least several days in a row, EDTA chelation, or penicillamine in any form. Supplementary cysteine, glutathione, or a "high sulfur" diet, or chlorella should not be used. All of these "therapies" will be very harmful to you.

The idea that essential minerals are depleted by chelation and require routine replacement via intravenous therapy is not correct. It is in effect a superstition believed among some in the "alternative medicine" community. This has been demonstrated both by direct measurements of blood levels and by mass balance calculations. DMPS and DMSA do not significantly alter the body's inventory of nontoxic materials under the conditions of use discussed in this book. Lipoic acid actually INCREASES the body's inventory of zinc and copper, and the chelation protocols as given here account for that fact. Oral supplementation of certain minerals is helpful in altering the body's metabolism in favorable ways or making up for common deficits - but they are not being administered to make up for materials removed by chelation and an increase in urinary excretion of a mineral during chelation is not an indicator it should be supplemented or injected.

DMPS and DMSA are used as described above in the early phase of detox to clear the bloodstream of mercury. Once blood mercury has been reduced adequately lipoic acid (LA) is added to remove mercury from internal organs - especially the brain.

Taking 50-100 mg of DMSA + 50-200 mg of LA every 3-4 hours will remove mercury from the brain and internal organs. You will want to do this for 3-4 days in a row and then skip several days. It removes about 1/2 to 1% of the mercury in the brain every day that you chelate. Thus in order to reduce brain mercury by 50%, you have to chelate for 70-140 days.

You can also take DMPS 50-100 mg ever 8 hours plus LA 50-200 mg every 3-4 hours. It is a bit more difficult to keep track of but works fine and feels a little better. Mercury is removed at about the same rate. You will want to do this for 3-4 days in a row and then skip several days.

If you can't get DMSA or don't want to, you can just use 25-200 mg of LA every 3-4 hours. You may want to do this for a week or so and then skip a week or so.

You do not want to chelate with lipoic acid more than half the time or your body levels of zinc and copper will increase a lot and other minerals may also go out of balance.

You select the dosages of DMSA and LA to use based on how you feel when you take them. Taking a high dose that makes you uncomfortable does not speed up detox all that much - it is best to select a dose that allows you to get on a schedule and do some chelation every week or two. You can raise the dose later if you become more comfortable as you detox.

Figure 15 earlier in the book gives a schematic illustration of where mercury comes out of and how you feel as this chelation process goes on.

For most people the proper chelation protocol using DMSA and LA is:

- Starting 4 days after the last filling is replaced, 50-100 mg DMSA every 4 hours (including getting up at night to take a dose) for 2-6 months, until urine mercury is reduced 80%.

- Then DMSA 50-100 mg + LA 50-200 mg every 3-4 hours (including getting up at night to take a dose) for about 3 days per week. When you feel all better, keep going for a few months. You may need to do this anywhere from 6 to 36 months depending on how sick you were to start and how hard your body holds on to the mercury.

- It is important to keep taking your supplements and medicines during the whole time you are chelating.

What to do about mercury poisoning

INTRAVENOUS VITAMIN C

Intravenous vitamin C is in vogue among alternative practitioners for mercury "detox." Since it is so commonly discussed for amalgam illness it bears discussing here. IV-C appears to help suppress mercury toxicity but it is NOT a chelating agent by itself. An IV of 20 grams of vitamin C substantially reduces symptoms for several days[1]. IV's of up to 50 grams are used by some practitioners. This is hard on the kidneys and should certainly not be used by those with low creatinine clearance or a history of kidney stones. Vitamin C IV's should not be given before dental procedures since they can interfere with local anesthetic action. A vitamin C IV given shortly after or during amalgam removal will eliminate the symptoms of increased mercury exposure that would otherwise occur regardless of how careful the dentist is.

Intravenous vitamin C is quite controversial in medicine today. If you and your doctor are not completely comfortable with it there is no need to use it. It is not an essential component of mercury detox, though it can make your life much more pleasant in certain situations.

The reason to administer vitamin C intravenously is that absorption from the gut is limited. Small amounts of vitamin C are absorbed efficiently, but large amounts are not. Even taking extremely large amounts of vitamin C orally, people absorb more or less 5 grams of it in a day. If it is administered intravenously much more than this can enter the body over an hour or two, leading to dramatically higher tissue concentrations. Since the amount of vitamin C required is large, it cannot be given as an intramuscular injection as, say, vitamin B-12 can.

Intravenous vitamin/mineral drips (putting a pint of vitamin solution into your vein over an hour or two) are a common form of therapy among "alternative" practitioners and very uncommon among "mainstream" physicians. It is safe in most instances and can be done easily at a medical office. These drips typically contain 20 to 50 grams of vitamin C.

First, the risks:

The two life threatening risks from intravenous vitamin C administration are:

1) Individuals with glucose-6-phosphatase deficiency (mostly black males) are believed to be at risk for a hemolytic crisis when vitamin C is infused properly; and

2) If the vitamin C solution is to be prepared in distilled water and the distilled water is inadvertently infused without mixing the vitamin C into it a hemolytic crisis will occur.

There is a further risk. Repeated infusions of large amounts of vitamin C, e. g. >50 grams, appear to carry a small risk of kidney stones. The more usual amounts of 20-30 grams used by many practitioners appear to not to have this risk even with frequent administration.

The merits of IV vitamin C, or IV vitamin/mineral drips (which contain 20-50 grams of vitamin C) are that they make pretty much anyone feel better. They are especially effective in controlling adverse reactions to improper use of chelating agents and helping people fight viral infections. Vitamin C injections were a well known therapeutic measure for inadvertent mercury toxicity in the past when mercury containing diuretics were commonly used. Thus the appropriate uses for vitamin/mineral drips are to:

- improve patient tolerance of amalgam removal

- improve patient response to infection early in detox if the immune system is compromised

- treat adverse reactions to chelating agents

---

[1] Since intravenous vitamin C makes people with a wide variety of conditions feel better, this cannot be used to test for mercury poisoning.

- strengthen the adrenal glands when they are stressed by high mercury exposure

- allow the patient to perform important tasks for several days if these cannot be delayed until later in detox

Vitamin/mineral drips should not be used routinely to allow improper use of chelating agents, nor should they be substituted for or delay detoxification.

The easy way for a physician not familiar with preparing intravenous vitamin C infusions to do so in the office is to add the desired amount of sodium ascorbate for injection - perhaps 20 grams or 3 30 ml vials of sodium ascorbate for injection - to Ringer's solution[1] and infuse this over 1-2 hours. The solution is hypertonic. More protocols may be found in an appendix.

TESTING TABLE AND SUGGESTIONS

Certain medical tests are likely to be helpful once a diagnosis of chronic mercury intoxication has been established as described in the DIAGNOSIS section above[2]. You and your physician should consider each of the following tests and think about whether you need to get the information it represents by performing it or in some other way in order to treat you properly.

- Great Smokies[3] Comprehensive Liver Detoxification Profile or equivalent;

- Digestive Stool Analysis (with ova and parasite exam, plus serum amoeba antibodies);

- Immunoglobulin E (IgE), RAST or prick allergy tests;

- Creatinine clearance[4];

- K, Mg and Cu in red blood cells (RBC's, erythrocytes);

- Autoimmune markers;

- Some sort of hormone profile including diurnal variations in cortisol, melatonin and sex steroids[5], appropriate testing of hormones and pituitary factors;

- Plasma amino acid analysis;

- Essential fatty acid profile;

- T, B and NK cell panel and IgG subclasses if appropriate;

- Check for infectious agents and parasites such as candida, giardia, amoeba, cryptosporidium, clostridia dificile, Lyme disease, mycoplasma, HHV-6, EBV, coxsackie virus, hepatitis, helicobacter pylori, chlamydia and HIV[6].

---

[1] Ringer's is suggested because it contains some magnesium and many mercury toxic people are low in magnesium. Saline and sterile water are also fine. Some mercury toxic people do not regulate blood sugar well so dextrose is undesirable.

[2] remember, it is what you think that is important. What the doctor thinks is only important if you believe it too.

[3] see appendix for information on some laboratories that offer useful tests.

[4] this is an indication of whether your kidneys are clearing your blood of toxins effectively. It is more sensitive than serum creatinine, which is also an indication of that. Since you will naturally end up with the information to have this number calculated it makes sense to do so.

[5] which measures the daily variation in cortisol, DHEA, the sex hormones and melatonin. Labs like Great Smokies and Diagnostechs offer useful tests. Daily amounts such as via Meridian Valley 24 hour urine hormone profile are also useful. See appendix.

[6] this is not an exhaustive list and which ones to test for should be guided by your physician's judgment. Tests should if possible include IgG and IgM or antibodies to assorted parts of the organism so some conclusion can be drawn regarding whether it is a current infection, evidence of a past infection, or a relatively high antibody titer due to chronic virus reactivation.

What to do about mercury poisoning

Some but not all of these tests are also useful in diagnosing amalgam illness.

The results of these tests may suggest other tests to perform. It is presumed things like a complete blood chemistry panel, blood count, etc. were run during diagnostic testing. If not, total cholesterol, triglycerides, sodium, potassium, magnesium, iron, ferritin, glucose, creatinine and sedimentation rate should be determined and a blood count performed[1].

A low sedimentation rate suggests testing for autoimmune antibodies[2]. A high sedimentation rate with symptoms of achiness suggests fibromyalgia as part of the symptom complex and suggests trial therapy with thyroid hormone even if tests show it normal. Low magnesium is another common cause and must sometimes be treated by injections for a while. These and other treatments for fibromyalgia, as well as diagnostic guidelines, are given by Teitelbaum (1996). Some treatments will also be discussed below.

Patient symptoms will suggest possible autoimmune problems to the physician and enough relevant antibodies should be measured to determine whether autoimmune disease is a part of the overall problem. If so, appropriate supplements and medicines should be used, and the autoimmune markers provide a good means of tracking progress. Certain types of autoimmune diseases, e. g. thyroid stimulating antibodies, require frequent attention since their effects wax and wane on a period of weeks to months.

If an infectious agent is identified, it must first be determined whether it is active or simply evidence of a past infection. Some labs test for a number of different antibody types which can be useful for this[3]. Then it must be determined whether this is simply due to mercury caused immunosuppression or the infection itself is actually causing most or all of the problem. Either way, it is likely to be helpful to suppress the infectious agent through appropriate therapy, if possible.

The creatinine clearance may conveniently be combined with other tests that doctors often like to order since it requires measurement of 24 hour urine creatine plus serum creatinine sometime during the 24 hour urine collection period. Those who are not eating much meat can use numbers from different days. Suggested tests to get CC are a very complete blood chemistry panel including CO_2, HDL cholesterol and magnesium as well as the usual 20 or so other things on these panels. A 24 hour urine steroid test (as through Meridian labs) or a 24 hour urine toxic and essential elements test (as through Doctor's Data) give creatinine numbers along with the other results[4].

The physician's role is not to deny you tests or to get you to order tests from a health plan lab that aren't really equivalent to the one you need, but instead to talk to you about what you are trying to figure out so that she can suggest the best approach to determining it. After all, the physician did spend years

---

[1] These are the kinds of things most physicians will order as screening tests if you press them to do something because you are sick. The "nothing is wrong, try some prozac" syndrome starts if these all come back normal.

[2] Many physicians test for these anyway. There are a very large number of autoimmune antibodies that can be tested for, so you need to depend on your physician to suggest a few that are most likely to be positive.

---

[3] For example, IgM is elevated in active infection along with IgG, but only IgG is elevated when the infection is over and you are immune to the agent. If only IgG can be determined, measuring it monthly will show a steady decline if the infection is recent, will show it going up and down if the infection is chronic, and will show it steady if the infection happened a long time ago.

[4] Your physician can do this using nomographs in standard books, or can ask a clinical laboratory to do it. They will need your serum and 24 hour urine creatinine values as well as your height, weight, and for some formulae, sex. If a surprising value results, check your 24 hour urine creatinine value with the formula in the appendix - it is not uncommon for labs to get this wrong due to sample mishandling.

and years learning about how your body works and what all the tests do. If she will work with you to understand why you think you need some testing she may be able to get you just the right test to figure out what is happening and get you well sooner instead of later!

Since chronic mercury poisoning has a broad effect on human physiological processes that is not covered during medical education, the physician will frequently be surprised when tests are abnormal that s/he was SURE would come back fine. When in doubt about what is happening to you, these tests are medically necessary because physicians will often be misled into overlooking problems if they rely solely on signs, symptoms, and your complaints[1].

FIBROMYALGIA

Fibromyalgia or generalized overwhelming achiness is most often relieved by supplementary thyroid hormone, even when thyroid blood tests are normal. On occasion it is relieved by certain antidepressants. Sulfur food exclusion diets will also often relieve it, but it does take about a week to clear up. Many people whose fibromyalgia is relieved by sulfur food exclusion do have low glutathione conjugation and must take NAC when they exclude sulfur foods. Excluding trans fatty acids (from partially hydrogenated vegetable oils) from the diet ends many people's

---

[1] It is necessary to have a physician who pays attention to you as well as to the piece of paper the lab sends them, because a lot of the tests they WILL think to order come back normal despite your having all of the symptoms of the condition they are testing for. In these cases treating the condition despite the lab test often makes all the symptoms go away and does not create any health problems or laboratory abnormalities. The informative tests are usually the ones discussed here that the physician is sure will come back normal when you have everything that suggests you do the test. It is not necessary or wise to treat all abnormalities or to not treat everything where the test comes back within normal limits - you and your physician need to exercise some thoughtful judgment here.

fibromyalgia, but it takes a month or two before this happens and puts most prepared foods off limits. People who have a rapid resting respiration rate for no apparent reason are good candidates to benefit from TFA exclusion. Guaifenesin also relieves fibromyalgia symptoms for some people after an initial period of one or two months of worsening them, as discussed widely on the internet. Magnesium deficiency is also a cause of fibromyalgia. Its diagnosis and treatment are described later. *Teitelbaum* discusses treatments for fibromyalgia.

A laundry list of things that might make you stop hurting if you have fibromyalgia is:

- Thyroid hormone. T4 + T3 or T3 alone. Not just T4

- Large amounts of supplementary magnesium

- Frequent magnesium injections

- Celebrex®

- Some powerful sleeping aid, e. g. Remeron® or Ambion®

- Tricyclic antidepressants

- Exclusion of trans fats (partially hydrogenated oils) from your diet

- Large amounts of flax oil, starting with a lot of fish oil the first month

- Coenzyme Q-10

- Acetyl-l-carnitine

- Ginger

- Correcting mild adrenal insufficiency (of the sort some docs may not notice)

FATIGUE

Many mercury poisoned people have chronic fatigue. The different treatments described here may correct it, it may respond

What to do about mercury poisoning

to the dietary manipulations, and it is likely to end once they are detoxified. In the meantime they may need medical help to have enough energy to cope with life.

Hydrocortisone 5 mg 2-4 times per day, or 10 mg with breakfast and 5 mg with lunch (and maybe 5 more mg with an afternoon snack) will alleviate fatigue if you have low cortisol levels due to hypoadrenalism - low adrenal function. This is discussed above in more detail.

Symptoms of feeling cold, lethargic, apathetic, sleepy and having a dark outlook on life may be due to low brain histamine. This can be corrected by taking the amino acid histidine. Response to 1/2-2 gram per day should occur within a few days.

Unrecognized hypothyroidism is a common source of chronic fatigue. See discussions in the pituitary and thyroid sections to decide whether a trial of thyroid hormone is appropriate.

Patients who must alleviate fatigue can use prescription medicines such as Cylert® and Ritalin® if less powerful (and less regulated) alternatives are ineffective. It is essential to use the lowest effective dose to prevent liver complications. Ephedrine several times per day is often effective. Pseudoephedrine also works for some people. If tyrosine was notably low on the plasma AA profile, supplementing it or phenylalanine may be energizing. Note that thyroid medication and cortisol make the patient more sensitive to the effects of these materials, and to their own epinephrine.

AMINO ACID ANALYSIS

Mercury poisoning impairs the body's ability to regulate the level of amino acids appropriately. It is very likely that giving you some supplementary amino acids will make you feel a LOT better, and that knowing which amino acids are available in what amounts will allow other biochemical abnormalities to be identified that can be treated. The plasma amino acid (AA) analysis is used to determine which amino acids to supplement (or increase through dietary modification) and which to reduce by looking at which ones are relatively high or relatively low compared to the others. This is NOT done by checking which ones are out of the normal range! Normalizing the amino acid balance generally relieves some symptoms and leads to an increased feeling of well being. This is "balancing" the metabolism. It may be desirable to supplement certain amino acids at high levels for pharmacologic reasons without regard for the AA results. This is most often done with arginine. Remember - neither you nor the food you eat contains a "perfect balance" of amino acids. The idea is to gently push certain things in the right direction, or to shove hard on other things that relate to specific problems you are having. There is no point in taking some special supplement to achieve "perfect balance."

Like all laboratory tests, the amino acid test is a way to get additional useful information. It is NOT a substitute for paying close attention to how you feel or what signs you have of problems. Many things can be figured out from signs and symptoms alone. Many things can't be figured out just from the test results.

Some people are very sensitive to supplements that directly affect brain chemistry. If you have had past experiences with these supplements that indicate you are sensitive, start with very small doses and increase them slowly when you try new things to change your brain chemistry. The specific amino acids of concern here are phenylalanine, tyrosine, tryptophan and histidine.

The AA analysis may provide insight into which therapeutic trials are unlikely to be productive - for example, selective serotonin reuptake inhibitors (SSRI's), 5-HTP and increased dietary tryptophan are unlikely to relieve depression in someone who already has fairly high plasma tryptophan, so other things should be tried first. Amino acids to pay special attention to are phenylalanine, tyrosine, tryptophan, taurine, cysteine (available from the gsdl comp liver detox test and on some aa panels, but not most of them), glutamine, and histidine.

Elevated cysteine indicates excess levels of thiol groups are available and these must be restricted in the diet and supplements. This can lead to excess cystine in the brain. Cystine activates the neuronal acetylcholine receptor causes central nervous system stimulation, depolarization and firing of postganglionic autonomic neurons, and adrenaline + noradrenaline secretion. Elevated plasma cystine will also have the same effect.

Elevated cysteine will often lead to excitement, elevated blood pressure, increased immune activity and allergy, excessive talkativeness, impaired judgment, and increased libido. There may also be periods of depression, weakness and incoordination. Poor blood sugar regulation is also possible. These problems can be reduced by a "sulfur food" restriction diet and by taking chromium picolinate with meals.

Low cysteine and glutamine may lead to hypoglycemia and asthma.

In fibromyalgia, tryptophan, histidine and serine are usually low. Teitelbaum (1996) provides a good description of fibromyalgia and its treatment. Fibromyalgia is often present in mercury poisoning.

A sleepily depressed person with hypothyroidism and fibromyalgia either has low phenylalanine or low tyrosine (amino acids) or is hypoadrenal and has low cortisol.

Taurine is necessary to prevent too much magnesium from being lost in the urine, and it also regulates the balance of magnesium, calcium, sodium and potassium inside and outside cells. Thus correcting low taurine is likely to improve electrolyte problems - especially those that have not responded to supplements. Intractable electrolyte problems suggest testing for plasma amino acids to investigate taurine. An anxiously depressed person with low taurine and possibly signs of hypothyroidism is hypoadrenal - that is, has

cortisol levels which are too low. This may not show up on tests for cortisol since the dynamic range of cortisol levels are so wide and people's individual needs for it vary so much.

Taurine also specifically scavenges the hypochlorite (OCl^-) anion. Sensitivity to chlorine as in swimming pool chlorine or bleach odor strongly suggests taurine deficiency.

Taurine is involved in proper heart function. Heart problems of any sort suggest a taurine trial unless it is known to be relatively high.

Women produce taurine less efficiently than men and are thus more likely to need to supplement it.

Deficient histidine can cause endocrine problems that resolve on supplementation. It can also cause immune system dysregulation. Some individuals experience schizophrenia when histidine falls low enough to reduce brain histamine below a critical level and can have it quickly put into remission with adequate supplementary histamine, but not by any other means.

Lysine improves concentration and if it is low concentration may be impaired and not responsive to other treatments.

Supplemental arginine (3-18 grams per day) without regard for the level found during AA analysis is helpful in healing leaky gut (along with glutamine), relieving angina, promoting growth hormone release, and generally promoting tissue formation and healing. It is often helpful in alleviating chronic fatigue.

A high ratio of glutamate to glutamine suggests adrenal insufficiency. Glutamine and GABA will be low in hypoadrenal people, which will lead to concentration difficulties and anxiety.

People with low histidine and high methionine cannot tolerate copper, have abnormal symptoms during allergy season (no runny nose itchy eyes as in typical histamine reactions because they have low histamine). People with elevated histidine and low methionine will have severe "normal" allergies and lots of colds. Meat is the primary source of methionine, and grains are a major source of histidine.

An upset stomach can often be calmed with glycine. Glutamine helps but not for hypoadrenal people. Glutamine also helps heal up the gut for people who are not hypoadrenal but have yeast, leaky gut, IBS, colitis, etc.

If you are exercise intolerant you may find that glutamine, BCAA's, and creatine taken 2 hours before and then just after exercise help if your cortisol levels aren't too low.

If you feel bad after taking glutamine or creatine you may have problems with the bacteria and yeast in your intestines making too much ammonia. These can sometimes be fixed by taking flora supplements like bifidobacteria and lactobacteria acidophilus in large doses (about 10 times what it says on the bottles).

If you have alcohol or sugar cravings you can cut them down by taking 1-4 grams of glutamine in divided doses before 4 PM.

Low tyrosine, phenylalanine, tryptophan or glutamine is often seen in depression, and supplementing helps. Glutamine is not helpful for hypoadrenal people unless they also take cortisol - which may make their glutamine normal anyway.

Brain levels of serotonin, dopamine, norepinephrine (noradrenaline), epinephrine (adrenaline), acetylcholine and histamine are known to depend on how much of the precursors (stuff they are made from) are in your diet. If you have a condition that suggests you have too much or too little of one, or are taking a drug to affect levels of one in your brain, you might want to try supplements or dietary modification. The precursors are:

phenylalanine and tyrosine ------>
     dopamine, noradrenaline, adrenaline

histidine --------------------------> histamine

tryptophan or 5-hydroxytryptophan ------->
     serotonin

choline or (better) phosphatidylcholine
or (best) DMAE
     --------> acetylcholine

Amounts of amino acid supplements that help many people:

Lysine 7-12 grams
Phenylalanine, men 4-7 grams,
     women and children 1-4 grams
Tyrosine, men 2-4 grams
     women and children 0.5-2 grams
Tryptophan, usually 3-4 grams,
     sometimes 1-6 grams
GABA, 1-2 grams

If you crave protein, take branched chain amino acids - this may be what your body is trying to get. If they don't help alone, take some cortisol (e. g. 5 mg 2-4 times per day) along with them and read the adrenal section. Other convenient sources of BCAA's may be found in the grocery store: whey contains high levels of BCAA's and sulfur amino acids (thus it must be excluded from the diet of people who are sensitive to "sulfur foods") and it is a common ingredient in grocery store bakery products like muffins and pound cake, some of which are also made with butter or vegetable oil instead of hydrogenated oils like margarine or vegetable shortening. Whey protein is also a common supplement available for bodybuilders. BCAA's themselves are also available from some supplement suppliers for those who are "sulfur food" sensitive. Whey is a component of milk, but not of cheese.

The AA analysis may also provide insight into whether magnesium is low, which is not apparent from serum levels and sometimes not even apparent from RBC levels. Indicators of magnesium deficiency are high phosphoserine with normal or low serine, high ethanolamine with low phosphoethanolamine, high citrulline, and low asparagine or arginosuccinate. Other indicators are low serum potassium, overly tense muscles (in extreme cases tetany with standard signs), anxiety, and heart disturbances.

MAGNESIUM, POTASSIUM, COPPER AND IRON

Many mercury toxic people have low magnesium. Since this is mostly stored inside cells other than blood, it is often not reflected in tests. In addition to the above amino acid indications, the problem should be considered if:

Serum magnesium is below 1.6
Red blood cell (packed erythrocyte) magnesium is low
Oral magnesium supplements have a laxative effect at or below a total magnesium content of 600 mg per day
You have fibromyalgia
You have angina
You have potassium wasting

A person with low adrenal function is also very likely to be magnesium deficient. Serum magnesium tests are not a reliable guide to magnesium status. Red blood cell magnesium is better but not definitive. Certain patterns in the plasma amino acid analysis, plus fibromyalgia, angina, muscle spasms, and finding oral magnesium supplements to be laxatives at doses below 600 mg of magnesium per day suggest magnesium deficiency. Oral or intravenous loading tests are difficult to interpret since magnesium could be low due to excessive loss through the kidneys, or due to inadequate intake.

Magnesium deficiency causes anxiety, muscle tenseness (in extreme cases, tetany), low potassium and inhibits some biochemical transformations. If you get muscle cramps, eat more potassium and magnesium to make them go away.

Magnesium deficiency can be treated with a variety of oral supplements. If there is difficulty absorbing magnesium adequately from the gut, epsom salt baths will get some magnesium into the system, and a magnesium sulfate cream compounded with DMSO is available by prescription from compounding pharmacies that causes a reasonable amount of magnesium to be absorbed through the skin. There are also protocols for administering magnesium by injection which are given in an appendix. Supplementary taurine, if deficient, may correct the cause of magnesium deficiency.

People who are magnesium deficient but respond poorly to it sometimes absorb and retain it better if they receive NAET treatment for it. If there is a practitioner in your area this should be relatively inexpensive, and you can decide later whether to do more NAET depending on how helpful this is.

Potassium deficiency often goes along with magnesium deficiency and sometimes must be corrected along with it.

Low potassium and sodium in hair or serum indicates primary adrenal insufficiency of some extent. Cortisol will also be lower than optimal. This will often lead to anxiety and depression[1] due to hypoglycemia. See the adrenal section for further discussion.

The problem is often due to poor magnesium absorption in the gut coupled with poor reabsorption in the kidneys. Supplementary taurine may help. Taking the magnesium supplement in the form of or along with aspartate or malate may also help. Magnesium helps potassium absorption.

Taking supplementary arginine, glutamine and taurine may help heal up the gut so that magnesium absorption improves. Taking alkaline supplements to keep the urine alkaline will assist in retaining magnesium. Caffeine accelerates magnesium excretion and should be avoided if you are low. Low thyroid reduces magnesium levels, which

---

[1] Almost always misdiagnosed as a psychiatric rather than a physical problem by physicians.

increase if thyroid supplement is given. Vasopressin, the antidiuretic hormone that your pituitary releases to keep your urine volume down, also helps your kidneys keep magnesium in.

People who have high-normal or high serum potassium and/or magnesium but low-normal or low red blood cell potassium and/or magnesium have trouble getting these into their cells. It is important that enough potassium and magnesium be inside the cells, so magnesium and/or potassium should be supplemented at fairly high levels under these circumstances despite serum or plasma levels. It is important to have potassium supplementation followed by a physician if it is done for this purpose since high potassium can cause dangerous heart conditions. If supplementing with more than 1 gram of potassium chloride per day physician supervision is mandatory for safety. If you keep taking the same amount of magnesium and potassium and your cells start to absorb them better your serum levels will go DOWN.

If copper or iron are elevated they should be excluded from diet and supplements and things taken to interfere with their absorption. The ideal levels of both are in the lower part of the normal range. Iron can also be lowered by giving blood regularly. If they are LOW, modest amounts of supplements should be given until they are normal. If you have rheumatoid arthritis or another inflammatory disease you might respond well to some supplementary iron even if your levels are normal. It has to be tried for a week to tell.

Copper increases the symptoms of PMS. Lowering copper levels will reduce PMS. Excluding high copper foods and taking 10-20 mg of zinc plus 250-1000 mcg of molybdenum with each meal will reduce copper absorption.

Many people have impaired excretion of copper. This may be genetic or acquired. Normally, 80% of copper excretion is via the bile, 16% via intestinal secretions, and 4%

via urine. Biliary and intestinal secretions are ultimately excreted in the feces.

A normal person's copper half life is about 35 days. For a person who is not excreting any copper in their bile, the half life increases to about 175 days and body concentrations of copper increase about 5 fold. This can bring copper levels into the toxic range. The symptoms are usually psychiatric.

In addition to genetic problems, anything that interferes with bile secretion, such as gallstones or other liver disease, will cause elevation of body copper.

Lipoic acid increases copper in urine and somewhat in intestinal secretions but eliminates copper secretion in the bile. Thus for a copper toxic person lipoic acid may be helpful or harmful, and the correct measurement is fecal copper[1] rather than urinary copper. If fecal copper increases with lipoic acid, it is helpful in clearing the body of copper, but if it decreases the LA is a hindrance and will further increase body levels.

The normal intake of copper is 2-5 mg per day of which 40-60% or 1-3 mg is absorbed. Someone who is not secreting copper in their bile needs to limit absorption to 0.2 to 0.6 mg daily to keep tissue copper within normal limits.

Vitamin C in large amounts, zinc, and molybdenum hinder copper absorption from the intestine. Taking 10-20 mg of zinc, 250-1000 mcg of molybdenum, 250-500 mg of calcium and 2 grams of vitamin C every time you eat will greatly reduce copper absorption. Taking zinc and manganese in a ratio of 20:1 will increase the urinary excretion of copper. High copper foods are given in the appendix.

Low levels of thyroid hormone increase body copper, and increased thyroid hormone as well as cortisol lower it. Ensuring that

---

1 This test is available from Doctor's Data, Inc. See appendix.

you have adequate levels of thyroid hormone and cortisol for your body's needs is important in making sure you excrete copper adequately.

Drugs which interfere with copper excretion are estrogens, thorazine, librium, norpramin, diuril, orinase, carbamazepine, tapozol and indocin.

While penicillamine is often given in standard medical texts as a means to increase copper excretion. many people respond very poorly to it. Anyone with elevated plasma cysteine or dietary thiol (sulfur food) intolerance will respond poorly, and many other people do so as well.

Copper helps make hemoglobin, red blood cells, and bone. Low copper reduces these and also leads to a reduced sense of taste.

Vitamins A, B3, B5, B6 and C antagonize the effects of copper, as does iron. Appropriate supplementation with these may reduce the the toxic effects of elevated copper levels.

FATTY ACIDS

The essential fatty acids (EFA's) both control cell membrane function and also serve as precursors for signalling molecules (prostaglandins, thromboxanes and leukotrienes) that are used to regulate immune function, blood clotting and other body functions. An excess of one EFA compared to the others can cause inappropriately high or low inflammation, immune response, etc. The relative amounts of fatty acids can be changed by changing the diet and taking supplements.

The most common problem is lack of omega 3 EFA's relative to omega 6 EFA's. This can usually be corrected by taking 1-6 tbsp a day of flax oil. The blood cells come into equilibrium with this in about 3-4 weeks, but it takes several years for all of the body tissues to equilibrate. It is helpful to take a loading dose of flax oil on top of the 1-6 tbsp

maintenance dose. This loading dose makes a good start on getting those body tissues in equilibrium. It is taken by consuming as much flax oil as you can in addition to the equilibration dose. The loading dose is 8 ounces of flax oil plus 1 tbsp for every pound you are over your "ideal" weight. For overweight people this becomes a LARGE amount of flax oil and may be impractical to consume in less than several months. 1 tbsp of flax oil = 1/2 ounce of flax oil = 14 one gram capsules of flax oil.

Some people do not convert the linolenic acid in flax oil to EPA and DHA. If skin dryness does not improve, inflammation continues at high levels, and nervous symptoms remain unabated, another fatty acid profile will reveal whether this is happening. If so either large amounts of fish oil must be taken (usually economically impractical), large quantities of mackerel and salmon consumed, or assorted means must be used to activate the conversion enzymes. This is discussed in many popular works and websites.

When flax oil is taken, 1-4 grams of borage oil should also be taken to maintain a balance of omega 6 oils containing gamma linolenic acid. Borage oil is the most economical source of that.

Meat, dairy products and shellfish are the major dietary sources of proinflammatory arachidonic acid and inflammatory conditions can be reduced by excluding them from the diet. To immediately reduce inflammatory conditions these may be excluded from the diet and 10-30 grams of fish oil taken per day for a month or so while the flax oil derived linolenic acid saturates the blood and starts to work on other tissues. Other antiallergy or antiinflammatory steps may be combined with this.

Acetylcholine increases arachidonic acid release. Thiamine mildly antagonizes acetylcholine receptors. Some of the tricyclic antidepressants like doxepin also are anticholinergic. People with multiple chemical sensitivities are often especially sensitive to acetylcholine.

What to do about mercury poisoning

Arachidonic acid is ultimately derived from the linoleic (not linolenic) acid in the diet, which comes from nuts and many vegetable oils high in polyunsaturates. The general rule is: oils from seeds are omega 6, oils from grasses are omega 3.

Cattle and sheep have microorganisms in their gut that hydrogenate the dietary fatty acids they get in their grassy vegetarian diet. Thus Beef, lamb and mutton are highly saturated fats with most of the EFA's in the form of arachidonic acid. Pigs and birds do not do this so their fats have more of the dietary unsaturated fats carried through. This also means that poultry fat, and especially lard, can form lipid peroxides during cooking and cause temporary immune activation which happens much less with tallow, sheep fat or butter. The really savory taste you get from frying things in lard is due to the lipid peroxides and other degradation products of those unsaturated fats.

When you want to fry or extensively cook things, butter or beef fat is preferred. If you otherwise want to eat animal fats, chicken (poultry) fat or lard has a better balance of unsaturated fatty acids in it than beef fat, lamb fat or butter. Anything you use is going to be better for you than frying in a polyunsaturated oil, which is marginally better than using margarine or vegetable shortening.

Taking borage oil (gamma linoleic acid, an omega 6 EFA) increases production of prostaglandin E1 for a few hours while it is being moved around the body. This increases urine volume significantly, and creates a warm and somewhat spaced out feeling. This can be prevented by taking 1/2 to 1 aspirin tablet with the oil.

The ultimate product of omega 3 fatty acid metabolism, docosahexanoic acid (DHA), is essential for nerve and brain cell membranes. The long term consumption of flax oil slowly repairs these and improves neurological function.

People with low pancreatic lipase won't digest these EFA supplements unless they take lipase. People with low bile secretion won't absorb them unless they take bile (often included in animal derived digestive enzymes). People with low albumin won't be able to move them around the body until they get enough protein in them, and get their liver healthy enough, to make adequate albumin.

Your metabolism makes the various EFA's from the linoleic and linolenic acid you eat. If you have a lot of insulin, as from insulin spikes when you eat lots of sweets and carbohydrates but don't take chromium, you make less EPA - the EFA that protects against blood clotting, heart attacks, and reduces blood pressure and excessive inflammation. If you have elevated cortisol naturally or from excessive stress, you make more arachidonic acid - the EFA that causes inflammation, blood clotting, etc.

OXIDATIVE STRESS

Markers of oxidative stress are given in assorted tests. Usually there are markers of stress in water compartments and oily (lipid) compartments. The goal of using antioxidant supplements is to push these markers down towards zero. One of the most fundamental ways mercury hurts you is to cause oxidative stress, so one of the most fundamental ways you keep yourself well while you chelate it out is to take water and lipid soluble antioxidants to keep oxidative stress low. These markers don't measure the whole body (e. g. the brain is not well represented), but they are an overall guide. If they are elevated, take more antioxidants. If they are low, you are taking enough.

HEART PAIN (ANGINA)

Some patients may experience angina (heart pain on exertion). This can be caused by fast liver phase 1 metabolism activating hydrocarbons, in which case it can be reduced by slowing down phase 1 metabolism, e. g. by taking 500-750 mg of niacinamide (not niacin) 3-4 times per day. It can also be treated directly with NO producing agents like nitroglycerin or arginine, and by beta blockers.

Coenzyme Q-10 improves heart metabolism and may eliminate angina. Co-Q-10 is highly recommended as it greatly reduces the chance of more serious ischemic heart disease which can lead to sudden death. Appropriate dosage is at least 200 mg/day.

Acetyl-l-carnitine 500 mg 4 times per day can improve the heart's ability to burn fat for energy and thus relieve angina.

Low magnesium and low taurine are other possible causes of heart pain. Low magnesium can cause changes in the electrocardiogram (EKG): T wave flattening or the very dangerous prolonged QT interval. Recall that serum and even red blood cell magnesium may be normal even when body stores of magnesium are low. Angina due to low magnesium will be promptly relieved by intravenous magnesium, thus a therapeutic trial may be the best diagnostic test.

Testosterone is known to be effective in relieving angina (Lesser 1946), has been shown to do so by preventing EKG ST segment depression (Jaffe 1977), and has been shown to correlate with heart disease along with high insulin and lipids (Lichtenstein 1987). In fact, high insulin correlates very strongly with ischemic heart disease. Thus taking chromium picolinate every time you eat, avoiding sweets, and not eating high carbohydrate meals will lower insulin and may help alleviate angina. Methylating agents to lower total lipid levels may also reduce angina. Angina is also known to correlate with low testosterone in men (Phillips 1994), suggesting that androgen supplementation to young adult levels may be beneficial for men and perhaps women with angina. Supplementation with transdermal gels or creams is more effective in restoring a normal physiological state for men and is essential in women to prevent fluctuations that might lead to masculinization. Elevated estrogens are known to correlate with greater incidence of

ischemic heart disease so estrogens should be lowered rather than raised.

If hydrocarbons, especially aromatic ones, are a problem, the patient may have slow phase 2 glutathione conjugation. This can best be corrected with N-acetylcysteine. Reasonable doses to clear such problems (and in general in multiple chemical sensitivities) are 1-4 grams per day. Some people also require additional glutamine and glycine to use NAC on for a prolonged period. Take 4 parts NAC to 2 parts glutamine to 1 part glycine for this purpose, and take it with a "B-50" or similar vitamin. Note that patients who have impaired metabolic conversion of cysteine to taurine and sulfate may respond negatively to NAC, though much less so than to cysteine itself. NAC is also much more effective in elevating liver glutathione than either cysteine or glutathione.

There is a particular syndrome due to what are called your alpha 2 adrenoreceptors being too active. It causes angina, difficulty thinking clearly and enunciating words, being tired and having fibromyalgia, and having hypoglycemia. This can be addressed by doing several things. Avoid alpha agonists, take forskolin, hydergine, flax oil all the time and fish oil 1-2 grams every 4 hours when you are having trouble, and avoid fried foods or anything containing polyunsaturated oils that were heated to cooking temperature.

Citrate solutions such as Alka Setzer Gold® may provide temporary relief of angina in some circumstances.

Your angina is not due to anxiety. You may have anxiety stemming from the same thing that is causing the angina, or you may quite understandably be very anxious about the frightening heart pain you are experiencing. Some physicians may find it too difficult to diagnose what is causing the problem so they will say it is caused by anxiety. If you are told this, don't bother to get upset or argue. Go find a real doctor who knows enough medicine to be able to solve the problem instead of blaming it on you.

KIDNEYS

The kidneys are a target organ for ACUTE mercury poisoning. They are NOT a target organ in CHRONIC mercury poisoning. If you are chronically poisoned your kidneys will usually be fine. If your kidneys are actually responding to mercury poisoning with nephrotic syndrome (blood in the urine, death of kidney tissue) it is crucial you figure out where your source of mercury exposure is - and it is a big one - and end that exposure immediately.

Creatinine clearance is a sophisticated and sensitive measure of kidney function that can be easily determined from other tests you will be doing. If the creatinine clearance is low, be very careful with chelating agents and with anything else that puts stress on the kidneys and do more kidney tests to figure out WHY[1]. Supplements such as taurine may be used to help the kidneys heal.

If kidney problems are due to deposition of immune complexes on the glomerular filtration membranes, administration of intravenous immunoglobulin is very helpful.

Kidney problems are often accompanied by magnesium wasting. Excessive magnesium supplementation may also place a strain on the kidneys. Care must be taken to ensure that the patient receives an appropriate level of magnesium. If the kidneys are healthy magnesium can be given orally to bowel tolerance without problems.

A large source of the solute load[2] on the kidneys is the amount of protein in the diet. If the patient is hypoglycemic, the total amount of protein can be restricted somewhat if supplementary branched chain amino acids are given in reasonably large amounts (e. g. 8

---

[1] Your physician will know how to do this or will refer you to a urologist who does.
[2] The amount of material dissolved in the urine, which the kidneys must work to rid the body of.

grams per day) along with glutamine. It is important to ensure that the BCAA's are given in the proper ratio - 1 part isoleucine to 2 parts leucine to 2 parts valine. The BCAA's are not helpful to people with any degree of adrenal insufficiency until they also receive supplementary cortisol. Your body also may not be able to use them if you are poisoned by arsenic.

Androgens specifically promote growth and healing of the kidneys. Recall that hypoadrenal (and thus hypoglycemic) women will be androgen deficient.

If you are urinating a lot, and producing an unusually large volume of urine each day (more than 2 quarts and 3 cups) it is unlikely your kidneys are the problem. Your pituitary is most likely the problem. It lets out a special hormone that tells your kidneys not to make too much urine. There is a special test for this where you don't drink any water for 12-16 hours, give urine and blood samples to measure what is called the osmolality, and then take a special medicine called DDAVP and give another urine sample. The first two numbers get plotted on a special chart in Harrison's in the section on diabetes insipidus.

Some physicians may think that urinating a lot is because you drink a lot of water for psychiatric reasons. If this is so then the test above will show everything is normal and it should be ordered regardless of why the physician thinks you are urinating so much since it will distinguish among all the possibilities - psychiatric problems, pituitary disease and kidney disease.

DIGESTIVE TRACT

Digestive stool analysis is used when there is evidence of malabsorption, such as low essential hair or urine elements across the board, digestive problems, or other generally recognized symptoms. High food intake while remaining thin is more likely due to adrenal insufficiency. Malabsorption can be due to flora imbalance in the gut, parasites, excessive gut inflammation -

possibly due to allergy, gluten intolerance[1] (celiac disease), or a combination of these. Correcting malabsorption is the first order of business since supplements become expensive sewage and don't do you any good if you don't absorb them. There is much medical art on how to treat candida, parasites, and excessive gut inflammation so I won't go into them specifically here, though they are discussed as appropriately throughout the book. The most useful things I can say are that in rebalancing intestinal flora it is often helpful to use much more "probiotic" material than is usually indicated on supplement bottles, and that a number of parasites are surprisingly difficult to identify through testing so they may need to be treated "blind" if symptoms suggest them and other approaches are not solving the problem.

Supplements which help heal the intestines are glutamine, glucosamine, arginine, gotu kola and flax oil. Some supplementary cortisol is also necessary for people with low cortisol (hypoadrenal people).

Ginger can reduce intestinal (and other) inflammation as well as stimulate the appetite and suppress nausea. If you are having trouble getting those supplements down - or keeping them down - ginger may allow you to do it.

Patients who have severe malabsorption may require a series of vitamin/mineral drips with additional "probiotic" components to heal their GI tract sufficiently so that nutrients and supplements can be administered orally. Arginine is available for intravenous infusion and is effective for this purpose. As a rule these patients will have low tissue magnesium and will benefit from its inclusion in the IV. The focus of such a therapeutic regimen should be on prompt healing of the GI tract since prolonged intravenous therapy is expensive, time consuming, uncomfortable, carries risks, and does not address the underlying problem of mercury poisoning.

If you are magnesium deficient you will have sensitive veins which spasm enough to make it difficult to administer large volumes of fluid intravenously. Correcting the magnesium deficiency and keeping it corrected allows other materials to be administered IV. Local anesthetic in the IV material helps counteract vein spasms, but affects you systemically.

The amount of minerals administered in an IV is seldom significant compared to the total amount normally in the body. Exceptions are potassium, which must be done with great care since this is potentially quite dangerous, and magnesium. Administering large amounts of magnesium intravenously can also be dangerous so it is done following a proper protocol in a physician's office or hospital while the patient is carefully watched. See the appendix.

If a significant number of meat or vegetable fibers pass through into the stool, or there is much undigested fat in it, you should take animal derived digestive enzymes and use betaine hydrochloride or take your vitamin C as ascorbic acid with meals in order to provide the acid your stomach may not be making.

An alkaline stool indicates poor acid production. Alkalinity also fosters yeast growth. One possible cause for poor acid production is lower than necessary cortisol levels. Since low cortisol both reduces immune response to yeast and increases pH which favors yeast it needs to be addressed. See the adrenal section for further discussion of cortisol. Betaine hydrochloride can be taken to increase stomach acidity.

Malabsorption can be due to food allergies. A RAST test for foods, particularly one including IgG sensitivities, can be informative. In case of food allergies make reference to the allergy section and take betaine hydrochloride or take your vitamin C in the acid form with meals, plus either plant

---

[1] check promptly with saliva or blood test for antigliadin antibodies.

What to do about mercury poisoning

or animal derived digestive enzymes to digest antigens before they set off an immune reaction.

The stool analysis indicates whether the intestinal flora are imbalanced or digestion is impaired. This can be addressed with supplements, diet and sometimes with medications. It also shows whether secretory IgA is low. If sIgA is low, unrecognized giardia or other parasitic infection is likely. The symptoms of chronic gut parasitic infection are often much more subtle than in acute infection. Giardia can be treated with metronidazole, which is metabolized by those phase 1 enzymes to some extent but also slows them down. Thus people who are slow phase 1 metabolizers need to watch their dose carefully if they take metronidazole. Giardia can also be eliminated with black walnut and tea tree oil. These herbals are themselves powerful medicines and must be used with care. Chronic infections often require repeated treatment augmented with digestive enzymes taken on an empty stomach.

Giardia and other intestinal parasites are very easy to come by, hard to test for, were only discovered to be a problem recently, and are thus often ignored by "mainstream" MD's. While many "alternative" practitioners believe EVERYONE has them and EVERYTHING is due to parasites, I simply note that a lot more people have them than are going to get diagnosed by their health plan MD, and it pays to consider them when you are having some intermittent abdominal and excretory problems that your MD thinks you should just ignore and hope they get better. If you do have and get rid of assorted parasites, make sure to treat any pets, family members, etc. who might have them too so you don't pass them back and forth. All that healthy food and all those good supplements you take don't do much good if parasites eat half of it and your body uses the other half up fighting them.

Yeast is a common complication of mercury. A low sulfur diet may suppress yeast. A high sulfur diet will feed it, as will one high in sugar and carbohydrates. There

are also assorted medical and dietary approaches. Of all the systemic antifungals, Terbinafine is by far the easiest on the liver. The other antifungals block phase 1 metabolism and should not be used by people in whom it is already slow.

Coffee is a "sulfur food." Tea has yeast killing tannin. If you have a yeast problem, take your liquid stimulant in the form of strong black tea instead of coffee.

There is ample literature on yeast treatment. It is well summarized in appendix D of Teitelbaum (1996). Appropriate treatment is MERCURY REMOVAL and anti-yeast agents like nystatin and nizoral or lamisil. Appropriate diagnostic testing is to look for levels of anticandida IgG and IgM, or to look for circulating yeast immune complexes. There are also protocols for a therapeutic trial of nystatin to induce "die off" symptoms. Yeast should not be a diagnosis of exclusion, routinely treated in the absence of positive evidence it is present.

Note that people with low cortisol (due to low adrenal function) are MORE susceptible to infection than normal people. Cortisol doesn't just suppress the immune system - it suppresses inflammation, and the proper level of cortisol is required for the immune system to function. People with low cortisol levels are likely to have yeast problems, and may benefit from 5 mg hydrocortisone 2-4 times per day. This is contrary to popular wisdom among both mainstream and alternative MD's, but it is both what their books say and what is observed in people who try this.

Intestinal yeast overgrowth can crowd out the bacteria that produce vitamin K, which is essential for blood clotting. Vitamin K can be administered orally or by injection.

Excessive yeast growth can also interfere with vitamin D metabolism in the liver and kidneys, affecting calcium metabolism. Vitamin D can be taken orally.

SKIN

Skin infection with yeast or fungus is common. (e. g. athlete's foot). If systemic treatment is administered for other reasons that may be sufficient. Otherwise topical treatment should be used. Many OTC products are effective. The prescription drug Nystatin® is also inexpensive and effective. Combining products (e. g. Nystatin® mixed in an OTC product) is especially effective. Since there may be substantial difficulties with dry skin some care must be taken to check patient asserted "resistant" fungal infections to ensure that they are not uninfected dry skin. Also, some care must be taken to ensure that a "treatment response" is not simply improvement of uninfected dry skin due to the antifungal vehicle rather than the medicinal agent.

Fingernail and toenail fungus are only easy to treat topically if the infection is recent and has not penetrated into the nail, and can be treated only with liquid agents. Persistence with fungal tinctures containing urea, undecylic acid and tea tree oil (twice daily application for 6 months) may be effective.

Repeated reappearance of skin dryness, hyperkeratosis or other irritation over areas where mercury containing antiseptics have been applied in the previous few years is not uncommon and should not be confused with yeast or fungal reinfection.

The skin of mercury toxic people becomes quite sensitive to irritation. Control this by using safe hand lotion, not bathing too often, using a mild, unscented soap sparingly, using washing soda or Arm and Hammer® detergent, taking off socks in the house, being aware of more or less irritating types of clothing, etc. The herbal supplement Gotu Kola is also very helpful.

ALLERGY

Immunoglobulin E, IgE, is "allergy globulin." Mercury toxic people can have vastly elevated IgE without having classic symptoms like a runny nose - rhinitis. Someone with elevated IgE but no rhinitis will still experience much lethargy, fatigue and malaise which can be ameliorated. Finding an antihistamine that is tolerated, using leukotriene inhibitors, and taking vitamin C, magnesium, flax oil, borage oil, silymarin, alpha and beta agonists, and forskolin will help with these symptoms. If IgE is elevated, allergy testing is helpful as avoiding foods related to inhalant allergens works well to reduce symptoms (despite what allergists say, e. g. that people who react to olive pollen can safely eat olive oil, which is often not true). It is possible to have asthma and allergies without very high IgE numbers - as always, it is the patient who must be treated, not the lab results.

There are also allergies caused by IgG. These cannot be treated by "conventional" or "mainstream" methods and their existence may be disputed by people who use such methods. IgG allergies can be tested for with RAST tests. They are often more of a problem with foods than with inhaled or contact allergens.

Food allergies, of whatever kind, may be treated by identifying and not eating the offending material, using the techniques described under malabsorption to heal up the gut so that food derived antigen does not make it into the bloodstream where most antibodies are (especially for IgG allergies), and by taking either plant or animal derived digestive enzymes and extra acid in the form of betaine hydrochloride or take your vitamin C in the acid form with meals to digest the antigen before it finds antibodies and triggers of an allergic reaction.

When you are experiencing serious allergy problems or have just been exposed to a lot of dust or pollen, take a shower. It can be very short and you don't have to use soap, but it is very helpful to rinse your hair out.

Conventional allergy shots are generally not worthwhile given the time they take compared to the time it takes a detoxification program to lower allergies (6 months to 1 year). They may also contain the mercury salt thimerosal as a preservative.

The "alternative" therapy of Enzyme Potentiated Desensitization (EPD) works well for some people giving fairly prompt relief from allergic symptoms. Some care must be taken to find an experienced practitioner who is able to sort out the allergens without excessive testing and who does not charge exorbitantly. EPD therapy consists of a special allergy injection given once every 2 months or so, with substantial restrictions on what you may eat, contact and do for the few days around the injection.

Acupuncture and related techniques such as NAET can be very effective at reducing or eliminating allergy problems in relatively short periods. NAET is highly recommended for people who have a few especially troublesome allergies as it works one allergen at a time. NAET is described by Ellen Cutler in her book *Winning the War against Asthma and Allergies* and on the web at www.allergy2000.com as well as www.naet.com. It works very well for many people, but does not work for everyone. Unfortunately some practitioners (including some certified ones) claim to offer NAET but do not perform treatments according to the proper protocol. In this case allergy relief is temporary and sensitivity returns in some months. It can be relieved again by retreatment - permanently if retreatment is performed correctly.

Sublingual allergy drops are effective at reducing allergy response and clearing symptoms. Few practitioners prepare these nowadays due to some poorly designed placebo controlled trials which incorrectly concluded they were not effective. Unlike allergy shots they can be used to stop or clear allergic reactions, and they can be used when

needed since the patient self-administers them. It is unclear whether they reduce long term allergy response like injections do, but amalgam removal and mercury detox are so much more effective than allergy injections that the real issue is to suppress allergies for the year it takes them to dwindle away during chelation.

With messed up metabolism and an intoxicated brain, mercury victims may have to try a large number of antihistamines before finding one that is nonsedating and not depressive. Allegra seems to be the one to try first. If that doesn't work, try zyrtec and claritin. Be careful with hismanal - the other antihistamines can be depressives, but hismanal can lead to psychotic-like behavioral disturbances. Alpha and beta adrenergic agonists are often helpful in controlling allergy symptoms. The OTC ones are (alpha) pseudoephedrine, (beta) ephedrine and epinephrine sulfate. The tricyclic antidepressants - especially doxepin - have antihistaminic activity as a side effect. Doxepin as distributed has large amounts of sulfite in its formulation. Vitamin C is also a mild antihistamine.

If the allergic response does not contain a large component of drippy nose, tearing eyes, and other inflammatory components, then taking the amino acid histidine to make more histamine can paradoxically IMPROVE allergies. Histamine not only causes these symptoms, but also regulates the immune system by, in effect, saying "ENOUGH ALREADY!" Increasing available histamine downregulates allergic response if it is deficient. You can take lots of extra histidine along with antihistamines to tell your immune system to calm down without experiencing any worse allergy symptoms than you are now.

Conjugated linolenic acid (CLA) reduces IgE while increasing other immunoglobulins, and it also reduces some of the lipid mediators of allergic reactions. These lipid mediators cause much of the long term wooziness, spaciness and lethargy you experience after allergic exposures as well as keeping the immune system in an allergically sensitized state.

Cimetidine (Tagamet®), famotidine (Pepcid®, Mylanta AR®), nisatidine (Axid®), and ranitidine (Zantac®) are histamine H2 blockers which are used to reduce stomach acid. These drugs also block the histamine H2 receptors on immune system cells. This causes a reduction in the number of T suppressor cells, and tells the immune system to be especially ready to sensitize to new antigens, and to make especially large amounts of IgE. Stomach acid also destroys antigenic molecules before they get into the intestine where allergies to them might develop, so it is not a bad thing. Stomach acid can often be reduced by eating primarily meat and vegetables, and leaving grain and grain products like bread out of the diet without having to rely on H2 blockers. This diet also works pretty well in reducing fibromyalgia and hypoglycemia, which are common complications of mercury poisoning. Grains are the primary dietary source of histidine, so this diet is decreasing histidine intake and histamine levels. If that is not desirable then old fashioned calcium carbonate antacids can be used.

Much allergic reaction, inflammation and asthma is caused by the release of the essential fatty acid arachidonic acid to form proinflammatory signalling molecules. Leukotriene inhibitors directly interfere with the effects of some of these signalling molecules. In addition to prescription leukotriene inhibitors, ginger also interferes with the formation of leukotrienes. Acetylcholine can stimulate the release of more arachidonic acid. Thus DMAE, lecithin or phosphatidylcholine may worsen asthma, allergy and inflammation in susceptible individuals.

Arachidonic acid makes other signalling molecules that aspirin, Celebrex® and similar drugs as well as ginger slow the formation of. Glucocorticoids like cortisol interfere with the release of AA. EPA from fish oil and GLA from borage oil interfere with the metabolism of AA to these pro-inflammatory mediator molecules. Methylating agents make the interaction between acetylcholine and AA less. In the long term, taking flax oil replaces some of the AA in your cell membranes with DHA so that less pro-inflammatory mediators are formed.

The pro-inflammatory mediator molecules from AA cause lethargy, fatigue and difficulty concentrating as well as the more obvious symptoms of allergy, asthma or inflammation. They also make you more sensitive to pain.

If IgE RISES as therapy proceeds, one should suspect the Helminth class of parasites. IgE's rising to over 800 are a strong sign of this. Liver function will decline and jaundice will eventually develop. Many helminthic parasites are safer to treat for blind than to diagnose since diagnosis is usually performed on a wedge biopsy specimen of the liver. There are blood tests, but these have a significant false negative rate and should not be used to exclude helminths in the face of an otherwise unexplainable rise in IgE with uncharacterized liver disease.

If you have elevated plasma cysteine you will find your allergies dramatically reduced by going on a sulfur food exclusion diet.

Tryptophan containing foods can trigger asthma in susceptible individuals. Such foods are enumerated in the appendix.

AUTOIMMUNITY

Mercury poisoning can cause autoimmunity. If you have autoimmunity from mercury poisoning it will probably go away when you get detoxed. Some physicians will think you have autoimmunity INSTEAD of being mercury poisoned, but they don't think autoimmunity is curable. It is up to you to decide whether you have incurable autoimmune disease or whether you have autoimmune disease as a symptom of mercury poisoning.

What to do about mercury poisoning

Autoimmune disease can be ameliorated with DHEA, niacinamide, forskolin, flax and borage oil in addition to the usual therapies. Androgens may suppress autoimmunities and should thus be replaced in both men and women if they are not well into the normal range APPROPRIATE FOR YOUR AGE. Most lab ranges are for the aged and are not applicable to generally younger mercury toxic patients. Some people prefer to raise androgen levels to the high end of normal for young adults regardless of patient age. The use of supranormal amounts of DHEA (100-250 mg 4 times a day) for lupus is well known. A few physicians believe DMSA and perhaps DMPS may exacerbate autoimmune disease.

People with a high ratio of CD4 T helper cells to CD8 T suppressor cells are "universal reactors" and will rapidly sensitize to new antigens, including self antigens. Supplements to raise CD8 and lower CD4 cells are appropriate - e. g. histidine, forskolin.

SUSCEPTIBILITY TO INFECTION

People with low NK cells have trouble clearing viral infections and are more prone to cancer. Echinacea 1 week per month, ginseng, inositol and its hexaphosphate, alpha agonists like sudafed, etc. boost NK cell number and function.

Other things that help fight viral infections are supplementary lysine (2-4 grams per day), with a SMALL amount of copper for a short time if the infection is a real problem, grapefruit seed extract, elderberry extract, and the prescription drug ribavirin. There are some other prescription drugs that help fight certain classes of viruses, like flumedyne for influenza B.

Arginine helps the immune system fight bacterial infections but makes it more prone to viral infections. Taking lysine with the arginine allows antibacterial activity to be enhances without reducing antiviral activity.

Vitamin A also enhances overall immune competence at 25,000 IU per day, which may be taken continuously by an average sized adult[1]. Doses of 50,000 IU per day may be taken for up to a month - but if continued indefinitely at this dose there is substantial risk of toxicity. A few days at 100,000 IU can be used at the onset of illness to rapidly activate the immune system.

IMMUNE FUNCTION

Deficiencies in certain immune system cells may be seen on a blood count. There are some supplements and medicines which can address some of these problems, such as using antioxidants and alpha agonists to increase neutrophil function, iron to activate neutrophils and macrophages, glutamine feeds macrophages and lymphocytes, or forskolin to activate lymphocytes and deactivate neutrophils.

Cell mediated immune response - inflammation, NK cell activity, etc. as opposed to just having antibodies - is influenced by noradrenergic nerves in the spleen and lymph nodes. It is possible to increase cell mediated immunity by taking selegiline[2] or by taking alpha agonists.

Exercise (within the limits of appropriate adrenal response) enhances immunity. Sleep deprivation and depression reduce natural killer cell activity. CD4+ T helper cells are affected by the level of plasma thiols, being elevated as they rise and depressed as they fall. Optimism and trust enhance immune response. Anxiety, anger and sadness reduce immune response. So the prescription you don't need a doctor to write or to gulp a lot of pills for if you want to boost your immune function is to be happy, trusting, optimistic, exercise regularly and get enough sleep.

---

[1] Adults under 120# should use 20,000 IU, and those under 100# should use 15,000 IU.

[2] ThyagaRajan et al. 1998.

LIVER METABOLISM

The liver detox test will tell you whether to exclude sulfur foods from your diet (if cysteine and glutathione are high or high normal), which supplements might help you specifically, and whether you are a 'fast' or 'slow' phase 1 metabolizer[1]. Slow phase 1 metabolizers will have trouble with colorings (natural and artificial) and spices in foods, partially hydrogenated vegetable oils, and will take a while to clear out chemicals they are exposed to. They need to be especially restrictive with their diet. Fast phase 1 metabolizers will make certain classes of compounds MORE toxic. If these people are also slow phase 2 metabolizers they will have multiple chemical sensitivities and experience great toxicity from, for example, paint fumes. At the time of this writing, the Great Smokies Diagnostic Laboratory Comprehensive Liver Detoxification Test (different from the standard liver detox test) appears to be unique and to provide information not otherwise available.

Phase 1 and 2 metabolism are described in detail in the physiology section. An iron deficient person with fast phase 1 enzymes might get worse when she corrects her iron deficiency, and someone with slow phase 1 enzymes would be well advised not to eat a box of grocery store sugar cookies (so as to avoid the large amounts of sugar and partially hydrogenated fats). Opportunities also exist to tailor diet, supplements and medications to push phase 1 rates in the proper direction.

Cruciferous vegetables increase many phase 2 rates and can be used if sulfur food exclusion is not required. Ellagic acid from red grape skins also does this, as do rosemary and soy. The sulfate pathway in particular can be overloaded. Acetaminophen depletes sulfate, and the Feingold diet controls dietary materials requiring sulfation.

---

[1] the test only checks one of the many phase 1 enzymes, so it may not accurately reflect what your liver is doing. As always, it is one piece of information to be combined with everything else you know about your body.

If it is not practical to test phase 1 and phase 2 metabolism, some inferences can be drawn from observation and other tests. Multiple Chemical Sensitivities often goes along with fast phase 1 and slow phase 2. Anxiety sometimes accompanies fast phase 1. Needing high doses of anti-anxiety or antidepressant drugs or of analgesics or painkillers also fits fast phase 1. Slow phase 1 implies increased sensitivity to such things, as well as with being sensitive to antibiotics in meat and to partially hydrogenated oils.

Phase 2 metabolism has many parallel paths. One of them is glutathione conjugation, which removes hydrocarbons from the body as well as heavy metals. It also reflects the amount of glutathione available in the cells as an antioxidant. If the patient is sensitive to hydrocarbons, the preservatives BHT and BHA, and feels bad on penicillin or tetracycline she may have impaired glutathione conjugation. Sulfation will show up most notably if the patient does well on the Feingold diet, or if she responds poorly to DHEA supplementation. Impaired methylation leads to slow clearance of epinephrine, norepinephrine and dopamine, which would exacerbate agitation, anxiety and "psychotic" symptoms. Elevated bilirubin on standard blood chemistry tests may indicate impaired glutathione conjugation and/or glucuronidation.

Many people with multiple chemical sensitivities are unusually sensitive to acetylcholine. Thus if they supplement with DMAE they will require much smaller doses than other people. They may also be quite sensitive to choline, phosphatidylcholine and lecithin. Thiamine may reduce this excessive sensitivity to acetylcholine. Excess acetylcholine sensitivity also affects arachidonic acid release as discussed in the fatty acids section.

Impaired methylation can be corrected with choline, trimethylglycine, folic acid and vitamin B-12. S-adenosylmethionine is a very effective but more expensive way to increase methylation. Improving methylation often reduces fibromyalgia symptoms.

If glutathione conjugation is slow it will slow the liver's excretion of heavy metals in the bile. This is best corrected with N-acetylcysteine.

People with defects in sulfation (a phase 2 reaction) are likely to have an aberrant response to DHEA supplementation. The response to oral DHEA will be brief and greatly exaggerated. Breast tenderness or pain is common in women with this problem. Taking sulfate (magnesium sulfate, glucosamine sulfate, magnesium sulfate injections) may correct these problems.

If you have a history of odd reactions to drugs, foods, and apparent trouble with chemicals your own body makes, go over the phase 1 and 2 liver metabolism information in figures 11 and 12. Your doctor simply doesn't have the time to pore over these looking for all the things you have ever had trouble with. Once you get an idea of what is wrong, mark up the figures and make sure you don't take things that you can expect to have trouble with. Show the figures to your doctor and talk to him about them when she is discussing drugs or nutritional supplements for you.,

SULFUR METABOLISM

High plasma cysteine means thiol containing foods and certain supplements must be rigorously limited. See appendix for a list.

Many people experience temporary relief of allergy, autoimmune or fibromyalgia symptoms for a few days to a few weeks by excluding sulfur foods regardless of their cysteine status.

If you have high plasma cysteine your urine may frequently have a "coffee" or "asparagus" smell.

Those who have low glutathione or glutathione conjugation on the liver detox test are likely to benefit from N-acetyl cysteine (NAC) 600-4,000 mg/day.

Supplementary glutathione itself is of very little value since your gut should digest it. If your gut is not digesting it you will soon start taking other things to MAKE your gut digest it because letting undigested things like glutathione into your bloodstream will soon cause major allergy problems.

Low sulfate indicates a need to supplement it (e.g. by eating 1/4 - 1/2 tsp epsom salts, or a gram or two of glucosamine sulfate, sodium sulfate, etc.), Do not take any sulfate containing supplements at the same time as calcium supplements because they will form insoluble precipitates. Sulfate can also be supplemented by taking epsom salt baths. Those with very low sulfate will not metabolize oral DHEA properly, and poor response such as a woman experiencing breast pain from 10 mg a day of DHEA indicates phase 2 sulfation should be investigated. Molybdenum supplementation may help the body make more endogenous sulfate.

Elevated plasma cysteine, sulfur food reactions, or reduced magnesium or sulfate levels indicate plasma taurine levels should be investigated. If they are low supplementation will relieve anxiety, improve toxin excretion in the bile, assist digestion, etc. The taurine level is determined as part of most plasma amino acid tests.

HYPOGLYCEMIA

Many mercury toxic people have trouble regulating their blood sugar. This may be in combination with adrenal problems (discussed below) or may be an independent problem. Hypoglycemia is characterized by craving sweets and carbohydrates, coffee, feeling anxious, and "crashing" a couple of hours after meals. In many states, blood glucose levels are one of the few lab tests a patient can order for themselves. In many states it is possible to buy a home blood glucose meter without a prescription. The meters are usually cheap - the refill measurement strips are where the cost is. Using these meters requires pricking your finger with a lancet and putting a drop of blood on the strip.

Reactive hypoglycemia occurs when blood sugar plummets a few hours after meals. This is because the body gets overly active about pulling food derived blood sugar out of the bloodstream and doesn't stop after the food is digested. This can often be controlled by taking 200 mcg chromium picolinate with meals, eating a high protein diet, taking branched chain amino acids, including a lot of fiber with meals, or eating small, frequent meals.

In reactive hypoglycemia if you make it past the 'trough' your blood sugar eventually comes back up to some reasonable level. In regular hypoglycemia your fasting blood sugar remains low once your meal is digested. Regular hypoglycemia is often associated with adrenal insufficiency. Hypoglycemia associated with adrenal insufficiency can be corrected by proper use of glucocorticoids or other means of correcting the adrenal problem. Otherwise, eat a high protein diet, take glutamine and eat frequent meals. People with adrenal insufficiency can't metabolize BCAA's to make blood sugar.

If regular hypoglycemia is NOT associated with adrenal insufficiency, then something is causing excess insulin production and this cause should be sought (and in the meantime take 2-3 grams per day of niacinamide in case it is an autoimmune problem). Try taking 200 mcg of chromium picolinate with meals to reduce the amount of insulin your body needs in order to metabolize the meal, eat a high protein diet, take branched chain amino acids (in the proper ratio), take gluamine, and eat frequent meals. Adrenally insufficient people will not benefit from BCAA's unless they take cortisol, but do need glutamine. People who are poisoned by arsenic may not benefit from BCAA's.

Reactive hypoglycemia can be directly measured by a glucose tolerance test, in which a large amount of glucose is consumed and blood is then drawn for glucose determination at frequent intervals. This is a standard test done to pregnant women nowadays and it is sometimes used to screen for diabetes. The test can be done informally by eating a sugary meal (e. g. pancakes with a lot of syrup) and having blood drawn to check glucose 2 hours later. These tests can be done by a lab or with your own (or a friend's) blood glucose meter. The blood sugar level should be between 80 and 145.

The extent to which hypoglycemia has occurred to someone over time can be determined using the same test that is used to check how much hyperglycemia diabetics have been experiencing - hemoglobin A1C. People whose HbA1C is below the lower normal limit (between 4.5 and 5.4 depending on the exact method the lab uses) spend a significant amount of their time with their blood sugar below normal levels. A high protein diet, frequent meals, supplementary glutamine and supplementary branched chain amino acids helps with generalized hypoglycemia.

Generalized hypoglycemia is a strong indicator of adrenal insufficiency or unidentified liver problems.

The regulation of insulin and blood sugar is under some control by the central nervous system, though this regulatory mechanism is poorly understood and thus generally ignored by physicians. However it is well known that people with strokes, Parkinson's disease, etc. regulate their blood sugar poorly. Thus in the long term any materials that improve brain function or protect the brain against oxidative stress will also improve blood sugar regulation. These are discussed in the brain function section, and for practical purposes start with you taking 3-5 mg of hydergine® 3 or 4 times per day. Better blood sugar control leads to better brain function, and better brain function leads to better blood sugar control. This system will be much easier to get properly adjusted if you work on both parts at the same time.

HORMONE PROFILE

A hormone profile allows one to determine if any of the body's endocrine hormones need supplementation. Even if they are normal, some mercury toxic people have hypothyroid symptoms which can sometimes be relieved with modest doses of T3 + T4 (NOT T4 alone) which do not raise the blood levels of the hormones out of the normal range, nor suppress TSH below the normal range. Doses of 50-100 mcg T4 plus 15-30 mcg T3 or 2-3 grains of armour thyroid are typical. Ideal target ranges for blood test results are: T3 - 120, free T3 - 3.0 and free T4 - 2.1. Seriously toxic patients may require supraphysiological doses of thyroid to achieve a clinically euthyroid state. Some physicians choose to treat the patient rather than the lab report and select dosage based on clinical response - the correct dosage is that which alleviates hypothyroid symptoms without causing any signs or symptoms of thyrotoxicosis. Signs of thyrotoxicosis that you can monitor for yourself are diarrhoea, weight loss and a fast resting heart rate. People with low thyroid are constipated and get an orange coloration to their palms and soles due to beta carotene. People with the right amount of thyroid don't have orange palms and soles unless they take truly exceptional amounts of supplementary beta carotene.

Mercury poisoned people will often be low in DHEA and pregnenolone and will benefit from bringing these up to normal values for young adults rather than just to the age related norms. Women must limit their intake of these substances to avoid masculinization. 100 mg pregnenolone plus 50 mg DHEA daily are usually safe oral doses.

PMS is sometimes made worse by a dominance of estrogens over progesterone during the relevant part of the menstrual cycle. Factors that encourage this are increased copper and lower than necessary cortisol. Lowering copper, increasing cortisol, and increasing progesterone will lessen PMS and are well worth doing if you find it to be troublesome.

PITUITARY

Many patients have partial diabetes insipidus (DI) since mercury concentrates in the hypothalamus and pituitary. This is usually not bad enough to require continuous treatment, but the drug DDAVP should be used to permit the patient to sleep through the night and should be available for the patient to use to make travel comfortable and for use in business or social situations where frequent urination and intake of water is not feasible (e. g. air travel). Even mild dehydration causes fatigue and increases susceptibility to disease - appropriate control of partial DI is not solely for patient comfort.

Many men who get up at night to urinate are told it is due to prostate problems. This is not always true. Their kidneys may make more urine than their bladder can hold. A 24 hour urine collection should be less than 2.5 liters (2 quarts and 3 cups). Anyone who pees, goes to bed, and makes more than 500 ml (2 cups) before waking up has a really big bladder if they can hold it in. Just because a doctor blames something on the prostate doesn't mean the prostate is the real problem. Leave a container by the toilet and check volume for a few nights.

The paradoxical fall of ACTH in response to stress that is discussed in the adrenal section happens in the hypothalamus and pituitary. The adrenal gland actually does what the brain tells it to do - the problem is the brain tells it to do the wrong thing and you are very sick as a result. This problem and how to test for it is discussed in the adrenal section.

It is important to determine whether the way your hypothalamus and pituitary are controlling your hormone producing glands is messed up because most of the tests that doctors, especially endocrinologists, use to decide how much of a hormone to give you

Amalgam Illness: Diagnosis and Treatment

are useless for that purpose if your hypothalamus and pituitary aren't working right. If you know that any of the pituitary's controlling hormones are not working appropriately it is pretty likely that none of them really are. So all of your hormone therapies have to be adjusted and controlled on the basis of how you look, and feel, and how tests of things the hormone in question controls comes out.

Clues that something is wrong with the pituitary:

* Inadequate antidiuretic hormone (high urine volume)

* Paradoxical ACTH response to stress

* TSH and thyroid hormone both towards low end (see figure in appendix)

* Low IGF-1 (SMC) or prolactin

* Men: testosterone and LH/FSH both towards low end

* Women: menstrual cycles without ovulation and low-end LH and FSH surges. Irregular menstrual cycles or cycles of unusual length or shortness.

Pituitary problems are very difficult to recognize unless they are extreme. Modest pituitary problems are very common in mercury poisoning. It is very important to recognize if you have them because you will not have appropriate levels of hormones regulating your body. If you supplement these hormones your health will improve dramatically and you will be able to live your life a lot better while you detox, as well as healing a lot faster as detox goes on.

If your pituitary is not working exactly right you may need to supplement many of your hormones - even the ones in the normal range. Also, measurements of pituitary factors like TSH, LH and FSH, GH and ACTH will not be helpful in determining whether you are taking the proper amount of hormone.

Tests that are valuable in helping to decide if the pituitary is not working right:

* Urine osmolality response to dehydration, ADH versus serum osmolality.

* ACTH response to stress.

* considering measurements of a large number of hormones and a large number of pituitary factors in comparison to each other[1].

Mercury poisons the pituitary and hypothalamus and slowly attenuate their response to appropriate stimulation. Provocative endocrine tests will often come back "within normal limits" even when things are so poorly adjusted as to leave you very ill. Provocative endocrine testing is suitable for identifying dramatic abnormalities like hyperactive tumors or half dead pituitary glands. It should not be used as the basis for deciding that there is no pituitary problem. It is of limited utility in mercury poisoning.

If in doubt as to whether the hypothalamus and pituitary are functioning exactly right, your doctor should decide how much of each hormone to give you the old fashioned way - by paying attention to hormone levels and how you look and not using the modern tests for pituitary factors to make dosage decisions.

When the hypothalamus or pituitary are not controlling the hormone producing endocrine system properly you have to pay special attention to the hormone interactions described below since your hypothalamus and pituitary may not naturally and automatically adjust all of the rest of your hormones when you start taking supplements of one.

---

[1] There is no standard way to do this. You and your doctor will have to look at your test results, the charts in the back of this book, the charts in medical textbooks, and your doctor will have to use the judgment she has hopefully gained by seeing a lot of people and their test results over the years.

What to do about mercury poisoning

HORMONE INTERACTIONS

Discussion of thyroid, adrenal and androgen deficiency and supplementation follow. There are important interactions between these hormones as well as between liver metabolism and steroid metabolism. Androgens increase thyroxine binding globulin and may reduce the effective level of available thyroid hormone - especially in people receiving thyroid medication. Thyroid medication increases the level of sex hormone binding globulin and thus reduces the effective amount of free androgens available. Thyroid medication also increases hepatic (liver) metabolism of steroids like androgens and cortisol. The most serious potential hormone interaction is that thyroid supplementation may worsen adrenal insufficiency. When hormones are being administered rather than produced by the body their levels will not naturally adjust to compensate for changes in the others. Other agents that accelerate liver metabolism, such as carbamazepine, can have similar effects.

As is evident from the descriptions below, mercury poisoning causes many problems by interfering with thyroid hormone and cortisol (an adrenal hormone) metabolism. These problems can be corrected by proper treatment of the thyroid or adrenal problem. The most common treatment is to supplement one or both hormones. As discussed above, they interact with each other and with other possible treatments. These interactions must always be kept in mind. These are discussed in standard medical texts like *Harrison's*, *Cecil*, and *Williams*, as well as by *Teitelbaum*.

An important hormone interaction to remember is that pregnant women have much higher levels of total T4 - one of the more common blood tests - than nonpregnant women and this is perfectly normal. They do not need to reduce their dosage of thyroid hormone as their total T4 rises during pregnancy, since it will naturally do this.

THYROID

During mercury poisoning, there are usually symptoms of low thyroid (hypothyroidism) despite normal lab tests. These symptoms include tiredness and lethargy to the extent of making it difficult to complete a full day's work, difficulty concentrating, depression, drowsiness, puffy face, especially puffiness around the eyes, dried sticky greenish mucus between the eyelids on awakening that is difficult to rub out, coarse dry skin, hair loss - especially of the outer third of the eyebrows, brittle nails, cold intolerance, tiring easily, constipation, a feeling of not having passed the whole stool when defecating even though you have, reduced senses of taste and smell, a deep, hoarse voice, high cholesterol, slow heartbeat, dry, scaly skin with a "puffiness" to it (called myxedema). Appropriate supplementation should correct everything but the eye changes. Apathy, listlessness, and a loss of interest in work and the environment are often misinterpreted as "depression" though they respond poorly to tricyclic antidepressants and are cured by thyroid supplement. A general dulling of the intellect occurs along with repetitive thought patterns. Mucus collects in the eyes and the lids are often stuck together on awakening. Stiffness and aching muscles may occur. Basal body temperature is usually subnormal[1] (<97.5 on awakening before any activity). Treatment is best guided by symptoms rather than lab work or body temperature. Mainstream physicians who are not experienced at this should at least be comfortable prescribing levels of thyroid supplement that make the patient feel better but do not move the blood hormone levels outside of the normal range.

The low thyroid due to mercury poisoning may be caused by what is called Wilson's Syndrome. Aberrant thyroid metabolism in this condition is due to the liver not converting T4 to T3 properly. It can be treated by special protocols of raising and

---

[1] There are many reasons for subnormal body temperature. Low thyroid is only one of them.

115

lowering T3 levels or thyroid supplement can simply be taken until the mercury is gone. Wilson's Syndrome is viewed skeptically by "mainstream" physicians.

"Alternative medicine" treatment of Wilson's Syndrome is by administering T3 (usually time release) and then discontinuing in hopes the liver can be coaxed into increasing its conversion of T4 to T3. Treatment may have to be tried repeatedly to be effective. Typical treatment is to get 7.5 mg 12 hour time release T3 from a compounding pharmacy, take it every 12 hours for a month, then stop it. Sometimes it is necessary to work up to 15 mcg every 12 hours, then go down to 7.5 for a couple of weeks, then drop to zero. Some physicians use much higher doses, or much more rapid cycle times. Subjective feelings of energy, overall symptoms and basal body temperature guide treatment. More information is available in books and on the web.

Physicians who are experienced at hormone replacement and at treating amalgam illness find their patient's clinical response to natural products like Armour® thyroid or Westhroid® to be superior to response to equivalent doses of synthetics like Thyrolar® or Levoxyl® plus Cytomel®. The reason for this is clear from figure 16. Bunevicius *et al.* showed that their hypothyroid patients had more symptoms alleviated by replacement therapy with thyroxine plus triiodothyronine than by thyroxine alone. The figure shows the normal range for T4, T3 and the relationship between T4 and T3 in euthyroid subjects (diamond - from data published by Larsen), the normal relation between T4 and T3 in T4 replaced hypothyroid subjects (shaded region - from data published by Ingbar *et al.*) and the average values of T4 and T3 for Bunevicius' *et al.* patients on T4 alone (circle), or T4 + T3 (square). Since it is known that there are different nuclear receptors for thyroid that have different relative affinities for T3 and T4 it is clear that this ratio has physiological significance and T4 is not just a reservoir form of thyroid hormone.

Bunevicius *et al.* show that therapy which provides a more physiologically natural relationship between T4 and T3 is more effective at alleviating hypothyroid symptoms. This would appear to resolve the debate over treatment of hypothyroidism in favor of those using combinations of T4 and T3 rather than T4 alone. The typical "4:1" combination products containing both T4 and T3 provide about twice as high a ratio of T3 to T4 as Bunevicius *et al.* used, which would be expected to place their total T4 and T3 values in the middle of the physiologically normal range as shown by the cross.

Excessive thyroid hormone supplementation can lead to thyrotoxicosis, which has signs and symptoms identical to those of hyperthyroidism[1]: weight loss, fatigue, heat intolerance, increased sweating, nervousness, restlessness, frequent defecation, rapid heartbeat, bug eyed stare, a fine tremor of the hands and fingers when they are held out, a euphoric feeling of energy during which the patient doesn't manage to focus and get things done, and in women menstrual irregularities. If treatment is not guided by laboratory test results, it must be guided by a careful consideration of the signs and symptoms of hypothyroidism and thyrotoxicosis to ensure that the patient ends up in between them - normal, or euthyroid.

Recent research shows that there is a cell surface receptor that pumps T3 into cells, keeping the intracellular T3 concentration above the serum concentration. If this pump were to stop working due to some pathological process, it would be necessary to elevate the serum T3 concentration above the normal range to achieve the euthyroid state. Surprising discoveries about thyroid hormone metabolism continue to be made. It is not appropriate to be dogmatic about what treatments "must" help or "must" be

---

[1] In medical terms, thyrotoxicosis is when you are poisoned by too much thyroid hormone, and hyperthyroidism is when your thyroid gland is making too much thyroid hormone and you are giving yourself thyrotoxicosis naturally, instead of by taking pills.

What to do about mercury poisoning

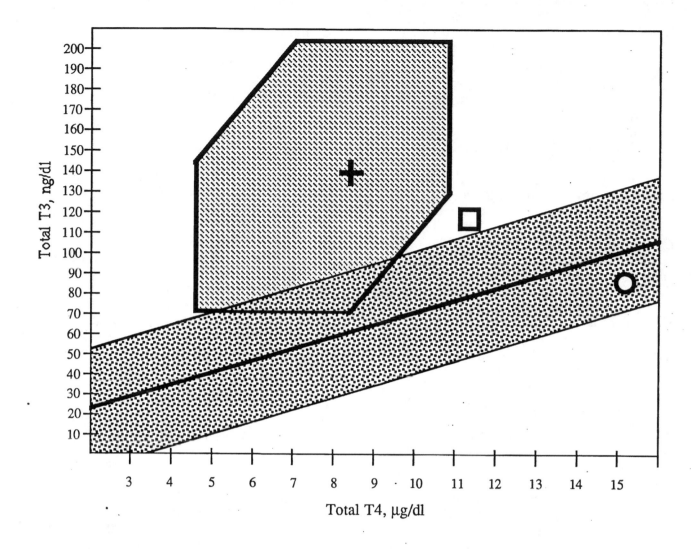

inappropriate based on our incomplete theoretical understanding. It is appropriate for physicians to treat the human being in front of them until signs, symptoms, subjective feelings, and assorted direct and indirect tests for the most part agree they are healthy rather than refusing them treatment because one particular test isn't in the range where it is "supposed" to be. This common sense guideline is almost universally ignored by "mainstream" physicians in the treatment of hypothyroidism in favor of making one particular piece of paper that comes from the laboratory have "good" numbers on it while the patient suffers in ill health.

WILSON'S DISEASE

Wilson's syndrome is not to be confused with Wilson's disease, a rare aberration of copper metabolism described in standard medical textbooks that has symptoms similar to amalgam illness. In Wilson's disease, hair, urine and RBC copper will be greatly elevated, but serum copper and serum ceruloplasmin will be low. Treatment is with penicillamine (conventional), DMPS or lipoic acid, for life. Taking 100 mg zinc + 1 mg molybdenum daily to reduce copper absorption is also expected to be helpful. Taking antioxidant supplements as for amalgam illness is expected to reduce symptoms promptly while tissue copper levels are reduced to safe levels.

ADRENAL INSUFFICIENCY

Many mercury toxic people (more common in women than men) are hypoadrenal. This is sometimes primary and sometimes secondary. It will seldom show up on an ACTH stimulation test. An insulin induced hypoglycemia test is NEVER appropriate for mercury toxic people since it places oxidative stress on the cerebellum, which is already a target for oxidative damage in mercury intoxication. The most reproducible laboratory test is a fall in ACTH after exercise. Draw blood for ACTH, have the patient perform at least a half hour of heavy exercise beginning within 15 minutes, and draw another sample for ACTH 15-30 minutes after the exercise is over. Both anaerobic and aerobic exercise are fine. ACTH should rise substantially - to high normal or high. A decline of ACTH following exercise is pathological.

An anxiously depressed person with low taurine and possibly signs of hypothyroidism is hypoadrenal - that is, has cortisol levels which are too low. This may not show up on tests for cortisol since the dynamic range of cortisol levels are so wide and people's individual needs for it vary so much.

People who do not sweat much and have this defect in ACTH regulation have an autonomic nervous system biased one way. People who sweat a lot and have this defect in ACTH regulation have their autonomic nervous system biased the other way. The "sweaters" will be helped overall by the drug carbamazepine since it pushes the ANS the other way. The "nonsweaters" may have positive and negative effects from carbamazepine. Administration of intravenous procaine as for cardiac problems will push the ANS towards the "sweating" side. The ACTH response is unlikely to be changed. "Sweaters:" high average cortisol[1], DHEA at reasonable levels, some energy, immune system sensitizes to everything. "Nonsweaters:" low cortisol, low DHEA, very weak, low energy, immune system nonreactive, pupils dilated. "nonsweaters" are much sicker than "sweaters."

Carbamazepine is well described in many medical books. For this use dosage is slowly increased and the test repeated (either with lab work or by subjective patient experience of increasing dose until the patient does not "hit the wall" and become de-energized with increased allergy symptoms 2-4 hours after exercising, but rather feels energized). Doses should be given every 8 hours or the extended release type used. The effective dose is often close to that which begins to induce clumsiness, slowing of reflexes, slurring of words, etc., so the daily dose should be adjusted up and down in 100 mg increments to find the lowest effective amount.

A very good guess about adrenal status can be made by evaluating symptoms. Frank hypocortisolism causes weakness, anorexia, malaise, apathy, fatigue, somnolence, nightmares, depression, increased sense of taste (e. g. to salt and sugar solutions), smell and increased pain sensitivity. Low cortisol causes body fat to be on the arms and legs with a thin abdomen. High cortisol causes thin arms and legs and a fat abdomen. Low cortisol for a long time leads to being quite thin and being unable to gain weight. Women with this lose the "baby fat" under their skin and begin to have more male like contours of skin following their muscles and bones, as well as wearing a smaller bra size than they used to since their breasts aren't as full as before. Thin, stress intolerant, high strung chemically sensitive women are almost certain to benefit from supplementary cortisol. Symptoms clear with adequate replacement therapy, and reappear if the

---

[1]which doesn't increase in response to stress, which is very important. The body's adaptation of maintaining a high average level is better than leaving it low but still very unhealthy and you will spend most of your time woozy and tired.

patient's glucocorticoid requirement increases and becomes larger than the dosage used.

If adrenal insufficiency is due to adrenal gland problems, mineralocortocoids will also be deficient and the patient will be intolerant to potassium (as in lite salt or salt substitute). Supplementary glucocorticoids aggravate this. Potassium intolerance is corrected by epinephrine and mineralocorticoids. Pregnenolone may help make a little extra of both glucocorticoids and mineralocorticoids. Such a person should be tested for antiadrenal antibodies. Someone who has low glucocorticoids but needs extra potassium has a hypothalamic or pituitary defect, may respond to carbamazepine, and will show up as normal on an ACTH stimulation test (a test which endocrinologists unfortunately worship as definitive). Centrally mediated[1] hypofunction of all other endocrine glands should be carefully considered in this case.

The combination of symptoms of anxiety, fear, depression, agitation, crying, sweating, palpitations and blood pressure spikes from a low base level is a consequence of cortisol insufficiency. First, low blood sugar (hypoglycemia) occurs due to low cortisol. Then adrenaline shoots up to mobilize glucose. Since adrenaline can't do this very well without adequate cortisol, vast tidal waves of it wash over you and the "psychiatric" symptoms occur. Just like they do in people injected with tons of adrenaline. Just like they do in people who got the old fashioned insulin induced hypoglycemia test and had their blood sugar pushed through the floor on purpose. This whole problem can be made worse by hyperinsulinism. If your body has too much insulin floating around, it can't get rid of the stuff so there is insulin making your cells suck up blood sugar and keeping it low. In order to prevent this, you can limit your insulin levels by not eating sweets, sticking to modest size low carbohydrate meals, and taking 200 mcg of chromium picolinate with them. The rest of the symptom complex can be controlled by

---

[1] that is, pituitary or hypothalamic.

giving your body what it needs to make blood sugar on demand - eating frequent, small, high protein meals and taking hydrocortisone 5 mg 2-4 times per day (or 10 mg with breakfast and 5 mg with lunch). Branched chain amino acids are not helpful and glutamine is of limited utility unless you take enough hydrocortisone.

If you have a paradoxical stress response, using hydrocortisone 5 mg 2-4 times per day as needed to get rid of spaciness and brain fog will get you re-energized and let you get a lot more done. This is a controversial therapy since some physicians believe there is a risk it may lead to adrenal suppression, while others believe it has no such effect. This is a silly argument. In a very important way you already ARE adrenal suppressed - since "adrenally suppressed" means your cortisol doesn't go up like it is supposed to during stress.

If you and your physician decide to use hydrocortisone (cortisol)[2], pay attention to what is happening, how much of the stuff you take, etc. and ask your physician about whether you should wear a medalert bracelet. If you use carbamazepine to normalize the paradoxical response you are in effect "un-suppressing" your adrenal responses. Folklore has it that taking 5 mg hydrocortisone 2-4 times per day can lead to increased yeast problems. People with mild adrenal insufficiency[3] will feel MUCH better and be MUCH more functional if they do something to address it. They will also experience a reduction in yeast problems since both high AND low cortisol increase susceptibility to infection.

A prednisolone or hydrocortisone taper every 2-3 months lasting no more than 10 days is another possible approach to ameliorating the effects of a paradoxical adrenal response. This regimen is generally

---

[2] hydrocortisone and cortisol are different names for the same hormone.

[3] A "mainstream" physician would say subclinical. An "alternative" physician would say adrenally impaired.

accepted as presenting minimal risk of adrenal suppression.

The textbook rules of thumb for treatment with glucocorticoids (hydrocortisone and medicines that act like it) are that large doses for less than a month do not generally lead to long term adrenal suppression. Tapers for 5-10 days every 2-3 months do not lead to significant suppression even if large doses are used. Daily doses up to the equivalent of 20 mg of cortisol over long time periods lead to measurable suppression that is not clinically significant. Some conservative physicians believe that 20 mg with breakfast and 5 mg with lunch - shown to be helpful in chronic fatigue - leads to enough suppression to be clinically significant.

Taking supplementary glucocorticoids early in the day is less suppressive than taking them later. This is because they mimic the body's natural rhythm this way.   If possible it is best not to take them after 4 PM, or to take the smallest possible doses in the later parts of the day. One very common dosing strategy is to take 2/3 of the daily dose in the morning and 1/3 in the early afternoon, e. g. with breakfast and lunch.

Suppressed patients or those on replacement therapy must have steroids available for stress or trauma, must know when to take them, and must have a syringe with injectable steroids available which they and their family members know how to administer. They also must wear a medical alert device[1]. In the case of any infection, the steroid dose is immediately increased by the equivalent of 100 mg of cortisol (20 mg prednisolone/prednisone) - which calls into question the idea that adrenal steroids will be harmful for people with chronic yeast problems. A person who has had significant adrenal suppression requires 9 months to fully recover proper adrenal function. Some physicians believe it can take as long as 2 years, but studies with seriously ill people who were given large amounts of glucocorticoids did show them returning to

normal within 9 months, and it is these studies that are shown in endocrinology books which provide literature citations and republished graphs in support of their assertions.

The most common error in supportive treatment for mercury toxic (and chronic fatigue) patients is failure to treat adrenal insufficiency. The symptoms are debilitating yet readily controlled. Dosages for tapers are given in an appendix.

One   practical   advantage   of methylprednisolone is that it comes in dosepacks which are arranged to provide a proper   taper   automatically. Methylprednisolone is about ten times more expensive than prednisolone[2].

A positive response to the trial is obviously improved mood, energy and well being during the following week.

Your doctor or someone who has experienced it needs to explain gastroesophageal reflux to you repeatedly so you will remember and realize what is happening if you experience it. On the higher dose days of a taper, the stomach makes a lot of acid. During sleep, the valve at the top of the stomach can let the acid into the esophagus and throat where it will try to digest you. This is very painful! You will wake up with a burning pain in the chest and throat, which can be quite frightening if you don't realize what it is. The pain can best be dealt with by sipping on 1-2 tsp. baking soda dissolved in water and sitting upright. It takes about an hour for the pain to subside to tolerable levels. You should sleep upright for the rest of the night if possible. Residual discomfort will be noticeable for a day or two. To reduce the chance of reflux, you should not eat any food for 2-3 hours before bedtime. You may also wish to take H2 blockers for a few days[3], take a lot of

---

[1] MedicAlert® or Medalert® bracelet or pendant.

[2] perhaps $50 worth of medication for a taper instead of $5.

[3] A few days will not have a substantial effect on the immune system but may have a very substantial

What to do about mercury poisoning

calcium carbonate antacid tablets, and eat a high protein diet.

Proper immune function depends on appropriate glucocorticoid levels. An adrenally insufficient patient with yeast problems will do better in controlling the yeast if glucocorticoids are replaced at the appropriate level.

Long term replacement of adrenal steroids is possible and will make a hypoadrenal person feel MUCH better, but requires careful monitoring, immediate medical attention after stress or trauma, wearing a medalert bracelet, etc. It also takes nine months to to be safely weaned off glucocorticoids once once you stop using them when the mercury is gone and the endocrine system capable of operating on its own.

The major problem with simply giving up on your adrenal glands for a while and taking however much cortisol you need is that this changes so much from day to day. If you are able to keep your body responding to your changing needs, even if poorly, by just taking some supplementary cortisol, you won't have to spend lots of time thinking and worrying about exactly what the proper dose to take today is. Thus the discussion here is based on preserving as much natural adrenal function as possible, augmenting it with tegretol and pregnenolone, and using supplementary hydrocortisone 5 mg 2-4 times per day (or more in the morning, such as 10 mg with breakfast and 5 mg with lunch to mimic your body's natural rhythm), and occasional prednisolone tapers to clear out accumulated stress effects. If this just isn't doing it and you need to take a replacement dose, it is usually 25-37.5 mg a day in a normal unstressed state, typically 2/3 in the morning and 1/3 at lunch or in the early afternoon. Most mainstream physicians will

---

effect on your comfort if you need them to avoid gastric reflux. Do remember that, like any other drug, if you react to a lot of things you do have a good chance of reacting to these and will need to decide whether to take your chances on them or on stomach acid.

know how to do this and know the standard textbook precautions you need to be aware of.

Hypoadrenal people may not wish to embark on long term supplement therapy (which should use cortisone or hydrocortisone or prednisolone but not prednisone) but may need occasional 'tapers' to respond to stresses. The antiepileptic drug carbamazepine increases the body's cortisol response to stress at doses similar to those used to treat epilepsy. NB the 'phase 1' liver detoxification interactions with carbamazepine. Carbamazepine may also be helpful in patients who have certain personality disorders (most likely caused by mercury intoxication, but quite real until detox is complete). It does have significant toxicity and side effects.

The hypoadrenal symptom complex of depressed mood, listlessness, lack of energy, apathy, low motivation and weakness or tiredness is likely to respond positively to a prednisolone taper regardless of whether laboratory tests show frank hypoadrenalism. Apparently the effects of stress never get cleared out and just pile up even though the adrenals do their day to day job otherwise.

Hypoadrenal females will be deficient in androgens, since half (premenopausal) or more (postmenopausal) of their androgens are of adrenal origin and these are produced in response to ACTH just like cortisol is. Administration of DHEA and androgens should be routinely considered in hypoadrenal and hypoglycemic women. This should be done orally or transdermally. It will lead to an increased sense of well being, a more well regulated immune system, and an increased libido.

Some people have normal to high cortisol at rest but have ACTH and cortisol fall in response to stress. Carbamazepine will often normalize baseline cortisol and restore the stress response. This is quite dose sensitive and the dose must exceed a certain threshold for there to be much effect. ACTH response to exercise stress should be determined in

121

anyone for whom fatigue, lethargy, allergy or stress intolerance is a problem, especially if they are overweight.

Both men and women can have normal cortisol levels yet very low DHEA. DHEA is an important hormone and should be replaced to normal levels for young adults - not for age. Target blood levels of DHEA-S (measured in the AM about 4 hours after the morning dose) are: men, 700-900 mcg/dl. Women, 300-400 mcg/dl. Oral dosing is with meals, with about half the daily dose at breakfast. Transdermal creams are also available and some people like them better. Creams are usually applied twice per day. Oral doses in excess of 50 mg/day have some potential to exert virilizing effects on women, and to lower their HDL cholesterol. Some women respond poorly to modest doses of DHEA even if they are low. In such cases phase 2 sulfation status should be investigated.

Like cortisol, DHEA has a daily cycle, being high in the morning and low in the evening. It is best to use dosing strategies that mimic this most of the time.

While pregnenolone is the precursor to cortisol and DHEA, and taking supplementary pregnenolone will raise these two hormones, it will not greatly increase them. It will also not correct problems with a lack of response of ACTH to stress. It is worth taking pregnenolone as it will help. Much of the benefit of taking pregnenolone is that it is also used by the brain and the major reason to take it is indeed to help the brain work better.

SEX HORMONES

Hypogonadal people may benefit from supplementary sex hormones. Pregnenolone, DHEA and androstenedione (all OTC in the US, though DHEA at least is a controlled substance in Canada) can substitute to a certain extent. Men can take androstenedione at bedtime to mimic the diurnal pattern of testosterone production. Hypoadrenal women also have low levels of androgenic

hormones since these come from their adrenal glands, and they will benefit greatly from supplementary DHEA or androgens. Women who take too much DHEA can increase their androgen and estrogen levels too much.

Women with excess estrogens will have a tendency towards inflammation problems, severe PMS, and a high risk of breast cancer. High estrogen levels can sometimes be reduced with folic acid, SAMe, or other methylating agents.

Some researchers have found that women with chronic fatigue syndrome who have low testosterone can benefit from replacement to appropriate female levels, which is usually done using a transdermal patch. When greater anabolic effects are appropriate in women than a "feminine" dose of testosterone is likely to provide, decadurabolin is the preferred therapy since it has the highest ratio of anabolic to androgenic action of any available steroid.

Appropriate male doses of testosterone creams and gels are about 400 mg of testosterone applied daily. Appropriate female doses are roughly 50 mg applied daily.

The injectable forms are: testosterone cypionate in linseed (flax) oil, and testosterone enanthate in sesame oil. Someone who has dietary problems with one of these oils would be wise not to inject it. Blood testosterone levels fluctuate substantially when it is given by injection.

While medical sources are unclear on how to use testosterone without suppressing endogenous production, anyone politically incorrect enough to read bodybuilding sources quickly sees that trial therapy for men lasting less than 2 months with a 3-6 month break afterwards does not suppress the body's natural secretion rate and may thus be used to see how the patient responds or to try to 'kick start' the system without making a long term commitment to therapy. Testosterone cypionate or enanthate given by injection is much easier on the liver (a target organ for mercury poisoning) than are oral

What to do about mercury poisoning

preparations. Women have less liver trouble from oral preparations because they require much less than men. There are transdermal patches, though most people eventually develop allergies to them. Compounding pharmacies can make transdermal creams which are less expensive and less irritating than patches. Patches and creams deliver testosterone in a MUCH more physiological manner and also avoid the need for deep intramuscular injections using large bore needles.

Some men may appear to have normal testosterone levels but will lack the diurnal variation characteristic of a healthy endocrine system (testosterone should be highest in the AM) and will feel better if this rhythm is restored by using patches or cream.

Androgens are mildly immunosuppressive. They reduce inflammatory and other immune responses and may ameliorate allergy or autoimmune symptoms in some individuals.

The libido of both men and women is controlled by androgens. Estrogens have nothing to do with it. Greatly reduced libido in either sex is a sign that androgens are very low. Libido is not strongly or precisely controlled by androgens so it can neither be used as a precise measure of dosage, nor can androgens be used to 'fine tune' libido.

Androgens are also mildly mood elevating and lead to an increased feeling of well being. This is true in both sexes.

GROWTH HORMONE

While currently expensive, growth hormone therapy is likely to lead to greatly increased feelings of well being. Growth hormone must be administered by injection. There are sublingual preparations claimed to have similar effect but this is not well established. There are approaches to increase growth hormone using nutritional supplements, such as consuming large amounts of arginine at bedtime[1]. Testing for IGF-1/SMC (growth hormone markers) is worthwhile since some mercury toxic patients who appear on physical examination to be low in growth hormone actually have enough - they just have other problems.

SLEEP

Most mercury poisoned people have difficulty getting to sleep, staying asleep, and keeping their body clock in phase with the rest of the world.

Melatonin in doses of 3-20 mg per night can be used to relieve insomnia, which mercury toxic people usually have. It is also a good antioxidant, especially for the brain[2]. It also helps protect the brain's hormone regulatory system[3] from "adrenal alerts," stress spikes in cortisol that some people with chronic fatigue experience. Taking some immediate release and some time release melatonin seems to be most effective. If melatonin is not completely effective adding some GABA at bedtime may help. GABA stimulates the same receptor benzodiazepines like Valium and Klonopin do. Melatonin (and serotonin) are derived from tryptophan.

- Some people find that small doses of antidepressants also improve sleep

- It is also worth trying thiamine (B-1), niacin, niacinamide, and inositol

- All anxiolytics may help with sleep

---

[1] There are many OTC products to increase growth hormone production. One of the more conservative and old fashioned recipes is 4-12 grams arginine, 2-6 grams ornithine, and 1-3 grams lysine at bedtime on an empty stomach, or 1/2 to 1 hour before intense exercise. This does cause nausea. Obviously the exercise prescription is not appropriate for people who have a paradoxical adrenal response to stress.
[2] *Journal of Physiology and Biochemistry* 53 301-305 (1997).
[3] the hypothalamus and pituitary.

- Drugs which may increase melatonin are fluvoxamine, desimipramine, most MAO inhibitors

- Herbs which may raise melatonin levels are Hypericium perforatum (St. John's Wort), cannabis sativa (marijuana)[1]

- Vitamin B-12 may also increase melatonin

- Foods high in melatonin and tryptophan are given in the appendix

BRAIN FUNCTION

One of the most obvious brain problems is a migraine. Ginger may relieve these. Arginine can aggravate them.

Many cognitive or emotional problems that come and go are due to dietary components. If you have such problems you may be able to sort them out by keeping a food diary. Few MD's will be familiar with the possible correlation of different dietary components with brain function so you will need to find some kind of health care practitioner who is or sort it out yourself.

Many of the problems mercury causes in the brain are simply because it makes it harder for the brain to get oxygen and glucose to turn into energy. This in turn makes it harder for your brain to make the neurotransmitters it needs to function properly. Both Hydergine® and vinpocetine increase brain oxygenation and blood flow, and may generally improve your mood and brain function.

You can make some good guesses about your brain chemistry by paying attention to sleeping and waking activity patterns.

---

[1] Which is illegal for this use even in those few states that have passed "medical marijuana" initiatives. The author highly recommends you stick to legal means of treating your medical problems.

Dreaming involves cholinergic and dopaminergic mechanisms. Not dreaming indicates that choline precursors are needed. People with low B-6 don't remember their dreams.

Being able to concentrate and pay attention is also cholinergic. Attention deficit also indicates cholinergic precursors are needed. DMAE is an excellent acetylcholine precursor, and lecithin or phosphatidylcholine works as well. Choline itself has a hard time getting from your body into your brain.

Waking up stiff and unrefreshed with no dreams indicates too little dopamine. This can be helped with GABA and taurine (which are relaxing as well as raise dopamine levels) in addition to the more obvious approach using tyrosine or phenylalanine.

The depression mercury toxic people usually have is caused by some underlying pathological alteration in how their body works. This pathological process must be corrected to really get rid of the depression. Antidepressants are only useful for controlling it while the underlying pathology is corrected. Antidepressants should not be considered as a real treatment for the problem, but rather as "mental aspirin" while the "broken brain" heals up. The ultimate solution is mercury detox. Often some intermediate solution like correcting hypoglycemia can be found.

Choline can deepen depression in depressed people - their response should be checked and if they can't tolerate it TMG may be used as a methyl donor (for liver health and sometimes antidepressant action) instead.

Mercury poisoning causes a lot of symptoms that are considered "psychiatric problems." Despite the fact that the symptoms are "behavioral" and a lot of people will think they are "all in your head," you may have a real physical need for "psychiatric" drugs due to your mercury poisoned metabolism. Don't live in misery by trying to "think happy thoughts" or some such silly thing! If mercury poisoning is

What to do about mercury poisoning

causing a metabolic defect that makes you suffer by making your brain work funny, take drugs or supplements that make your brain work properly until you are detoxed, just like you would do for your kidneys or liver.

Depressed people often have much lower levels of pregnenolone in their cerebrospinal fluid than normal people[1]. Blood levels can be tested, but some depressed people have normal blood levels of pregnenolone despite low levels in the CSF. Supplementary pregnenolone may help ameliorate depression and should be considered regardless of blood levels.

Mercury poisoned people are usually depressed. Depression is a classic symptom of hypothyroidism. Blood tests are notoriously unreliable in telling whether mercury toxic people are hypothyroid. In addition, it is well known that refractory depression which does not respond to antidepressants will often respond if some T3 is also administered. A trial of thyroid hormone should be given for depression unless it is clearly unnecessary based on symptoms rather than blood tests.

Since the depression mercury that toxic people experience is biochemically based, talk therapy is unlikely to help. The goal of alleviating depression is to reduce the number of crying bouts, lessen the heavy feelings of sadness and demoralization, create more interest in areas unrelated to the illness, reduce suffering, and let the patient lead a more normal life now rather than a year from now. It is especially important to treat depression if thoughts of hurting yourself or even of committing suicide sometimes come to mind. Depression is best treated by taking drugs or supplements to correct the metabolic problems in your mercury poisoned brain. No therapist is going to be able to talk the mercury atoms into being nice and coming out.

---

[1] Don't go get pregnenolone or anything else tested in your CSF unless you absolutely have to.

While many people do not find talk therapy helpful, some are able to use it to relieve their suffering while detoxing, to help them exercise good judgment, and to let go of the trauma this serious illness - mercury poisoning - caused when they are finally well. If talk therapy helps you by all means use it. But don't replace drugs or supplements with it.

Many patients find adequate relief from herbals and supplements in adequate dosages. St. John's Wort, niacinamide, acetyl-l-carnitine and methylating agents may also be helpful for depression.

Appropriate supplementation of amino acids often solves the problem - phenylalanine, tyrosine, histamine or tryptophan being the most common choices. The plasma amino acid analysis is helpful in selecting amino acids to try as well as antidepressants.

If you are taking amino acids to affect your brain chemistry they have a lot more punch if you take them on an empty stomach.

When treating depression it is best to start at lower than normal doses of antidepressants to see if the patient tolerates the drug since they often don't. These tolerance trials do not need to be long - the goal is not to see if the low dose is therapeutic but only to find a tolerated dose and effective therapeutic agent. Selegiline or other MAO inhibitors are usually helpful. Tricyclics sometimes work. Many patients do not respond at all to the SSRI drugs. It is often necessary to try several antidepressants to find one that works. Ask your physician to start with drugs that take effect promptly. Even with slower acting drugs, if nothing is happening after three weeks, try another drug. Hydergine typically improves mood somewhat and should be administered for other reasons anyway.

Some antidepressant biochemistry: the MAO inhibitors phenelzine and tranylcypromine elevate all the neurotransmitters that might be involved in the problem. They act FAST and have lots of side effects. If the problem is only serotonin, trazodone and the SSRI's work. If it is norepinephrine, the secondary amine tricyclics do it. If the problem is serotonin + norepinephrine, the tertiary amine tricyclics do it. If the problem is dopamine, bupropion, amoxapine and selegiline do it. If the problem is histamine you have to take histidine - there is no appropriate prescription drug. Phenylalanine and tyrosine elevate norepinephrine and dopamine. Tryptophan and 5-hydroxytryptophan elevate serotonin. Alpha agonists and to a limited extent ephedrine mimic norepinephrine.

Mercury toxic people often suffer from things other than depression. Agitation, anxiety and emotional changes that in the extreme appear to be schizophrenia do occur.

Anxiety and agitation are usually due to hypoglycemia or environmental chemicals that your liver is not detoxifying rapidly enough to keep them from building up in your body. The best treatments are to correct the hypoglycemia and support liver metabolism as discussed in the relevant section. Anxiety and agitation can also be controlled directly.

Having too much or too little cortisol or not having it at the right times also affects how your brain and emotions work. See the adrenal section.

Taking 1/2 gram of tryptophan 4 times per day on an empty stomach will sometimes reduce agitation. Taking large amounts of choline (3-10 grams) or of phosphatidylcholine (5-15 grams) can stop mania.

The standard anti-anxiety drugs are the benzodiazepines (Valium® etc.) and the newer Buspar®. The benzodiazepines are addictive and sedating. The antidepressant Trazodone also reduces anxiety. See discussion in the section on therapeutic agents. Natural alternatives are GABA, gotu kola, vitamin B6, niacinamide, and taurine.

Kava kava is popular but may not be appropriate for mercury toxic people[1].

If you are having a lot of anxiety and anger, do NOT take phenylalanine, tyrosine, alpha or beta agonists or other things that elevate noradrenaline and adrenaline. Reducing your protein intake to reduce phenylalanine and tyrosine may be helpful.

Mercury poisoning can also cause subtle emotional changes that affect how you relate to other people. If you find yourself becoming more distant from people and more socially detached it may be how the mercury feels - not you.

Severe mercury poisoning can push your emotions farther and farther from where you would normally be - eventually getting to the point where you feel like "that's not really you," where you have difficulties relating to other people and figuring out what they want, and you experience anxious feelings of emptiness and meaninglessness, and eventually where you become so poisoned that you exhibit schizophrenic behaviors[2].

There are several treatments in addition to those offered by conventional medicine which might help you ameliorate these symptoms while you detoxify and get well.

Things that are common in mercury poisoning which can cause this are low thyroid, poor methylation (usually due to folate and B-12 deficiency), out of control allergies (including to gluten in grains), yeast infections and sleep deprivation. Correcting these in the course of supportive treatment for your mercury poisoning may also make you feel a lot better emotionally.

---

[1] It is a central nervous system depressant and has side effect similar to common mercury poisoning symptoms.
[2] and psychiatrists who don't believe in amalgam illness would diagnose you as schizophrenic, or schizotypal, or schizoid instead of as mercury poisoned.

What to do about mercury poisoning

Of course, mercury directly poisons your brain so you may continue to have problems even after dealing with all of the things in the last paragraph.

Some people with these problems feel better and behave more normally when they have a fever. These people will benefit from taking borage oil - without aspirin - and perhaps also penicillin. Borage oil causes the formation of a particular prostaglandin, as does penicillin. This prostaglandin both elevates your temperature and affects how you feel. Some people don't have enough of it in their brains because the mercury chews it up.

Some people have excessively low histamine (as shown in a blood test or by symptoms). In this case you will benefit from vitamins B-12 and C, zinc, niacin, folic acid, pantothenic acid, a high protein diet, supplementary histidine, and you should consider taking modest amounts of manganese to get your levels above average although mercury poisoned people should otherwise avoid manganese. You will also likely have relatively high copper levels in your serum and hair and will benefit from strictly excluding copper from your diet and supplements. If you do need prescription medicines, phenytoin will be bad for you and neuroleptics will work well.

Some people have the opposite problem - excessively high histamine (as shown in a blood test or by symptoms). Your serum and hair copper will be normal. You will have special problems with suicidal depression, having your mind go blank, and being very sensitive to pain. You may have allergies and they will make your nose run and eyes itch like mad, as will colds. You will respond well to calcium, methyl sources except folate, zinc, and antihistamines that make you feel drowsy[1].

If allergies are causing these emotional problems, you will be able to relieve them by fasting. You will often have daily mood swings. You will have low blood histamine and your pulse will be rapid when you are having problems. You will need to identify the foods that you are allergic to by eliminating them from your diet one by one. Vitamins B6, C, calcium and potassium will be very helpful. Leukotriene inhibitors may also help.

Other possible metabolic aberrations can cause emotional difficulties. Vitamin B6, zinc and hormone supplementation as appropriate will often help alleviate them.

The Pfeiffer Center is experienced at treating schizophrenia and related conditions and finds that they are often caused by the kinds of things discussed above, and are readily cured by appropriate medical treatment (but that psychiatric treatment never solves the problem). They both accept patients and will often consult with your doctor on the phone to help him find the best treatment for you. They can be reached at:

Pfeiffer Center
1804 Diehl Road
Naperville, IL

(630) 505-0300.

Before the initial visit it is helpful if you can have the following tests available so they can determine whether they can get insurance to cover your treatment, and get some idea of what you have: Zinc, copper, lead and manganese in blood and a hair analysis heavy metal screen, kryptopyrrole urine analysis, blood histamine, thyroid panel, ABO blood type and an extensive blood chemistry panel equivalent to Chemzyme® Plus.

Discussion of things to do to help reduce excessive copper levels and compensate for their effects are given above in the section on magnesium, potassium iron and copper.

Drugs which themselves can cause schizophrenia like paranoid reactions at high enough dosages are bromides, glucocorticoids, levodopa, monoamine

---

[1] including diphenhydramine (Dramamine®).

oxidase inhibitors, tricyclic antidepressants, amphetamines, and drugs that act similarly to dopamine.

All of these emotional, or "psychiatric" problems will be cured when you finally detoxify your brain enough by using lipoic acid. Everything else you do is to help make you happier and more comfortable until that is finally done.

Mercury can do enough brain damage to create standard neurological problems. Hearing loss, tremor, and difficulty concentrating are the most bothersome. Tremor is the most obvious sign and anything that controls it will likely help with the others. Note that the tremor mercury poisoning victims experience is not caused by anxiety - even if they are anxious at the time - so if you find yourself arguing with a physician who insists your tremor is just anxiety and all you need to do is go talk to a psychiatrist, what you really need to do is find a doctor less brain damaged than you who will figure out something to help.

Tremor, particularly intention tremor, can be controlled by the prescription drug hydergine® (generic: ergoloid mesylates) in doses of 15-20 mg/d rather than the 3 mg/d more typically used in US practice. If you find hydergine helps with tremor, concentration, depression, etc. but you need further improvement, try increasing your dose.

Tremor is also a symptom of Parkinson's disease, caused by oxidative stress as it is in mercury poisoning. Drugs such as selegiline that are effective in that case are helpful for many mercury poisoned people as well.

Other things that may control tremor are glycine, and eating a ketogenic diet - one of the low carbohydrate, high fat, high protein diets that used to be popular for weight loss. E. g. steak, salad, no bread or potatoes.

Some people find they can control tremor or peripheral neuropathy by eliminating wheat and gluten containing foods from their diet. This can be explored by measuring anti-gliadin antibodies, and if they are not unequivocally low, eliminating these foods from their diet for a week long therapeutic trial.

If you are very poisoned, you may have extreme problems with how your brain controls your body. During serious chronic mercury toxicity autonomic nervous system dysfunction is common. This causes you to have cold, sweaty hands and feet, a fast heartbeat (tachycardia) alternating with a slow one (bradycardia), not to sweat, to have low immune reactivity, and to find even the lightest activities overwhelmingly fatiguing. These can be brought under control for a period from days to weeks, and sometimes permanently corrected, by administration of large amounts of procaine. The most effective protocol involves intravenous administration of enough (e. g. 10 cc 1% procaine) to promptly render the patient unconscious for a period of time. Intramuscular administration of 3-5 ml of (epinephrine and preservative free) procaine may lead to an improved feeling of well being for a few days.

Mercury causes chemically induced brain damage. This is why amalgam illness victims have emotional changes, memory problems, and endocrine problems. Once the mercury is gone, there are a number of things that can be done to promote brain healing. Taking steroids like pregnenolone and DHEA which are involved in brain development and function is helpful, as are ergoloid mesylates, and vinpocetine. Learning something completely new and different is also helpful. Activities that involve active use of balance are help too, as do certain types of vision therapy (offered by developmental optometrists). Cranial sacral therapy by an experienced therapist (a DO or a chiropractor trained in it with some experience) is also effective. Speculative medical therapies that leading evidence in the literature suggests may be effective are relatively high doses of lipoic acid, androgens[1], and materials that increase the formation of cyclic AMP and cyclic GMP in brain tissue, such as forskolin, or ginkgo biloba and arginine.

A lot of spontaneous brain healing will take place as you remove mercury and provide the essential substrates to rebuild damaged neurons, like omega 3 essential fatty acids. If you attempt to regenerate and repair your brain before you removed enough mercury and got enough healthy material into you any improvements you make will quickly be taken back by continuing pathology. The most important part of brain healing is detoxification and supplementation. Work on that first and add other stuff later if you don't like where you are going.

SIDE EFFECTS AND ADVERSE REACTIONS

If you unexpectedly start to react to a drug, supplement, or herbal, it may be something in the formulation. It is not necessarily the supplement itself. Try a different brand or have that substance specially compounded without additives if it is important to your treatment protocol.

Mercury toxic people have a high incidence of side effects and adverse drug reactions, yet end up taking a lot of different things. Try to stick to things that are widely used and have a low adverse reaction rate. Don't change brands or formulations unnecessarily. Try new things gingerly - and pre-test them if they might have to be used in an urgent situation. Do not automatically assume all worsenings or adverse reactions are caused by the most recent material introduced. Keep careful track of problems to look for commonalities. After one material has caused significant problems, do not try similar materials unless necessary.

There are some things that as a rule are contraindicated in mercury toxic people. These are:

- HMG Co A reductase inhibitors (cholesterol drugs)

- Pennicillamine

- Dimercaprol (BAL)

- H2 blockers (to reduce stomach acidity)

- Sulfites (preservatives in many local anesthetics)

- Supplementary cysteine

- Supplementary glutathione

- Chlorella or other algae, especially in large amounts

- Dandelion/Beet green/Lemon juice/Olive oil liver flushes

The HMG co A reductase inhibitors are a common class of cholesterol lowering drugs that work by interfering with a particular part of the liver's biochemistry that really needs to be left functional because it also produces metabolic intermediates crucial for other life processes. These drugs are fluvastatin (Lescol[®]), lovastation (Mevacor[®]), pravastatin (Pravachol[®]) and simvastatin (Zocor[®]). Do not get distracted from the important health issue of mercury detox, but if you feel you need to lower cholesterol, bile acid binding resins, fiber, and the reasonably high doses of antioxidant supplements you need anyway will reduce cholesterol substantially. And remind your doctor that low thyroid levels cause high cholesterol, so if you are worried about cholesterol and haven't tried some thyroid hormone yet, perhaps you should.

Mercury toxic people can and do independently have other common problems (e. g. they may come down with a cold or flu and spend several days trying to figure out which drug or supplement they are reacting to this time). Do not become too fixated on mercury as the root cause of every single new problem you have.

---

[1] above the normal male physiological range.

HOSPITALS AND AVOIDING HARMFUL CARE

Mercury toxic people will not receive proper care at hospitals and it can be life threatening for them to be involuntarily retained at a hospital and treated by a physician who does not believe in 'amalgam illness.' Such a physician will refuse them necessary medicines and supplements while administering medications which the patient has a high probability of experiencing adverse reactions to[1]. Mercury toxic people should be routinely instructed by their physician in what to say, or not to say, in order to obtain appropriate care and prompt release if they unexpectedly find themselves in this situation.

Many laymen are not aware that hospitals only let physicians who have privileges at that particular hospital participate in patient care there, or that getting such privileges is rather political so that it is uncommon for physicians who believe in amalgam illness to have hospital privileges anywhere. Once you are hospitalized is unlikely you will be under the care of the physician treating you for amalgam illness.

Your friends and family must have it impressed on them how important it is not to call 911 under all but the most dire circumstances. They are generally unaware that calling 911 sets a bureaucratic process in motion that cannot be stopped. The ambulance crew has some legal ability to strap you to the stretcher and take you to the hospital if they think you need to go regardless of what you say, and the hospital has some legal ability to hold you and treat you against your will if they think you are not making rational decisions.

---

[1] See Lazarou, Pomeranz and Corey, 1998, where the incidence of adverse drug reactions in hospitalized patients is studied and found to be disturbingly high. This is for patients who mostly DON'T have amalgam illness and have normal metabolisms!

PSYCHIATRIC EMERGENCIES

Mercury toxic people whose symptoms or history include psychiatric manifestations should be provided with appropriate medications to control these symptoms IMMEDIATELY if chelation or other events bring them on. The patients, their friends and family should be instructed as to how and when to use these medications. The medications should be pre-tested to assure they are safe by trying them at some convenient time in slowly increasing doses. Everyone concerned needs to understand that calling 911 has a high probability of leading to a few days of involuntary confinement at a psychiatric hospital during which the patient will not receive appropriate medication, supplements or diet. It will also cost several thousand dollars which insurance does not as a rule reimburse.

If you ever think of suicide or of hurting yourself and you need to talk to people about it (often a good way to distract you from doing it) make sure you have some friends and family members who understand they MUST NOT call 911 about this unless you really are going to do yourself in this instant and they can't stop it. The same problem as above occurs - you get dragged off and may be involuntarily committed, you don't get your supplements, medicines or diet for several days, you may get harmful medications forced on you, and your insurance company may not pick up the bill.

If you ever find yourself in this unfortunate position, the first priority is to get let go. Refusing to talk to the doctor about your problems will most likely result in your being held. You want to convince the doctor that what they perceive as the "precipitating problem" is over. Try to relate to the doctor. Don't talk about how "special" your other health care providers are - that is interpreted as a sign you are delusional. But do be aware that if you go on in too much detail and give them full access to your medical records they may decide you are delusional for thinking you have amalgam illness, and may also turn your doctor in to the licensing authorities. Within reasonable limits, try to be cooperative. If they try to talk you into voluntary commitment, don't agree. If they are going to commit you involuntarily, neither sign nor refuse to sign agreements[1]. Then tell them you can't decide whether to sign or not without having your attorney go over it with you - and write that on the forms. Don't let them give you an attorney 'for free.' You can always take them up on that later if you wish to. The point now is to tie their hands as much as possible so it is inconvenient to hold you and convenient to let you go. If they say you "have" to take some medicine, ask what happens if you refuse. Ask why you have to take it. Be very reasonable. A lot of times you don't actually have to take it, they just say that because they want you to go along. If they don't want to let you go after the minimum hold period and you can't wait out their statutory maximum hold time, having an attorney sue the doctor who committed you (and the one who can release you, if different) personally for violating your civil rights may be necessary to convince them to let you go right away.

People who talk about suicide are not likely to commit it unless they can answer all the following questions: when are you going to do it, how are you going to do it, where are you going to do it, what means do you have right now to do it with? Make sure people you might talk to when you are feeling really really down know to ask all these questions before deciding whether to call 911.

WHAT WILL HAPPEN - PROGNOSIS

Both you and your doctor need to know how long it takes before you get well, and what do you expect along the way.

---

[1] If you refuse to sign things the doctors usually gain a lot more legal leeway than if it is left ambiguous. If you don't REFUSE to sign, but simply demand your legal right to counsel before deciding, it gives them less freedom to do what they want to you.

Using a proper protocol, e. g. DMSA every 3-4 hours on alternate weeks: 2-6 months to feel better. Then DMSA + LA every 3-4 hours 3 or 4 days every week or two to clear the brain and internal organs, 2-6 months to feel better. Continue supplements and diet control with continuing DMSA + LA chelation while healing takes place, another 4-30 months to good physical and mental health. Total time: 1 to 4 years if you stick with the program.

The big determiner of how long it takes is the DMSA+LA phase. That depends on how seriously poisoned you got.

- You feel depressed, tired, icky. You are moderately poisoned. 6-11 months of DMSA+LA treatment will be required. You will FEEL cured immediately if you take the right supplements and medicines, but you have to chelate to get rid of the mercury.

- You are starting to get stuff like chronic fatigue, fibromyalgia, environmental sensitivities, severe allergies or asthma, emotional disturbances. 14-25 months of DMSA-LA will be required. You will feel MUCH better with the proper supplements and medicines and be able to get on with life pretty quickly.

- You have multiple chemical sensitivities, chronic fatigue syndrome, serious emotional disturbances. You really are not able to participate in life. You are very seriously poisoned. You will need 20-36 months of DMSA+LA to get well. You will need proper supplements and medications to be at all functional and will need to pay careful attention to continuing them and adjusting them for 2-3 years until you are detoxed enough that your health isn't coming out of a pill bottle.

If you continue to chelate with DMSA+LA for 6 months to a year after you are sure you are well you will remove more mercury from your brain and greatly reduce the chances of future problems, neurological disease, or premature aging.

Amalgam Illness: Diagnosis and Treatment

If you follow a standard "alternative medicine" or "witch doctor" protocol, e. g. DMSA every other day or DMPS injections monthly: you will get worse for 6 months to one year, then slowly get better for another several years - but behavioral and coordination problems are exacerbated by this therapy and emotional symptoms are not alleviated. There is also a substantial risk of psychiatric illness. Total time: a year of misery, 5 years to feel better, but you never will be completely well.

If you drill out your fillings then do nothing: about the same thing will happen as with the "witch doctor" protocol, but without the side effects, expense, or risk of insanity.

What to take for mercury poisoning

The different categories of therapeutic agents are listed here. These include prescription drugs, over the counter drugs, drugs not yet approved in the United States but available in foreign countries, vitamins, herbs, and nutritional supplements.

I have provided a table of everything I list and what it is useful for - with the pages in the text where it is mentioned, plus lists of what things fall under each general category. Each material I list is then described appropriately to let you know what it is useful for in treating mercury poisoning and consequent conditions. Greater detail can be found in other sources.

This is my best understanding. It is not perfect. I have certainly left out things you can take[1], and not put down useful properties or hazards of some things in the tables. It is up to you what to take. You may find things that are not in these lists are very helpful to you. They are here to help you, not limit you. But do be careful to understand what you are taking and why - there are many things that can be harmful to you and they are often suggested as helpful instead until a lot of people get hurt by them[2].

Those things I thought you should not take are shown in ~~strikethrough~~ letters - in the overall list if most people should avoid them, and in the conditions lists if they should not be taken in specific circumstances.

---

[1] My coverage of prescription drugs is pretty limited. There are good lists of these broken down by class of drug in *Martingdale's*, *Mosby's*, *Drug Facts*, but not in the *PDR*. There are discussions of what to use for certain conditions in *Harrison's* and *Cecil*.

[2] The most obvious examples being the large number of drugs the FDA approves and then later pulls off the market.

The things I think everyone should strongly consider taking right away have a dot • to the left of them.

Things that are prescription have (Rx) after them. Things not available in the US have (~~US~~) after them.

What you need to do is pick the things that you need to help solve your particular problems. Read about them here and in other sources. If you are familiar with one and already know you tolerate it, use it first. If you are very sensitive to foods, supplements, etc., start at very low doses and use mild agents. If you are not so sensitive, just start trying things at doses high enough you will know if they work.

Start with the things everyone is likely to need. Then add things to fix the specific problems you have. The first thing to fix is problems with your digestive system so you can actually get things into you. Next, take care of your liver so it can do its job of getting rid of toxins and keeping your body clean. If your adrenals or thyroid is not performing you have to help them as early as you can - especially since they affect the liver and digestive tract. After this, start to work on your other problems in the order you think important.

CONSIDER TAKING THESE:

- Vitamin C: 4-12 grams
- Vitamin E 1000+ IU
- Coenzyme Q10 100-400 mg
- Carotene 7.5† mg
- Milk thistle extract - equivalent to 250-750 mg silymarin
- Ergoloid mesylate (Rx) (trade name Hydergine®) 10-20 mg/day
- Flax oil 15-50 g
- Borage oil 1-4 g

- Inositol or inositol hexaphosphate 2-12 grams
- Lysine 2 grams
- Arginine 6 grams
- Magnesium 750 mg
- Chromium 1,000 mcg
- Acetyl-L-carnitine 1-2 grams
- "B-100" multiple B vitamin supplement
- Zinc 50-100 mg
- Molybdenum. 1,000 mcg

Unless you know you don't need them or shouldn't take them, you should also try forskolin, DHEA, pregnenolone, cortisol (Rx), desiccated thyroid (Rx), vitamins B-6 and B-12, folic acid, trimethylglycine, histidine, Accolate® (Rx) and taurine.

If you have a REALLY restricted budget and can't get a doctor to do anything for you, see if you can do this each day:

- Vitamin C: 4 grams, 1 with each meal, 1 at bedtime.
- Vitamin E 400-800 IU
- Milk thistle extract one capsule with each meal
- Flax oil 1 tbsp
- Magnesium 1/4-1/2 tsp epsom salts with each meal
- "B-50" or "B-100" multiple B vitamin supplement
- Zinc 50 mg
- Molybdenum 250-500 mcg
- Chromium 200 mcg with each meal
Vinpocetine 5 mg 3 times a day

If you have a specific problem they would help, consider l-carnitine, forskolin, DHEA, pregnenolone, vitamins B-6 and B-12, folic acid, trimethylglycine, histidine, and taurine.

CHELATING AGENTS

BAL or dimercaprol (Rx)
Cilantro
Citrate
Cysteine

DMPS (Rx[1]) or Dimaval® (US) or Unitiol® (US)
DMSA or Chemet® (Rx)
DMSO
EDTA (Rx)
Lipoic acid or alpha lipoic acid or LA
MSM
Penicillamine or Cuprimine® (Rx)

PAIN RELIEF (ANALGESICS)

Acetaminophen or Tylenol® or paracetamol
Aspirin
Celebrex®
Ibuprofen
Magnesium

ANTIOXIDANTS

- Carotenes (beta, alpha, etc.)
- Coenzyme Q10
Garlic
Lycopene
Selenomethionine
Selenite
- Vitamin C
- Vitamin E

ANTI-ANXIETY AGENTS (ANXIOLYTICS)

Benzodiazepines: Diazepam (Rx) or Zanax® (Rx) or Klonipin® (Rx) or Valium® (Rx) etc.
Buspar® (Rx)
Desyrel® (Rx)
GABA
GHB - gamma hydroxybutyrate
Gotu kola
Kava kava
Niacinamide (Vitamin B-3)
Taurine
Vitamin B-6

---

[1] Not fully FDA approved. Currently an investigational new drug.

What to take for mercury poisoning

IMPORTANT NOTE: Anxiety is often caused by hypoglycemia. If so, the agents above won't help much.

LIVER SUPPORT

Curcumin
Folate
Gamma oryzanol
~~Glutathione~~
~~Liver flushes~~ using: ~~dandelion~~ or ~~beet green~~ or ~~lemon juice~~ or ~~olive oil~~
~~Methionine~~ - the M in SAMe
Methyl donors.
• Milk thistle extract
NAC (N-acetylcysteine)
SAMe - S-adenosyl methionine
Taurine
Trimethylglycine (TMG)
Vitamin B1 or thiamine
Vitamin B2 or riboflavin
Vitamin B3 or niacinamide
Vitamin B3 or niacin
Vitamin B5 or pantothenic acid
• Vitamin B6
Vitamin B12

DIGESTIVE TRACT SUPPORT

Arginine
Forskolin
Glutamine
Yarrow

To reduce nausea:
Ginger
Glycine
<u>Anti-yeast (candida)</u>

Amphotericin B (Rx)
Bifidobacteria and lactobaccilus acidophilus
Caprylic acid
FOS - fructooligosaccharides.
Fluconazole or Diflucan® (Rx)
Ketoconazole (Rx)
Nystatin (Rx)
Terbinafine or Lamisil® (Rx)
<u>Anti-parasites</u>
To kill the parasites:

Black Walnut
Bromelain and papain or digestive enzymes
Metronidazole or Flagyl® (Rx)
Tea Tree Oil

To increase secretory IgA:
Vitamin A

ANTIDEPRESSANTS

It is of course important to recognize things that can CAUSE depression or can MAKE IT WORSE. These include: metronidazole, indomethacin, aspirin, phenacetin, birth control pills, estrogens, progesterone, carbamazepine, benzodiazepines, GABA, ~~GHB~~, ~~Tagamet~~® and ~~penicillamine~~.

5-HTP (5 hydroxytryptophan)
Acetyl-l-carnitine
Folic acid, SAMe, any methylation metabolism enhancer.
Phenylalanine
Pregnenolone
St. John's Wort (containing hypericin).
Thyroid hormone - triiodothyronine (T3) and thyroxine (T4) (Rx)
Tryptophan
Tyrosine
Vitamin B3 (as niacinamide)

There are three basic classes of antidepressants and three "atypical" or one of a kind agents. The classes are the SSRI's, the tricyclics and the MAOI's. Within the tricyclics there are subclasses - secondary amines and tertiary amines. If you try one drug in a class and it does nothing, go to another class. If it helps but has side effects, try others in the same class.
Selective Serotonin Reuptake Inhibitors (SSRI's) Prozac®, Paxil®, Effexor®, Serzone®, and Zoloft®.
Tricyclic antidepressants (Rx): doxepin, amitriptyline, desipramine, nortriptyline
Monoamine oxidase inhibitors (MAOI's) (Rx)
Eldepryl® or selegiline or Deprenyl® (Rx)

Other antidepressants (Rx: bupropion (Wellbutrin®), nefazodone (Serzone®), and trazodone (Desyrel®))

Manic depression (bipolar disorder)
Carbamazepine or Tegretol® (Rx)
Lithium (Rx)

BRAIN SUPPORT

Dimethylaminoethanol (DMAE)
• Ergoloid mesylate or Hydergine®
Ginkgo biloba
Glutamine
Histidine
Methylating agents
NADH
Niacin (not niacinamide)
Omega 3 essential fatty acids
Omega 6 essential fatty acids
Neuroleptics
Phosphatidylserine
Piracetam (~~US~~)
Schizandra
Vinpocetine

Note: Dreaming involves cholinergic and dopaminergic mechanisms. Not dreaming indicates that choline precursors are needed. People with low B-6 don't remember their dreams. Being able to concentrate and pay attention is also cholinergic. Attention deficit also indicates cholinergic precursors are needed. Waking up stiff and unrefreshed with no dreams indicates too little dopamine. This can be helped with GABA and taurine (which are relaxing as well as raise dopamine levels) in addition to the more obvious approach using tyrosine or phenylalanine.

IMMUNE SUPPORT

~~Copper~~
~~Iron~~
Antioxidants (see above)
• Arginine
Astragalus
Cat's claw (una de gato).
Dimethylglycine (DMG)
Echinacea

Forskolin
Garlic
Ginseng
Goldenseal
~~Histamine H2 blockers Tagamet, Zantac, Pepcid Axid.~~
Histidine
• Inositol or inositol hexaphosphate
Intravenous immune globulin
Leptotania
• Lysine
Quercetin
Suma
Vitamin A.
Zinc

ASTHMA/ALLERGY SUPPRESSION

CLA (conjugated linolenic acid, see essential fatty acids)
Forskolin

Hydrocortisone (cortisol, Cortef®)
Inhaled glucocorticoids
Licorice
• Magnesium
Mullein
~~Prednisone~~ prednisolone
Vitamin C

Cromolyn or Gastrochrome® Nasalchrom®
Leukotriene inhibitors: Accolate® Singulair®
Antihistamines: Chlor-trimeton® and its generics[1], Benadryl® and its generics, as well as Tavist® and its generics. The prescription ones are Allegra®, Claritin®, Zyrtec®, and Hismanal® doxepin

ADRENAL ISSUES

Carbamazepine
DHEA
Ginseng
Hydrocortisone, cortisol
Licorice
Pregnenolone

---

[1] brompheniramine maleate as well as chlorpheniramine maleate.

What to take for mercury poisoning

HYPOGLYCEMIA

Branched chain amino acids (leucine, isoleucine and valine)
• Chromium picolinate
Glutamine

BLOOD PRESSURE

High:
• Arginine
Beta blockers
Calcium channel blockers (flunarizine, nifedipine, nicardipine, and verapamil)
• Coenzyme Q-10
Forskolin
Garlic
• Magnesium
• Omega 3 essential fatty acids
• Vitamin C

Low:
Everything under Adrenal, plus:
Alpha agonists like: pseudoephedrine, Adrafinil, or Ordinal
Beta agonists like: ephedrine, epinephrine, or albuterol
Ginseng
Phenylalanine or Tyrosine

Warning: alpha and beta agonists can cause anxiety and induce psychotic behaviors in susceptible individuals when used in high doses.

HORMONES (ENDOCRINE SYSTEM)

Androstanediol
Androstenedione
Decadurabolin
Desiccated thyroid
Estrogens
Growth hormone
Progesterone
Testosterone
Thyroxine (T4)
Triiodothyronine (T3)
~~Yohimbe~~

INSOMNIA

All anxiolytics
Catnip
Chamomile
Inositol
Melatonin
Passion flower
Skullcap
Valerian
Vitamin B1
Vitamin B3 (both forms)
Vitamin B12

ACHINESS OR FIBROMYALGIA

Aspirin
Celebrex
Guaifenesin
• Magnesium
Omega 3 essential fatty acids
Omega 6 essential fatty acids
Phenylalanine
d,l-Phenylalanine
SAMe
Thyroid hormone as combined T3 and T4
Tyrosine

ENERGY IMPROVEMENT

• Acetyl-L-carnitine or l-carnitine
Alpha agonists like: pseudoephedrine, Adrafinil, or Ordinal
Beta agonists like: ephedrine, epinephrine, or albuterol
• "B-100"
Calcium
Conjugated linolenic acid
Forskolin
Ginseng
Octacosanol
Phenylalanine or Tyrosine

Warning: alpha and beta agonists can cause anxiety and induce psychotic behaviors in susceptible individuals when used in high doses.

Amalgam Illness: Diagnosis and Treatment

In the book *Betrayal by the Brain*:[1] Jay Goldstein, MD suggests the following list of drugs as having potential utility against chronic fatigue syndrome:

Acetazolamide, ascorbic acid, baclofen, cannabinoids, ergoloid mesylates, felbamate, gabapentin, lamotrigine, glycine, histamine-2 receptor antagonists, hydrocholorothiazide, oxytocin, pentazocine, pindolol, risperidone, spironolactone, sumatriptan, tetrahydroaminoacridine, tacrine, venlafaxine, and TRH mixed with saline for use as a nasal spray.

Dr. Goldstein finds that a given patient will respond well to one or two and have no beneficial response - or even a negative response - to the rest. He keeps trying things (these plus others) until one works, instead of deciding it is too hard to actually help people and giving them psychiatric diagnoses for which no effective treatment is known.

ANTI-MERCURY SUPPLEMENTS

~~Copper~~
~~Manganese~~
• Molybdenum
Selenomethionine
~~Selenite~~
• Zinc

[1] not clearly written enough that I recommend reading it.

HEART

For all conditions:
• Acetyl-l-carnitine or l-carnitine
• Coenzyme Q-10
• Magnesium

Angina:
• Arginine
Beta blockers
Ginkgo biloba
Nitroglycerin
Testosterone

Arrythmia:
Fish oil
Selenomethionine
Taurine
Vitamin D3 1000 IU
Vitamin E
~~Vinpocetine~~ may worsen arrythmias in some cases

~~Lipoic acid~~ is sometimes recommended for the heart. DO NOT USE IT FOR THIS PURPOSE if you are mercury toxic!!!!!!! It will move mercury all over the place and make you incredibly sick! You have to use it in a careful and controlled manner as a chelating agent at the appropriate time!

SUMMARY TABLE OF THERAPEUTIC AGENTS

Agent	Uses	Pages
5-HTP	antidepressant that works via serotonin	95, 135, 156
Acetyl-l-carnitine	improve angina, depression, memory, energy	68, 94, 102, 125, 135, 137, 143
Adrafinil (US)	improve mood and energy	137, 164
Alka seltzer gold	clears reactions and problems quickly	102, 143
Alpha agonists (Rx)	increase energy, improve mood, immune function	67, 95, 106, 109, 125, 126, 137, 143
Amphotericin B (Rx)	anti yeast drug	135, 143
Androgens	Male hormones having effects like testosterone	33, 47, 103, 108, 115, 122, 123, 128
Androstanediol	androgenic or anabolic steroid	144
Androstenedione	androgenic or anabolic steroid	92, 122, 137, 144
Antihistamines	allergy relief from runny nose, itchy eyes, etc.	107, 127, 136, 144
Antioxidants	protect the body from oxidation, promote healing, improve immune function	30, 66, 101, 109, 134, 144

What to take for mercury poisoning

Arginine	improve immune function, growth hormone levels	67, 68, 96, 98, 101, 104, 109, 123, 124, 129, 135, 136, 144
Astragalus	immune system stimulant, especially NK cells	67, 68, 136, 145
BAL (Rx)	obsolete chelating agent with extreme side effects	129, 134, 145
Benzodiazepines (Rx)	anti-anxiety drugs like valium	100, 126, 134, 145
Beta agonists	things that act like adrenaline	106, 126, 137, 145
Beta blockers (Rx)	things that oppose the action of adrenaline	46, 101, 137, 146
Bifidobacteria	"good bacteria" that help your intestines function	68, 97, 135, 146
Black Walnut Hulls	kill of intestinal parasites	105, 135, 146
Branched chain amino acids	amino acids that help your liver make blood sugar and prevent hypoglycemia, also build muscles	67, 70, 97, 103, 112, 119, 137, 146
Bromelain/papain	enzymes to digest proteins, kill intestinal parasites	135, 146
Bupropion (Rx)	antidepressant that works through dopamine	136, 147
Buspar® (Rx)	anti-anxiety drug	126, 134, 147
Calcium	important for nerve and muscle performance	105, 111, 127, 137, 147
Calcium channel blockers (Rx)	blood pressure reducing drugs that interfere with calcium movement. Side effects common	41, 137, 147
Caprylic acid	anti yeast agent	135, 147
Carbamazepine (Rx)	corrects adrenal crashes after stress, also calming	100, 118, 119, 121, 136, 147, 181
Carotenes	lipid soluble antioxidants that make vitamin A	67, 134, 147
Cat's claw	immune enhancer for viruses and inflammation	136, 147
Catnip	sopoforic	137, 147
Celebrex (Rx)	anti-pain drug that may work well for fibromyalgia	94, 108, 134, 147
Chamomile	sopoforic, anti-anxiety	137, 148
Choline	improves liver handling of fats, methyl source	67, 68, 110, 124, 126, 136, 148
Chromium	improves blood sugar metabolism	67, 101, 102, 112, 119, 137, 148
Cilantro	may remove mercury from the brain	134, 148
Citrate	mild chelator, clears "brain fog," reactions	87, 102, 134, 148
Coenzyme Q-10	improves heart, brain and immune function	67, 68, 94, 102, 134, 148
Conjugated linolenic acid	an essential fatty acid that reduces allergy globulin	107, 137, 152
Copper	an essential mineral related to mercury	30, 53, 66, 90, 96, 99, 100, 109, 113, 117, 127, 136, 138, 148, 178
Cortisol (Hydrocortisone Rx)	a hormone that controls immunity and blood sugar	47, 59, 92, 95, 96, 97, 101, 103, 104, 105, 108, 113, 115, 118, 119, 120, 121, 122, 123, 126, 136, 156
Cromolyn or Gastrochrome	allergy desensitizing materials	136, 149
Curcumin	may improve liver function, bile flow, GSH level	135, 149
Cysteine	an amino acid that may have to be limited, not a chelating agent and dangerous if used as one	51, 95, 96, 100, 108, 111, 129, 134, 149, 184
Decadurabolin (Rx)	anabolic steroid that is least masculinizing	122, 137, 149
DHEA	improves well being, immune function	59, 67, 68, 92, 108, 110, 111, 113, 118, 121, 122, 128, 136, 149, 186

Dimethylamino-ethanol (DMAE)	Improves concentration	68, 108, 110, 124, 136, 149
Dimethylglycine	Improves blood oxygenation	136, 150
~~Disulfiram~~ (Rx)	can move mercury to the brain, inhibit enzymes	150
DMPS (Rx)	Mercury chelating agent	15, 54, 55, 66, 76, 82, 83, 86, 89, 108, 117, 131, 134, 150, 180
DMSA (Rx)	Mercury and lead chelating agent	15, 54, 66, 76, 82, 83, 86, 88, 89, 108, 131, 134, 150, 179, 181
~~DMSO~~	not a chelating agent, not helpful for most things	150
Doxepin (Rx)	Tricyclic antidepressant that is an antihistamine	100, 135, 150, 164
Echinacea	Immune stimulant, especially of NK cells	68, 109, 136, 150
~~EDTA~~ (Rx)	an old intravenous chelating agent, not useful	89, 134, 151
Elderberry	extract is antiviral	68, 109, 151
Ephedrine	a natural compound similar to adrenaline	67, 95,126, 137
Epinephrine	adrenaline. The body's "get excited" chemical	40, 49, 97, 110, 119, 126, 137
Ergoloid mesylate (Rx)	a brain specific antioxidant	77, 102, 112, 124, 125, 128, 136, 151
Essential fatty acids	omega 3 and 6 fats mercury destroys that your body can't make. These fats are essential in cellular signalling, and in the proper function of cell membranes. When out of balance there are neurological and immune problems.	37, 94, 100, 101, 104, 107, 108, 129, 136, 151, 182
Estrogens and progesterone	female sex hormones	33, 47, 58, 92, 100, 122, 137, 152
Fluconazole (diflucan Rx)	an anti-yeast drug which gets into the bloodstream	41, 135, 152
Folic acid	part of methylation metabolism	67, 110, 122, 126, 127, 135, 152
Forskolin	increases the signalling molecule cAMP, reduces allergy, activates the brain and hormones	67, 68, 102, 106, 108, 109, 115, 129, 135, 136, 137, 152
FOS	feeds beneficial bacteria in the gut to fight yeast	68, 135, 153
GABA	a natural anti-anxiety agent similar to valium	67, 96, 97, 123, 124, 126, 134, 153
Garlic	a natural immune system stimulant	134, 53
Ginger	stimulate appetite, relieve nausea	67, 68, 94, 104, 108, 124, 135, 153
Ginkgo Biloba	activates the brain, relieves angina	67, 129, 136, 153
Ginseng	increases energy, adrenal function	43, 67, 109, 136, 137, 153, 195
Glucosamine	heals leaky gut	68, 104, 111, 154
Glutamine	feeds the brain, heals leaky gut	68, 95, 96, 97, 98, 102, 103, 104, 109, 112, 119, 135, 136, 137, 154
~~Glutathione~~	a body component that is not absorbed when eaten	111, 129, 135, 154
Glycine	anti-nausea, heals digestive tract, reduces tremor	97, 102, 128, 135, 155
Goldenseal	natural antibiotic	136, 155
Gotu kola	anti-anxiety, improves concentration, skin, tremor	67, 104, 106, 126, 134, 155
Grapefruit seed	the extract is antiviral and antibacterial	68, 109, 155

What to take for mercury poisoning

Growth hormone (Rx)	makes your tissues grow and heal	36, 47, 114, 123, 137, 155
Guaifenesin (Rx)	claimed to help with fibromyalgia	94, 137, 155
H2 blockers	stomach acid reducers that mess with immunity	107, 129, 136, 155
Histidine	may help emotional and allergy problems	68, 92, 95, 96, 107, 109, 125, 127, 136, 155
Ibuprofen	pain killer. Take aspirin or celebrex instead	134, 156
Immune globulin (Rx)	helps clear kidneys of immune complexes, blood of chronic virus infections	136, 156
Inositol or IP6	antidepressant, increases NK cell number	68, 109, 123, 136, 156
Iron	mineral used in blood cells and liver function	68, 99, 100, 109, 110, 136, 156, 178
Kava Kava	an anti-anxiety and sleep inducing agent	134, 157
Ketoconazole (Rx)	an anti-yeast drug that gets into the blood stream	41, 135, 157
Lamisil® (Rx)	an anti-yeast drug that is gentle on the liver and gets into the bloodstream	105, 135, 163
Leukotriene inhibitors	anti-asthma drugs that reduce allergic sensitivity	41, 106, 108, 127, 136, 157
Licorice	helps with asthma and respiratory infections	43, 67, 136, 157
Lipoic acid	chelating agent - removes mercury from the brain	66, 89, 90, 99, 117, 128, 131, 134, 157, 179
Lithium (Rx)	drug for manic depression (bipolar disorder)	58, 136, 157
Lycopene	lipid soluble antioxidant - the red color in tomatoes	158
Lysine	helps you concentrate, fights viruses	68, 96, 97, 109, 136, 158
Magnesium	helps metabolism, reduces pain and fatigue	67, 68, 92, 93, 94, 98, 99, 102, 103, 104, 106, 134, 136, 158, 177, 178
Manganese	controls tremors, blood sugar, copper levels	99, 127, 138, 158
MAO inhibitors (Rx)	antidepressants that increase adrenaline etc.	123, 125, 127, 158
Melatonin	natural sleep hormone and antioxidant	40, 70, 92, 123, 124, 137, 159, 195
Methyl donors	help with fat metabolism in liver, antidepressants	108, 110, 122, 125, 127, 135, 136, 145, 159
Metronidazole (Rx)	harsh but effective anti-parasite & anti-ameba drug	105, 135, 159
Molybdenum	mineral that helps with detox and enzymes	66, 99, 111, 117, 138, 159
Mullein	relaxes airways, slows heart, sedative	136, 159
N-acetylcysteine	NAC helps you make more glutathione	102, 111, 135, 136, 159
NADH	increases acetylcholine	136, 160
Nefazodone (Rx)	an antidepressant that works via serotonin	41, 135, 160
Neuroleptics (Rx)	anti-psychotic drugs that only control symptoms	41, 110, 127, 136, 160
Nystatin (Rx)	an anti-yeast drug that doesn't get into the blood	105, 106, 135, 160, 189
Octacosanol	increases blood oxygenation	137, 160
Ordinal (US)	helps with low blood pressure and fatigue	137, 143
Passion flower	sedative and anxiety reliever	137, 160
Phenylalanine	amino acid that makes adrenaline, dopamine, etc.	67, 70, 92, 95, 96, 97, 124, 125, 126, 135, 137, 161, 195
Phospatidyl-choline	improves liver handling of fats, methyl source, improves concentration	30, 51, 67, 68, 108, 110, 124, 126, 136, 161
Phosphatidylserine	improves memory and alleviates depression	30, 51, 67, 136, 161
Piracetam (US)	enhances memory and mental capacity	136, 161

Prednis(ol)one (Rx)	reduce immune activity, raise blood sugar, improve mood and energy	119, 121, 136, 161, 190
Pregnenolone	improves memory, mood, and adrenal function	67, 92, 113, 121, 122, 125, 128, 136, 161
Quercetin	antiviral and antitumor compound	136, 162
Schizandra	improves brain function	43, 162
Selegiline	antidepressant, improves brain function	109, 125, 128, 135, 158
Skullcap	sleep aid	137, 162
SSRI's (Rx)	antidepressants that affect serotonin metabolism	125, 135, 162
St. John's Wort	an antidepressant agent	67, 124, 125, 135, 162
Suma	immune system stimulant	136, 163
Taurine	anti-anxiety, improves liver and heart function.	51, 92, 96, 98, 102, 111, 118, 124, 126, 134, 135, 163
Tea Tree Oil	a natural but harsh anti-parasite agent	105, 106, 135, 163
Testosterone (Rx)	improves libido, tissue growth, well being	58, 92, 102, 103, 114, 115, 122, 137, 163, 186
Thyroid hormone (Rx)	treat thyroid problems. The most effective form contains both T4 and T3, e. g. desiccated thyroid. T4 alone, e. g. Synthroid is much less effective.	27, 31, 33, 46, 47, 50, 94, 95, 96, 98, 99, 113, 115, 125, 135, 137, 163
Trazadone (Rx)	an antidepressant that works through serotonin	135, 164
Tricyclic (Rx) antidepressants	antidepressants that work by inhibiting the reuptake of different neurotransmitters like norepinephrine	94, 100, 125, 135, 164
Tryptophan (Rx)	amino acid precursor to serotonin	51, 70, 92, 95, 96, 97, 108, 123, 124, 125, 126, 135, 165, 195
Tyrosine	amino acid that makes adrenaline, dopamine, etc.	67, 92, 95, 96, 97, 124, 125, 126, 135, 137, 161
Valerian	anti-anxiety and sleep aid	137, 165
Vinpocetine	improves brain function	124, 128, 136, 165
Vitamin A	stimulates immune function and controls scaly skin	100, 109, 135, 136, 165
Vitamin B1	helps some sensitive people with MCS	49, 100, 110, 123, 135, 165
Vitamin B2	prevents leaky gut and helps form blood cells	135, 166
Vitamin B3	affects liver and brain metabolism, anti-anxiety	67, 68, 100, 101, 108, 112, 123, 125, 127, 134, 135, 136, 166
Vitamin B5	helps liver, brain and adrenal metabolism	100, 127, 135, 166
Vitamin B6	anti-anxiety, helps brain function, helps PMS	67, 100, 126, 127, 134, 135, 166
Vitamin B12	helps with methylation and blood cell formation	67, 110, 123, 124, 126, 127, 135, 166
Vitamin C	protects against oxidation of proteins and DNA	67, 68, 77, 82, 83, 91, 99, 100, 104, 106, 127, 134, 166
Vitamin D	helps with calcium metabolism	66, 105, 167
Vitamin E	protects against oxidation of lipids	67, 68, 134, 167
Yarrow	heals mucus membranes	135, 167
Yohimbe	increases testosterone	137, 167
Zinc	improves mercury excretion and enzyme function	66, 67, 90, 99, 117, 127, 138, 167

Descriptions of stuff you can take (Materia medica)

Acetaminophen, Tylenol®, paracetamol - should only be taken if you are known to have adequate liver levels of glutathione, as verified by laboratory testing, and you have a good reason to avoid aspirin. Many mercury toxic people have low liver glutathione which can make even the usual therapeutic doses of acetaminophen toxic over a period of time. Acetaminophen causes oxidative stress on the liver, and your liver is already experiencing abnormal levels of oxidative stress due to mercury.

Acetaminophen is metabolized in the liver via the glutathione conjugation, sulfation and glucuronidation phase 2 pathways, and the 2E1 phase 1 enzyme.

• Acetyl-L-carnitine 1-2 grams - this helps move fats into the mitochondria where they can be burned. It helps give the body - and especially the brain and heart - more energy. It may relieve angina. It also gradually relieves depression over a period of one to three weeks. One of the things mercury messes up is the energy producing part of the metabolism that your mitochondria operate by burning sugar or fat with oxygen to make ATP. ALC makes it easier to get fat into the mitochondria and burn it. l-carnitine does about the same thing as Acetyl-l-carnitine but you have to take about twice as much for the same effect. Pick whichever one is cheaper per day - 1-2 grams of ALC or 2-4 grams of LC.

Adapin®. See tricyclic antidepressants.

Alka Seltzer Gold® - a mixture of sodium and potassium citrate in water (when dissolved) that is surprisingly effective at clearing up "brain fog" and "reactions" to environmental influences when you are having a bad time of it. Other forms of Alka Seltzer® also work but they have aspirin or tylenol in them as well.

Alpha agonists (pseudoephedrine, adrafinil) increase energy and reduce hypoglycemia, suppress histamine response, and activate neutrophils as well as increasing NK cell number. Alpha agonists also increase ACTH release[1]. They increase motivation but may also make you more argumentative and aggressive. They dry up the sinuses (their approved OTC use). They increase blood pressure.

Adrafinil - an alpha agonist which is not available in the US. Helpful for those with fatigue, as it acts directly on the brain centers that control alertness and does not affect blood pressure or heart rate much. It creates enthusiasm and optimism, ameliorating depression. After about 2 weeks you become more active. After 2-3 months your intellectual function is improved. Dosage is 300-600 mg four times per day. Higher doses should not be used. You should not use it if you have epilepsy, or liver or kidney impairment or are taking tranquilizers.

Ordinal - an alpha agonist which is not available in the US. Helpful for those with low BP and fatigue.

Caution: alpha agonists can cause anxiety and at high doses may induce psychotic behavior in susceptible individuals.

Ambion® (Rx). See zolpidem.

Amitriptyline (Rx). See tricyclic antidepressants.

Amoxapine (Rx). See tricyclic antidepressants.

---

[1] Alpha 2 blockers in theory have a similar effect do not in practice increase ACTH.

Amphotericin B - a very powerful yeast killing drug.

~~Anabuse®~~ (Rx). See ~~disulfiram~~.

Anafranil® (Rx). See tricyclic antidepressants.

Androstanediol - an over the counter supplement that is turned into testosterone by your body. It is not recommended for women unless taken with great care and appropriate testing. Neither sex should take this if they have not yet achieved their full adult height. Conversion is more efficient than with androstenedione, but it is also more expensive. See discussion under testosterone for effects.

Androstenedione 100 mg (men only) - is the immediate metabolic precursor to testosterone. It is not recommended for women unless taken with great care and appropriate testing[1]. Neither sex should take this if they have not yet achieved their full adult height. In fact, this is the major androgen naturally present in women and is made by their adrenal glands - which make a few milligrams per day. When taken by mouth androstenedione causes a substantial elevation in free testosterone - the most active form - for a couple of hours in men. Androstenedione is over the counter, cheap, and can be taken by mouth. And yes, this is the stuff Robin McGwire takes. See discussion under testosterone for effects.

Antihistamines (H1 blockers). Many of the prescription antihistamines are supposed to be nonsedating, unlike the over the counter ones, but mercury victims often find them sedating and depressive anyway. You may have to try them all to find one you can tolerate. Hismanal is not sedating but it can make you feel hyper and "nutso" you may wish to be careful with it if you have had psychiatric or behavioral problems. The over the counter antihistamines are Chlor-trimeton® and its generics, Benadryl® and its generics - by far the most sedating, as well as Tavist® and its generics. Dimetapp® is a combination product that contains an antihistamine related to Chlor-Trimeton® that some people respond better to, but it is almost always in combination products that contain other active ingredients as well. The prescription antihistamines are Allegra®, Claritin®, Zyrtec®, and Hismanal®. Also note that doxepin is an antidepressant that has strong antihistamine side effects.

Antioxidants like vitamins C, E, Se, etc. generally stimulate macrophages, natural killer (NK) cells and neutrophils. Aside from their obvious function in protecting your body against the oxidation that mercury catalyzes, they can improve your cellular immunity.

• Arginine 6 grams - this amino acid modulates the immune system to make it handle bacteria better, as well as stimulating growth hormone release (which helps keep tissues healthy despite mercury beating up on them). It can also heal up the holes in a "leaky gut." Arginine is an NO precursor and thus is helpful for heart pain (angina) that responds to nitroglycerin. Arginine can enhance the growth of herpes and other viruses. It is not recommended if there are lots of viral problems or a family history of lymphoma. In order to make the immune system handle both viruses AND bacteria, it is best to take arginine and lysine together. While your body ca make limited amounts of arginine from other things in your diet, it is actually an essential amino acid for children and during stress or illness when it promotes healing.

Asendin® (Rx). See tricyclic antidepressants.

Aspirin - is an excellent pain and fever reliever. It also reduces swelling. It reduces

---

[1] If women have androgenic hormones reach high levels in their bloodstream their body starts to develop masculine physical characteristics. Some of these changes do not reverse on discontinuing the androgen. Thus women who wish to use androgenic materials must do so with care and with constant attention to masculinizing side effects if large doses are used. 5 or 10 mg would be a 'feminine' dose of androstenedione. It is commercially available in 50 mg capsules.

Descriptions of things you can take

the blood's propensity to clot, and this blood thinning effect goes on for 2-3 weeks after the aspirin is taken. There is a lot of discussion in the US that taking a bit of aspirin every day thins the blood just enough to reduce the risk of heart attack and stroke. Many people do it. Mercury toxic people often have impaired clotting which this might make worse. Taking aspirin with omega 6 EFA supplements will reduce the formation of prostaglandins as the oils are digested and distributed systemically and thus reduce flushing, wooziness and urine volume.

Aspirin and other salicylates are metabolized in the liver via phase 2 glycine conjugation and glucuronidation.

Astragalus - stimulates cellular immunity, increasing NK cell number. It stimulates adrenal function and alleviates fatigue. It induces sweating. It should be taken only 5-7 days per month.

• B-50 and B-100. In the B vitamins there are standard products that simply have 50 or 100 mg or mcg as appropriate of all the B complex vitamins. These ensure that you get more than enough of all the B vitamins for normal metabolic needs. This way you will get all the bases covered and can focus your attention on those individual B vitamins you have a particular metabolic requirement for large amounts of. Timed release versions are desirable since these vitamins are excreted rapidly and some are poorly absorbed from a single oral dose. The best thing is to take a B-25 or B-50 several times a day. This is most economically done by cutting up a B-100 tablet rather than buying lower dose tablets. A few people with problems like MCS react oddly to enough supplements that they will need to supplement the B vitamins individually and only take the ones that agree with them. This is not very common.

BAL - an old injectable mercury and arsenic antidote. All patients experienced severe side effects from it and it may redistribute toxin to the brain. BAL is contraindicated as an injectable in all cases. BAL can also be applied as a skin cream, and it is then systemically absorbed and crosses the blood-brain barrier.

Benzodiazepines:
Diazepam/Zanax®/Klonipin® etc. are antianxiety medications and muscle relaxants. Dosages are given in the PDR and medical texts and vary with the drug. They also are believed to help correct the immune dysfunction in CFIDS to a modest extent. They reduce inhibitions and lead to more impulsive behavior, are addictive, and are metabolized by liver phase 1 enzymes though they do not induce enzyme activity. Klonipin is the least addictive of them. A typical dosing schedule involves a week or two of therapy and a drug holiday of a few days to a week to clear the system out and prevent addiction. In patients with symptoms similar to personality disorders careful consideration must be given to the tradeoff between increasing impulsive behaviors and reducing anxiety and agitation. GABA is the natural compound that is similar in action to these. These compounds are cross-tolerated with alcohol and cross-dependence can occur. If you have ever had a problem with alcohol you should be very careful with these drugs.

Benzodiazepines in large amounts may rarely induce psychotic behavior with suicidal ideation, depression, agitation, lowered inhibitions, etc. as can happen with alcohol, gamma hydroxybutyrate (GHB) and very rarely GABA.

Benzodiazepines are metabolized in the liver via phase 2 glucuronidation and phase 1 2C19 and 3A4's. Librium at least also reduces copper excretion.

Beta agonists (ephedrine, epinephrine, albuterol) are like adrenaline in making you feel excited, energetic, and resolving allergies and asthma somewhat. They also improve blood oxygenation and will sometimes ameliorate the condition where you are out of breath and have a high heart rate despite not having exerted yourself. They also increase blood pressure and heart rate.

Ephedrine - improves energy and reduces allergy symptoms. It is also anti-asthmatic and a weight loss aid. It is a beta adrenergic agonist which substantially increases the heart rate. Ephedra is discussed in more detail by Murray (1995).

Caution: beta agonists increase anxiety and may induce psychotic behaviors at high dosages.

~~Beet green~~ see ~~liver flush~~.

Beta blockers are the opposite of beta agonists. Beta blockers make you feel tired, depressed and make asthma worse. Beta blockers also relieve angina. In addition, they reduce blood pressure and slow the heart. They also reduce pooling of blood in the legs and (paradoxically, as they are used to reduce blood pressure) reduce posturally mediated hypotension. They are relaxing and reduce anxiety.

Bifidobacteria and lactobacillus acidophilus are "friendly bacteria" that live in your intestines. These are an integral part of the digestive process and help your body turn the food you eat into what your body needs. They are often lacking if you have yeast overgrowth (candidiasis) or other problems. If you don't have enough of them, you have to take mixtures of both of these in large amounts - typically 100 billion organisms daily - along with fiber, lots of water, and something like fructooligosaccarides or a bit of fruit to feed them. Typically you have to take 5-20 times as much as it states on supplement packages. Since these are cultured organisms, you do have to pay attention to what else is in with them if you have allergies. If you get enough of these growing in your intestines again they will naturally keep your yeast under control.

Black Walnut can be used to kill intestinal parasites. Despite being an over the counter nutritional supplement, it is "strong medicine" and needs to be used carefully under competent medical supervision such as that of a chiropractor or naturopath familiar with how to use it safely. Or your own if you really know what you are doing. But be careful.

Borage oil. See essential fatty acids.

Branched chain amino acids (BCAA's, leucine, isoleucine and valine) 5 g per day. These help the liver by making its metabolic job easier, and they also help support having healthy muscles despite other metabolic problems. The muscles hold on to these and send them to the liver between meals. The liver uses these to maintain a constant level of blood sugar. These are not helpful to people with adrenal insufficiency since hydrocortisone is what tells your liver to make the enzymes required to turn these into sugar, and also tells your muscles to make the enzymes required to turn the BCAA's loose. It is important to use these in the proper ratio of 1 part isoleucine to 2 parts leucine to 2 parts valine if you take more than about a gram of them a day as supplements. Bodybuilders also take these to make their muscles bigger. Whey is a source of branched chain amino acids as well as of large amounts of sulfur bearing amino acids. Whey protein powder is a common bodybuilding supplement, and also a common ingredient in bakery products in the grocery store. Whey is in milk but not cheese.

Bromelain and papain - these plant digestive enzymes are very high in sulfur and cause a 'sulfur food reaction' in susceptible individuals. Such people who also react to sulfur foods should take animal derived enzymes. They are otherwise helpful for people who have insufficient secretion of the protease pancreatic digestive enzymes. The pancreas also secretes other enzymes - lipases which digest fat and amylases which digest starch. Many people who need digestive enzymes will require animal derived products which contain all of these. Animal derived digestive enzymes usually work better anyway. Digestive enzymes reduce food allergy problems and increase the amount of nourishment available from protein foods. Protease digestive enzymes like these can be used to rid your digestive tract of chronic parasitic infections by taking them between meals. In this case only proteases are required as you are using them to digest the parasites. It is best to do this in combination with other antiparasitic therapies and to be careful how much you take since your intestines are made of protein just like the parasites are.

Descriptions of things you can take

Bupropion (Rx Wellbutrin®) is an antidepressant that works by inhibiting dopamine reuptake. Some people are depressed due to low levels of dopamine. Getting dopamine too high can cause schizophrenia like symptoms. See Goodman and Gilman for a useful summary table of antidepressants.

Buspar® (Rx) - a newer, less sedating, nonaddictive antianxiety drug that takes a while to take effect. It is usually given with one of the benzodiazepines for a month or two until the buspar starts working. Of course buspar doesn't work very well when the anxiety isn't psychological but is due to unrecognized hypoglycemia.

Calcium - 500 mg - a mineral important in nerve and muscle performance as well as in preventing bone loss. It helps you hold copper in and reduces histamine levels.

Calcium channel blockers (flunarizine, nifedipine, nicardipine, and verapamil, all Rx). Calcium channel blockers are used to control high blood pressure and heart pain (angina). Mercury and other heavy metal toxins (including methylmercury) interfere with calcium metabolism. Calcium channel blockers interfere with methylmercury toxicity in lab animal experiments under carefully controlled conditions. Many mercury poisoned people do poorly with these, but some tolerate them well. Magnesium is mother nature's calcium channel blocker and taking large amounts of magnesium often solves the problem the calcium channel blockers were prescribed for.

Caprylic acid reduces intestinal yeast. It also works on the skin.

Carbamazepine (Tegretol®) can be used to correct the "paradoxical stress response" problem where the brain doesn't tell the adrenals to make cortisol by emitting ACTH in response to physical or emotional stress. This often reduces the AVERAGE amount of cortisol secreted as well, which is also beneficial. It affects the autonomic nervous system by reducing sweating, contracting the iris, etc. It is somewhat sedating and reduces impulsiveness. It is used in psychiatry to reduce impulsive behaviors and as a treatment for manic depression. It induces phase 1 liver metabolism[1] and also reduces copper excretion. The side effects of carbamazepine are nausea, vomiting, ataxia[2] and lassitude which occur about one time in five. Slight clumsiness is usually the first sign. Carbamazepine levels are also usually measured directly by blood test as the dose gets established, and then periodically. Carbamazepine rarely induces agranulocytosis and aplastic anemia. It also reduces carnitine levels. Since carbamazepine causes the liver to metabolize it more rapidly, the dosage must be slowly increased from 200 mg per day when starting on it. Typically dosage will be increased by 200 mg per day every one to two weeks until the desired effect is achieved. When taking 1 or 2 200 mg tablets per day it is best to cut them up and take them in 3 or 4 divided doses.

Carnitine. See acetyl-l-carnitine.

• Carotenes (beta, alpha, etc.) 7.5+ mg - lipid soluble antioxidants that protect different things than vitamin E does. Beta carotene is the precursor to vitamin A, which is an immune system stimulant.

Cat's claw (una de gato) enhances the action of white blood cells. It is an anti-inflammatory. It is good for fighting viral infections. It should not be taken during pregnancy.

Catnip is a sopoforic. That means it puts you to sleep. It may help with insomnia, which means it also helps make you sleep soundly and not get up a lot at night.

Celebrex®. A new drug that inhibits a different version of the cyclooxygenase enzyme than aspirin and the other nonsteroidal antiinflammatory drugs do.

---

[1] specifically of the CYP3A4 enzyme.
[2] Lack of coordination.

Thus it inhibits the formation of prostaglandins which cause pain, fever and inflammation. It works for a surprising number of people aspirin etc. do not help. Celebrex® 1-2 capsules twice per day greatly relieves the pain associated with fibromyalgia for many people.

Chamomile is a sopoforic. That means it puts you to sleep. It may help with insomnia, which means it also helps make you sleep soundly and not get up a lot at night. In reasonably low doses it has antianxiety effects without being sedative. A sedative dose of tea is made from 1 heaping tablespoon of dried chamomile flower and is drunk shortly before bedtime. An antianxiety dose is made from 1 or 2 level teaspoons. For best effect it should be taken between meals.

Choline 1 - 2 grams - a methyl source and a precursor to the neurotransmitter acetylcholine. This helps the liver and body move fats around and lowers blood cholesterol. It also improves memory, attention and alleviates depression. It is not delivered to the brain very effectively in the choline form. Lecithin, phosphatidylcholine and DMAE are more effective at raising brain acetylcholine levels.

• Chromium picolinate helps with glucose metabolism by sensitizing the cells to insulin so less is required. Blood sugar metabolism is often deranged in mercury poisoning. Taking chromium prevents tiredness and crankiness and a need for a nap an hour or two after meals, and eliminates the need to eat frequently to keep blood sugar up. It is very effective at controlling reactive hypoglycemia. Take 200 mcg with every meal plus some extra for 1,000 mcg a day.

Cilantro - is reputed to be effective at removing mercury from the brain, but is not adequately well understood to determine an appropriate dosage or administration schedule. Current protocols were developed by people who developed protocols for other agents which were not properly optimized, so there is no reason to expect the usual cilantro protocols to be optimized either. The only reason I would suggest anyone consider cilantro is if they cannot tolerate lipoic acid despite repeated trials conducted with widely varying supplement/medication regimens and clearly need to get mercury out of their brain.

Citrate 5 grams - Chemically, citrate is a negative ion. One is needed for all that magnesium and calcium you ought to take as they are positive ions. Citrate is useful in that it reduces the risk of kidney stones and helps the body get rid of aluminum and of surplus iron. It also has a very mild chelating effect and may slightly reduce "brain fog" when it is most severe. It is the active ingredient in Alka Seltzer Gold®.

CLA. See essential fatty acids.

Clomipramine (Rx). See tricyclic antidepressants.

Clonazepam (Rx). See benzodiazepines.

• Coenzyme Q10 100-400 mg - protects the mitochondria from oxidative damage (which mercury causes) and helps them generate energy. It corrects many forms of heart disease, and also helps the brain make more energy, which improves mood and cognition. Co-Q-10 stimulates cellular immunity, and is used up at a high rate in fighting disease. It is made from dietary precursors by the healthy liver. Production may cease if the liver is poisoned, requiring supplementation. Many of the cholesterol lowering drugs (the Hmg Co A reductase inhibitors) greatly reduce co-q-10 synthesis rates and thus should not be used in mercury toxic individuals.

Coleus forskohlii. See forskolin.

Copper should not be taken by mercury toxic individuals except in small amounts if they are clearly deficient even though it is listed in many popular sources as stimulating immune function. It is desirable to take zinc and molybdenum to inhibit its absorption in most cases. You will feel best and be healthiest if your copper is towards the low end of the normal range.

Descriptions of things you can take

Conjugated linolenic acid. See essential fatty acids.

Cortisol. See hydrocortisone.

Cromolyn or Gastrochrome - antiallergy medicines that work by the unusual mechanism of stabilizing the cell membranes of mast cells so they don't dump out histamine when allergens happen by. While not generally accepted, some physicians have found that using gastrochrome (swallowable cromolyn) continuously will sometimes cause an overall downregulation of allergies that happens after 3 months or so. It is available over the counter as Nasalchrom® for nasal use, which can also be swallowed.

Curcumin - 500-2000 mg - increases biliary secretion. It may be helpful to those not secreting enough bile to get rid of their toxins who do not have an underlying cause for this such as low taurine. Use curcumin cautiously! It is also a liver antioxidant. Curcumin increases circulating levels of nonprotein sulfhydryl compounds and thus is likely not to be tolerated by individuals with high plasma cysteine or sulfur food reaction. Curcumin is discussed in more detail by Murray (1995).

~~Cysteine~~ - isn't really a chelating agent. It should never be supplemented. ~~Cysteine~~ is mentioned because some physicians who squeaked by in chemistry class many years ago don't understand biochemistry well enough to realize that this will redistribute mercury in the body rather than cause its excretion. Some mercury victims have defects in amino acid metabolism that elevate ~~cysteine~~ and they must exclude it, ~~methionine,~~ and other sulfur compounds from the diet as these things will hurt them a lot.

~~Dandelion.~~ See ~~liver flush.~~

Decadurabolin (Rx) - a synthetic androgen with a higher ratio of anabolic to androgenic effects than other available androgens. This is the preferred androgen for women to use who need to take relatively high doses.

Desipramine (Rx). See tricyclic antidepressants.

Dessicated thyroid. See thyroid hormone.

Desyrel® (Rx). See trazodone.

Diazepam. (Rx) See benzodiazepines.

DHEA 50 - 150 mg for men, 25-50 mg for women, none for children - increases serum levels of the steroid hormone dehydroepianosterone which is released by the adrenal gland and has some anabolic actions. It stimulates cellular immunity. People in their 20's usually have adequate amounts of the steroid hormones like DHEA. DHEA in particular declines with age. It is generally believed that women shouldn't take more than 30-50 mg a day of this as it has some slight androgenic action, though much higher doses have been used to treat lupus in women. It may also create an imbalance of the various steroid hormones and create unpleasant effects like breast pain in some sensitive women. DHEA and pregnenolone are also very important for proper brain function, though what they do is not well understood. Both men and women who take enough to raise their blood levels to high-normal levels for a mid 20's adult will feel MUCH better during detox.

Dimaval® (Rx). See DMPS.

Dimethylaminoethanol (DMAE) - a lipid soluble precursor of choline, which is MUCH more effective at raising brain levels of the neurotransmitter acetylcholine than are choline or phosphatidylcholine. This is helpful in correcting attention deficit such as the inability to concentrate on things, or to focus on tasks until they are done, or to shift mental gears and quickly pick up a new task when something is over. People with multiple chemical sensitivities are often overly sensitive to acetylcholine and need to use DMAE in very limited amounts. Such people may do well to take thiamine (vitamin

B-1) to reduce excessive sensitivity, and DMAE so that there is adequate acetylcholine around, but they will have to play off the proper dose of these two against each other.

Dimethylglycine (DMG) - reputed to increase oxygen utilization in athletics. DMG stimulates cellular immunity.

~~Disulfiram~~ (Rx) is used to prevent alcohol abuse. There are two reasons mercury toxic people should not take it. The first is that ~~disulfiram~~ is known to mobilize heavy metals and concentrate them in the brain. The second is that it inhibits the liver enzyme aldehyde dehydrogenase, and mercury poisoned people already have enough trouble metabolizing things without gratuitously blocking an enzyme. It is likely to already be working poorly enough due to mercury that drinking any significant amount will make you feel incredibly bad without the ~~disulfiram~~.

DMPS - chelating agent for mercury and arsenic. Currently investigational in the US. DMPS is a water soluble dimercapto chelating agent that stays outside the cells. It mops up mercury and suppresses symptoms very well. ~~Large doses~~ (e. g. 3 mg/kg ~~iv~~) have been associated with risks of liver damage, neutropenia, and other serious adverse reactions. Deaths may also have occurred. There are no statistics but best estimates are that the risk may be as high as 17% per patient undergoing monthly ~~DMPS therapy by injection~~. Lower intravenous doses appear to be safer, but not safe. ~~Intramuscular administration~~ appears to be associated with more severe side effects and a greater risk of adverse reactions. It is also painful. If yeast or fungus infection occurs or progresses during therapy, suspect neutropenia[2] . Agranulocytosis can occur[1] .When used properly by oral administration ever 8 hours DMPS is fairly safe and works very well. Proper use is described in the text. Orally administered DMPS relieves symptoms more promptly and completely than DMSA for the duration of therapy despite the fact that no more mercury is excreted. It is often tolerated by people who

do not tolerate DMSA, or has a similar side effect at a reduced level that may permit therapy. DMPS increases the excretion of mercury in the urine but not in the feces. It also increases the excretion of copper and other essential elements in the urine, but this does not significantly affect the body's balance since these are primarily excreted in the feces.

DMSA - chelating agent for lead and mercury. DMSA increases the excretion of mercury in the urine but not in the feces. It does not significantly affect excretion of essential elements. Single or repeated high oral doses are associated with adverse reactions. Doses given periodically at intervals longer than 4 hours (e. g 200 mg every other day) may produce motor and psychiatric effects. These may not be reversible. The frequency of adverse reactions on IMPROPER use is high. The frequency of adverse reactions on proper use is unknown but probably does not exceed 2%. If yeast or fungus infection occurs or progresses during therapy, suspect neutropenia[1]. Agranulocytosis can occur[2].

~~DMSO~~ may mobilize mercury and stir it around, but not a chelating agent in the proper sense and thus causes an increase in toxic damage from this mobilized mercury. Some people who are low in magnesium and not sensitive to DMSO may receive some relief from a magnesium and DMSO cream for transdermal absorption, but a LOT of it must be used.

Doxepin (Rx). See tricyclic antidepressants.

Echinacea - stimulates cellular immunity by increasing NK cell number. It also stimulates interferon production. Becoming allergic to echinacea is not uncommon. Echinacea should not be taken continuously. It should be taken for 5-7 days each month,

---

[1] a diminished number of neutrophils in the blood.
[2] low granulocytes in the blood, plus lesions of the mucus membranes and skin.

or when a viral infection is coming on. Echinacea is discussed in more detail by Murray (1995).

Ectasule® (Rx)   See beta agonists (ephedrine).

~~EDTA~~ - is an intravenous chelating agent for lead. It is not very selective and superseded for practical purposes by DMSA. ~~EDTA~~ is used by alternative physicians to treat coronary artery disease, intermittent claudication, and peripheral neuropathy with some success. It is not generally helpful for chronic fatigue and other mercury related symptom complexes. Physicians familiar with ~~EDTA~~ may not be aware that it is not the medication of choice to treat lead or mercury intoxication at present.

Effexor® (Rx). See selective serotonin reuptake inhibitors.

Elavil® (Rx).   See tricyclic antidepressants.

Elderberry - is an extract from berries of the elder bush which has antiviral activity. Elderberry jam and jelly also work fine for this purpose. They are available in grocery stores in certain parts of the United States. Take 1-2 times the dose suggested on the bottle if you get elderberry capsules. The darker and bluer the capsules are the more effective they are. Elderberry is typically taken during viral illness to suppress it, and not otherwise. It can be taken for several weeks to reduce an elevated viral load.

Ephedrine - see beta agonists.

• Ergoloid mesylate (Hydergine®) (Rx) 10 -20 mg/day taken in divided doses at least 3 times per day is a brain energy enhancer. It is also a brain specific antioxidant and there is no adequate over the counter substitute. Ergoloid mesylate increases circulation to the brain which improves mood, getting rid of lots of depressive thinking patterns. It also improves memory and cognition dramatically. About a month is required for it to take full effect. It is widely used to reverse and prevent the signs of brain aging.

Ergoloid mesylate stimulates attention, memory and intellectual activity. It may also stimulate nerve growth. It is somewhat helpful in suppressing allergy and post exercise asthma. The FDA approved dose is 3 mg. The typical dose used in Europe is 10-20 mg and is MUCH more effective, as many US physicians and patients have discovered. Many offshore pharmacies sell ergoloid mesylates by mail order to US customers for personal use at a much lower cost than it is available here. It is highly recommended for a therapeutic trial. Start with a low dose (2.5 mg/d) and slowly increase it over a period of days to prevent nausea and nasal congestion.

Eskalith® (Rx) See lithium.

Mercury accelerates the oxidative destruction of the essential fatty acids in your body. These are called "essential" because your body can't make more of them for itself - you have to eat them. You have to eat lots of EFA's now to replace all the EFA's mercury has destroyed inside of you over the years.

The essential fatty acids help with dry skin. Exceptionally dry skin is a common problem in amalgam illness - which goes away as the mercury does. Omega 6 EFA's also increase prostaglandin formation for an hour or two after they are taken in large amounts. This increases urine volume since prostaglandins interfere with antidiuretic hormone's action on the kidneys. Prostaglandins also reduce the ACTH response to hypoglycemia and stress. But these are listed here because the "dry skin" you see on the outside is like the "Dry brain" you CAN'T see on the inside. Your brain is the body organ with the most EFA's in it, and for which the EFA's are the most essential. Mercury messes up your brain by destroying the EFA's in your nerve cell walls. You have to replace those to make your nerves work right and heal up your brain.

• Flax oil 15-50 g - a source of linolenic acid - the the omega three essential fatty acid from which EPA and DHA are made. These are the part of the cell membranes which mercury accelerates the oxidation of. Your brain and nerve cells are very high in DHA.

Perilla oil - is another source of omega 3 linolenic acid. Flax oil is usually more economical.

Fish oil 2-6 g for the first month or two of supplementation - a source of EPA and DHA, other omega three fatty acids. Fish oil is known to lower risk of heart disease. It inhibits blood clotting. Your metabolism will start making EPA and DHA from supplementary flax oil after a month or two.

• Borage oil 1-4 g - a source of the omega 6 essential fatty acid gamma linoleic acid, which forms part of cell membranes, and which are also used in the production of prostaglandins that your body uses to limit and control inflammation, allergic response, etc.

Conjugated linolenic acid 2 g - helps transfer fat to the muscles where it gets burned and helps the body maintain a higher ratio of muscle to fat by building more muscles. CLA also reduces IgE while increasing levels of other immunoglobulins, and reduces the formation of certain lipid mediators of allergic reaction.

Evening primrose oil/black currant seed oil - other sources of omega 6 fatty acids, like borage oil. Borage oil is the most economical.

Menstruating women should take more omega 3 EFA's during the first half of their cycle and take more omega 6 EFA's during the second half (through the end of bleeding).

Taking aspirin with omega 6 EFA supplements will reduce the formation of prostaglandins as the oils are digested and distributed systemically and thus reduce flushing, wooziness and urine volume.

Estrogens/progesterone/etc - Many mercury toxic women have low female hormones and will be healthier and feel better if these are normalized. However, estrogens alone can be pro-inflammatory. Giving antiinflammatory progesterones allows your body to make however much estrogen it needs if the proper pathways are intact. Estrogens reduce copper excretion.

Fluconazole - Diflucan® (Rx) - a systemic yeast fighting prescription drug which keeps yeast from growing. Blocks phase 1 2C9 and 3A metabolism. Thus ketoconazole is preferable if you are also taking amitriptyline, fluoxetine or ibuprofen. Somewhat hard on the liver.

Fluoxetine (Rx). See selective serotonin reuptake inhibitors.

Fluvoxamine (Rx). See selective serotonin reuptake inhibitors.

Folate - 1.6-10 mg - is another part of methylation metabolism. Ten mg/day has been reported to alleviate depression by increasing serotonin via enhanced brain methylation. Such a dose is contraindicated in epileptics. Folate is generally safe and helpful and most people will benefit from 3 mg per day. Folic acid can also elevate histamine. Folic acid, SAMe, and any methylation metabolism enhancer may be antidepressive.

Forskolin. Coleus forskohlii extract equivalent to 80 mg forskolin - activates adenlyate cyclase thus forming the second messenger cyclic AMP throughout the body and brain as if a higher general levels of neurotransmitters and hormones were available. Mercury reduces levels of neurotransmitters and hormones as well as deactivating adenylate cyclase so this improves well being and suppresses symptoms. Forskolin may also be helpful in getting the brain to heal from the damage mercury does. cAMP is the second messenger that turns down the "allergic type" part of the immune response and turns up the other parts. It deactivates neutrophils and activates lymphocytes, but does not affect their number. Forskolin relaxes smooth muscle, such as that which causes bronchial spasms in asthma. It also increases thyroid hormone production, increases nutrient absorption in the small intestine, and stimulates lipolysis - fat burning. Forskolin generally makes you feel more together, less anxious, less volatile, etc. Forskolin does lower blood sugar which can be a problem for hypoglycemics. Forskolin antagonizes caffeine and theophylline at high concentrations (which both block the

Descriptions of things you can take

degradation of cAMP) so you may want to rely on one or the other type of stimulation. At low concentrations they appear to be synergistic. There is some brand sensitivity in how people respond to forskolin, so it is worth trying another brand if one doesn't seem to be helpful or is having side effects. Coleus forskohlii is discussed in more detail by Murray (1995).

FOS - fructooligosaccharides. This is food for the friendly bacteria in your gut. If your gut is acting up or your diet is very restricted it is a good idea to take supplements of this. Often taking several times the recommended amount is quite helpful in restoring normal gut flora and fighting yeast.

GABA 100-1000 mg - gamma amino butyric acid - is a neurotransmitter that has similar effects to valium and acts by the same mechanism. It is relaxing, anxiolytic, and sopoforic. It induces calmness and tranquility in mania, agitation, epilepsy and schizophrenia. It also increases prolactin levels. It may reduce the cortisol response to stress.

~~Gamma butyrolactone~~ is a precursor to ~~gamma hydroxybutyrate~~ that is legal in some places where ~~GHB~~ is not. It is not ~~recommended~~ as discussed below under GHB.

~~GHB~~ - ~~gamma hydroxybutyrate~~ - a natural compound similar in action to the benzodiazepines, alcohol and GABA. Duration of action is 3-6 hours and this substance is often used to induce sleep or to loosen inhibitions. There is much legal controversy about this substance and its legal status is changing rapidly from state to state. It is illegal in many places. Regardless of its actual status, the level of concern and misinformation among law enforcement authorities is high and it is best to stick with GABA or recognized prescription drugs for this reason.

Gamma oryzanol - increases cholesterol and therefore bile acids. It is useful for people who have low cholesterol for whatever reason. It also mildly encourages tissue building (anabolism). In addition it has a slight anti-anxiety effect.

Garlic - is rich in anti-oxidants. People with 'sulfur food' reactions will have trouble with it since these are sulfur antioxidants. It has some direct anti-yeast and anti-bacterial properties. It stimulates NK cells. Garlic is usually high in copper and should be restricted in people who need to reduce their copper levels a lot. Garlic is discussed in greater detail by Murray (1995).

Ginger - 1-5 grams of dried powder, or 25-75 grams of cooked root - has a variety of effects. Most well known is its anti-nausea effect, for which ginger ale is effective. Ginger can also be used to stimulate the appetite and increase food intake. It also blocks the formation of prostaglandins and leukotrienes, and is thus of value in allergy, asthma, and inflammatory conditions. It reduces pain in fibromyalgia and arthritis. It also alleviates migraines for some people. Ginger is discussed in more detail by Murray (1995).

Ginkgo Biloba - improves brain blood flow and thinking. It also activates the enzyme guanylyl cyclase which causes secretion of some hormones, and thus supports endocrine function. Ginkgo has some antidepressant effects. It is also useful in controlling heart pain (angina). It takes at least 2 weeks to achieve maximum effect. It may or may not be tolerated by any given individual. Ginkgo biloba is discussed in more detail by Murray (1995).

Ginseng - is an adrenal stimulant and general energy enhancer. It increases fat burning, increases energy, and lowers cortisol. It has estrogenic activity in women and may increase testosterone in men. People who are hypoglycemic or have high blood pressure should avoid it. It may elevate blood pressure and cause other effects in people taking MAO inhibitors. It also increases NK cell number. In addition it accelerates liver phase 1 metabolism. Ginseng should not be taken continuously. Take it for two weeks, then skip two weeks, then repeat. Ginseng is discussed in more detail by Murray (1995).

Inhaled glucocorticoids (Rx). One or two times the usual dose of a synthetic corticosteroid inhaler (up the nose) for sinus and lung allergy problems greatly relieves fatigue. Some people do not respond well to all the inhaled steroids. If one doesn't work or causes abreactions, try others. For those who don't get these on a prescription plan or who have a low annual limit on drug reimbursement, sniffing the steroid out of an inhaler is much cheaper than using nasal sprays for the same amount of steroid. These reduce the fatigue and lethargy experienced from allergen exposure quite a bit regardless of whether there is any inflammation or asthma associated with it. Symptom relief typically increases with dose up to 5 times the maximum recommended dosage. Using high doses is recommended. Adrenal suppression is very seldom observed.

Oral glucocorticoids (Rx). These can suppress the HPA axis and lead to a long term need to manage adrenal insufficiency. Excess glucocorticoids depress GH, TSH, LH and FSH release. They also increase the conversion of T4 to rT3 and decrease its conversion to T3. Glucocorticoids increase the number of beta adrenergic receptors and enhance the physiological effects of adrenaline (epinephrine - the body's natural beta agonist). The conversion of norepinephrine to epinephrine is reduced with low glucocorticoid levels and increased by high levels. High doses of glucocorticoids reduce prostaglandin synthesis and increase acetylcholine synthesis. Glucocorticoids also inhibit the enzyme that destroys cAMP and thus raise the level of this important signalling molecule inside cells. Glucocorticoids also inhibit the release of arachidonic acid from cell membranes, which greatly reduces the formation of inflammatory prostaglandins and leukotrienes. Some physicians find that allergy, fatigue, etc. can be reduced by 5 mg hydrocortisone or 1 mg prednisone or prednisolone 2-4 times a day with minimal HPA suppression. Hydrocortisone is believed to be less suppressing. "Tapers" of glucocorticoids of 5-10 days duration can be used every 2-3 months with minimal chance of HPA suppression and will greatly improve your subjective feeling of well being if you are hypoadrenal or have a paradoxical stress response. The adverse emotional effects most people experience with long term glucocorticoid therapy do not usually begin during the first two weeks. Tapers at relatively low doses (e. g. 20 mg prednisolone each day) increase immunoglobulin levels and reduce T suppressor cell numbers. Tapers at high doses (e. g. starting at 60 mg prednisolone each day) reduce immunoglobulin levels and reduce B cell number. Glucocorticoids are believed to increase neutrophil number and decrease lymphocyte number. Glucocorticoids also increase liver phase 1 metabolism.

Glucosamine 1-4 grams helps form connective tissue and mucus. It is useful for healing the gut, skin, and joints. It may assist with food and inhalant allergies if mucus secretions are thin and do not form as good a protective layer as they are supposed to. By healing the gut it may alleviate candida and food allergy problems.

Glutamine 1-4 grams helps keep the brain functioning, and is effective in suppressing "feeling crazy" (emotional problems or personality disorders) from mercury toxicity in people who are low in glutamine. It may also help heal the intestinal tract in "leaky gut" and keep bacteria and yeast from getting loose into the rest of your body. It feeds the immune system cells called macrophages and lymphocytes. It is used by the liver to make blood sugar. It is also one of the amino acids in glutathione, and those who need to boost their glutathione can best do this by taking 4 parts N-acetylcysteine to 2 parts glutamine to 1 part glycine between meals. It should not be taken by those who have elevated blood ammonia. Those with notable liver problems should ask their physician about the likelihood they have elevated blood ammonia before taking it.

Descriptions of things you can take

~~Glutathione~~ - those with demonstrated low blood glutathione and liver glutathione conjugation will raise them best with NAC. Those with elevated plasma cysteine and normal glutathione levels will find it harmful to try to elevate their ~~glutathione~~. Your digestive system should digest any ~~glutathione~~ that you take orally so that it is not absorbed undigested. If your digestive system is not doing so, you have a lot bigger problem than some ~~glutathione~~ is going to fix and you will be working on it.

Glycine - an amino acid with several functions. It will often reduce nausea (1-3 grams). It assists in healing the digestive tract (2-10 grams per day). It may also reduce tremor (2-20 grams per day). It is also one of the amino acids in glutathione, and those who need to boost their glutathione can best do this by taking 4 parts N-acetylcysteine to 2 parts glutamine to 1 part glycine between meals.

Goldenseal - is a natural antibiotic and also stimulates macrophages. In addition it causes the liver to secrete more bile. Goldenseal is discussed in more detail by Murray (1995).

Gotu kola - 60-180 mg extract - alleviates irritability and anxiety with no daytime drowsiness, sedation or blood sugar problems. It reduces tremors, and may make you feel more able to cope with life. Gotu kola increases your ability to pay attention and concentrate. It also enhances collagen formation and thus skin and joint healing, for which it is very effective. Gotu kola is discussed in more detail by Murray (1995).

Grapefruit seed extract - is an effective antiviral and antibacterial supplement. It strongly reduces liver phase 1 metabolism.

Growth hormone (Rx) - is sometimes deficient in amalgam illness. If deficient, supplementation makes you feel a LOT better. It promotes healing of tissue damage done by Hg. GH is presently quite expensive. It must be administered by injection. Administration of supplemental arginine and lysine may increase growth hormone secretion. Taking these amino acids at bedtime or before exercise is especially effective. Administration of benzodiazepines, GABA, and related compounds also stimulates growth hormone secretion for a while, though tolerance develops to this effect.

Guaifenesin (an expectorant) 300-1800 mg twice a day - may help reduce the symtpoms of fibromyalgia. Information is available from a variety of sources, especially on the web. It is prescription and sold at tablets in this strength. At lower strengths it is the active ingredient in many over the counter expectorant "XXXtussin" cough medicines.

~~Histamine H2 blockers~~ - reduce stomach acid. They also inhibit T suppressor cells and in theory should increase antibody production. They are ~~Tagamet®, Zantac®, Pepcid®~~ and ~~Axid®~~. These push the immune system in the direction of allergy, asthma and inflammation. The only real use you will have for these is if you use a steroid taper and want to take them on the high dose days to prevent gastric acid reflux.

Histidine - 0.5 to 2 grams - precursor to histamine, boosts T suppressor cell activity, helpful in rheumatoid arthritis. Histidine is needed in large amounts during stress. It increases liver phase 1 metabolism modestly. It stimulates the production of red and white blood cells. Histidine helps maintain the insulating myelin sheath around the nerves and deficiency leads to poor hearing. Some patients with low histamine (histapenia) will experience schizophrenia due to this biochemical deficit. In these patients histidine and other therapies to increase histamine can reduce or eliminate the behavioral and emotional disturbances. Since mercury is a D2 dopamine receptor activator such patients are likely to exhibit schizophrenia spectrum disorders and require supportive treatment until detoxification is complete. NB: certain "schizophrenic" patients have HIGH histamine (histadelia) and raising it exacerbates their symptoms. Some manic-depressive (bipolar) people also have elevated histamine and must avoid histidine.

Hydrocortisone or Cortef® (Rx), also called cortisol - is the natural glucocorticoid produced by the adrenal glands. It is involved in regulating blood sugar, energy, and immune response. It is antiinflammatory. It can cause increased appetite and weight gain. See the extensive discussion of its use and that of other glucocorticoids like prednisolone in the therapy section. Hydrocortisone for oral use is a prescription drug. However, it is the same stuff that is in hydrocortisone topical creams sold over the counter. Thus if you wish to take 5 mg 2-4 times per day and are unable to get this prescribed, 1/2 ml of 1% cream or 1/4 ml of 2% cream can be eaten (putting it on something or in capsules to avoid excessive exposure of the mouth). This should be done with careful thought and not randomly! However if, e. g. your old doctor used to prescribe this and it worked well but your new doctor won't give it to you, or if you have given very careful thought to the merits of self treatment this way and want to do it, or if you want to use it as a tool to get your doctor to help you instead of never doing anything by proving to him you can circumvent his control this is worth considering.

5-HTP (5 hydroxytryptophan) - the metabolic precursor to serotonin and melatonin. Unlike its precursor tryptophan, 5-HTP can easily be converted to serotonin in the body with reduced blood pressure and intestinal disturbances. It can be used with prescription decarboxylase inhibitors of the sort used with antiparkinsonism drugs (e. g. Carbidopa®), and a nutritional supplement mixture like this may be available. Those who respond to serotonin reuptake inhibitors may respond well to 5-HTP.

Ibuprofen - causes oxidative stress on the liver. It should not be taken by people who do not have verified normal levels of liver glutathione, and then not unless aspirin or other pain relievers are not appropriate. Ibuprofen will sometimes cause excessive immune activation or anaphylaxis and this occurs with reasonable frequency in mercury poisoned people. If this occurs Cytotec® (Rx) is reputed to turn off the reaction and reset the immune system, for which approximately one week of treatment is required.

Imipramine (Rx). See tricyclic antidepressants.

Intravenous immune globulin (Rx) - this is concentrated antibody and is very effective at creating a normal immune response in immune compromised chronic fatigue patients. Indeed, many of these patients have low IgG1, which is what suppresses viruses. Thus they may have chronic viral infections which IVIG will control. In order to clear the infections NK cell number and activity must be increased. Since IVIG provides a full spectrum of antibodies from healthy donors it will control chronic infections regardless of what they are - or whether they are identified. It will also often clear autoimmune diseases. Unfortunately it is expensive, often not available at all, must be used two or three times per month if maintenance is required. It is often not covered by insurance.

• Inositol or inositol hexaphosphate 2-12 grams. Inositol is an antidepressant in high doses (e. g. 12 grams per day). Both I and IP6 increase NK cell count. They help the liver move fat around and are involved in building cell membranes and in signal transfer at the membranes. They also help you sleep better. Most mercury toxic people need to lift depression, sleep better and raise the number of NK cells in their blood for at least the first 6 months.

Iron - stimulates neutrophils and macrophages. Iron deficiency slows down phase 1 metabolism. Iron deficiency leads to low energy, and is common in menstruating women. Iron excess is a common toxic condition in men. Iron catalyzes free radical production and low iron increases survival in experimentally poisoned animals. The best place for you to be is in the low end of the normal range. If you are low and have some

Descriptions of things you can take

symptoms of being low, take a bit of supplement. Otherwise avoid it.

~~Kava kava~~. take 45-70 mg kavalactones 3-4 times per day or for sedative use. Take 180-210 mg kavalactones 1 hour before retiring as a sleep aid. ~~Kava kava~~ reduces anxiety, induces muscle relaxation, and facilitates sleep. It does not act in a manner biochemically similar to GABA or benzodiazepines. People do not develop a tolerance to ~~kava~~ - it does not lose effectiveness with continuing use. Since ~~kava kava~~ is a CNS depressant and does have some side effects that are similar to common mercury poisoning symptoms[1], I recommend that you not use it unless you have used it recently and know you tolerate it, or the other medical and herbal options do not seem like they are appropriate for you. ~~Kava kava~~ is discussed in more detail by Murray (1995).

Ketoconazole - is a systemic yeast fighting drug which keeps yeast from growing. Strongly blocks liver 2C19 and 3A phase 1 metabolism. Thus fluconazole is preferable if you are taking tricyclic antidepressants or indomethacin. Ketoconazole is most toxic of the systemic agents. It is quite hard on the liver.

Klonopin® (Rx). See benzodiazepines.

Leukotriene inhibitors (Rx) - are considered antiasthma medicines. They also work against the inflammatory part of allergies. In some cases Accolate® appears to cause an overall down-regulation of allergies if taken for at least a month. When discontinued allergies may or may not remain reduced. Singulair® is the most popular but does not appear to downregulate allergies. It may however promptly relieve symptoms somewhat. These two are pretty safe and are well worth a trial in any patient with lethargy, malaise and fatigue that may be immune

---

[1] These include dry, scaly skin, a possibility of worsening depression, and accommodative and motor difficulties with the eye. It is also known to interact with other medications that cause lethargy and sedation.

mediated. Accolate® inhibits the liver phase 1 3A4 and 2C9 enzymes. Accolate®'s absorption is reduced about 30% if taken with food. Theophylline also decreases absorption about 30%. Aspirin increases absorption about 45%. Accolate® should be taken twice a day about 12 hours apart. Singulair® need only be taken once daily.

Licorice - adrenal (mineralocorticoid) stimulant. It loosens mucus and helps with asthma and upper respiratory infections. It should not be taken continuously. Licorice accellerates liver phase 1 metabolism. One week per month is appropriate. Licorice is discussed in more detail by Murray (1995).

Lipoic acid - also alpha lipoic acid - is a chelating agent able to cross cell membranes and remove mercury from the brain and internal organs. Side effects are reduced and mercury removal enhanced if it is used with a water soluble agent like DMSA or DMPS. It must be taken every 3-4 hours because your metabolism uses it up. LA is effective at removing intracellular arsenic as well as mercury. LA increases the liver's secretion of bile and nonprotein sulfhydryl groups. This is irritating to the bowel and anus, and may cause anal itching especially if hemmhoroids are present. Extra bile causes loose, dark stools. LA can exacerbate gall bladder problems or other bile duct blockages. Lipoic acid is sometimes recommended for the heart. DO NOT USE IT FOR THIS PURPOSE if you are mercury toxic!!!!!!! It will move mercury all over the place and make you incredibly sick! You have to use it in a careful and controlled manner as a chelating agent at the appropriate time!

Lithium (Rx). One of two effective drugs available for manic-depression (bipolar illness) or complications of other personality disorders characterized by euphoria alternating with depression. In these cases treating the depression alone is ineffective. Carbamazepine (Rx) is the other drug that is sometimes effective.

~~Liver flush: Dandelion~~ and ~~beet green~~ are often used in "~~liver flushes~~," as is a high intake of ~~lemon juice~~ and ~~olive oil~~. These liver flushes increase bile flow in an attempt to clear the liver of toxins. This places great stress on the liver. Healthy livers can tolerate such stress. Unhealthy livers - which almost all amalgam illness patients have - cannot. These "~~liver flushes~~" are invariably harmful for amalgam illness patients and make them very sick. Increasing bile flow with milk thistle and supplementary taurine (if appropriate, see under anxiolytics) is a safer alternative.

Ludiomil® (Rx). See tricyclic antidepressants.

Luvox® (Rx). See selective serotonin reuptake inhibitors.

Lycopene 5+ mg - is another lipid soluble antioxidant that protects against some things carotene doesn't. It is the red coloring in tomatoes.

• Lysine 2 grams - helps stimulate growth hormone release in combination with arginine. Lysine helps fight viruses by interfering with their replication and is especially effective against assorted herpesviruses (like cold sores). It also helps dissolve atherosclerotic plaques in combination with vitamin C. Mercury is believed to enhance formation of atherosclerotic plaque. Lysine also improves the mental ability to concentrate. It is low in vegetarian diets.

• Magnesium 750 mg - helps keep blood pressure down, reduces allergies and asthma, and supports antioxidant activity. No toxic effects are known, though at higher doses it is a laxative. The modern diet is often deficient in it. Fibromyalgia is often due to low magnesium. Heart problems can also be due to low magnesium. Adequate magnesium supplementation will often relieve heart pain (angina). Magnesium levels are not well reflected in serum and red blood cell magnesium tests. Its laxative effect begins at the level where you aren't absorbing any more. The aspartate and malate forms may be more easily absorbed than other salts.

~~Manganese~~ should only be taken by mercury toxic individuals in small amounts. If you are high or at the upper end of normal, you should stay away from it. ~~Manganese~~ helps control tremors and seizures, normalizes blood sugar and thyroid function, and is needed for the enzyme superoxide dismutase which protects you against one of the toxic effects of mercury. It also decreases copper levels. If you are having chronic or acute inflammation you should try taking a little to see if it helps. Use it with care since too much can cause lots of trouble, but don't be afraid to try a little now and then if the things mentioned are problems or your tests show you are low in it. Try to stick to normal "RDA" sized doses when you do try it.

Maprotiline (Rx). See tricyclic antidepressants.

The monoamine oxidase inhibitor drugs (MAOI's, Rx), phenelzine (Nardil®), tranylcypromine (Parnate®) and selegiline (Eldepryl®, Deprenyl®) alleviate depression by inhibiting the enzyme monoamine oxidase which destroys certain neurotransmitters like dopamine, norepinephrine and serotonin. Dietary restrictions are usually required when using these drugs, though they are not necessary for selegiline.

Selegiline is an effective antidepressant for some (and MAO B inhibitor) which is also an anti-parkinson's disease drug[1]. Selegiline works by elevating brain dopamine and norepinephrine levels. Selegiline does metabolize to amphetamine and methamphetamine in the body, which means anyone taking it will show up positive for them on a drug test. In theory selegiline may reduce phase 1 liver metabolism rates since amphetamines are known to do this. It does not usually do this at therapeutic doses. Selegiline may also increase cell mediated immunity. Dopamine receptors exist on mitochondria, so the effects of selegiline may be from enhanced intracellular signalling as well as intercellular signalling. Some

---

[1] Since mercury poisoning can be confused with Parkinson's disease it is probably a good choice.

people are hypersensitive to selegiline. Watch for excitation, agitation, anxiety, or other psychiatric manifestations. Selegiline may also increase testosterone modestly in men. In addition, selegiline increases levels of the antioxidant enzymes SOD and catalase in the brain. Effective antidepressant doses are often 1.25 to 2.5 mg (1/4 to 1/2 tablet) per day taken in the morning. Selegiline is used up to 10 mg per day in treating Parkinson's disease and it is reasonable to increase the dose to this level if it is improving the antidepressant action.

Some mercury toxic people find very prompt relief of depression from tranylcypromine. It is somewhat hard on the liver and the liver enzyme ALT is usually monitored by blood tests.

See Goodman and Gilman for a useful summary table of antidepressants.

Melatonin 6 mg immediate release + 3 mg timed release - Does away with sleep problems for many people! It is also an antioxidant - especially for the brain. Insomnia, inability to get to sleep at bedtime, waking in the middle of the night and being unable to go back to sleep, etc. are common mercury problems that melatonin often corrects. It does not work for everyone.

Methyl donors and compounds involved in methylation metabolism help the liver transport fats, help with one part of phase 2 metabolism, and have other effects in the body - most notably antidepressant effects through increased brain serotonin. They also reduce elevated estrogen levels in women, which cause inflammation and other imbalances. Methylation both increases and controls histamine levels. Your body cannot make methyl groups - it needs to get them from your diet. SAMe, choline, TMG, folate and B-12 all have similar effects via methyl metabolism, and lecithin, phosphatidylcholine and phosphatidylscrine can sometimes also act as methyl donors in the brain.

Methionine - the M in SAMe. Not recommended since it makes homocysteine and then cysteine after it gives up its methyl group. Elevated homocysteine causes atheroschlerosis. You can get methyl groups from other sources, you get adequate methionine from most diets, and if you really need it you can take SAMe directly. Methionine is no more a mercury chelating agent than is cysteine and can be very harmful if used as one.

MSM - may or may not mobilize mercury. There are some reports of adverse reactions to it indicating that it does so in some people. It is not a chelating agent in the proper sense and thus causes an increase in toxic damage from this mobilized mercury without helping get it out of the body.

Metronidazole (Rx) - Flagyl® - kills giardia, amebas, and certain other pathological organisms. Metronidazole may not cure long standing chronic infections if not used repeatedly. It strongly blocks phase 1 metabolism.

• Milk thistle extract - equivalent to 250-750 mg silymarin - is a very effective antioxidant specific for the liver. It also increases bile flow somewhat. It increases the growth of new liver cells and thus allows the liver to regenerate itself more rapidly. It inhibits the formation of leukotrienes, which are pro-inflammatory immune mediators produced from essential fatty acids. Milk Thistle is discussed in more detail by Murray (1995).

• Molybdenum - 1,000 mcg - the cofactor for three enzymes[1] often impaired in mercury intoxication. It may or may not improve their function. It inhibits copper absorption from the intestine. It also counteracts some effects mercury may have on gene expression.

Mullein - helps relax the airways, slows the heart rate, and has a mild sedative effect. It is helpful for asthma or sinus problems.

NAC (N-acetylcysteine) - 500-4000 mg - for those mercury victims who have low

---

[1] Sulfite oxidase, aldehyde oxidase, and xanthine oxidase.

blood glutathione or low glutathione conjugation in the liver, NAC may be helpful. Low liver glutathione conjugation (a phase 2 reaction) can best be corrected with supplementary NAC. It is much more likely to be helpful than glutathione itself or cysteine. People who are sensitive to paint fumes, exhaust, the preservatives BHT, BHA and TBHQ, and other hydrocarbons often benefit from NAC.

NADH - a form of B3 associated with enhanced acetylcholine metabolism.

Nardil® (Rx). See monoamine oxidase inhibitors.

~~Neuroleptics~~. Mercury is a D2 dopamine receptor stimulant. Many of the mental symptoms of mercury poisoning are similar to the symptoms of schizophrenia spectrum disorders such as borderline personality disorder. For patients who are troubled by these symptoms, or who do not have adequate social control and are having difficulties because of these conditions, low doses of neuroleptics may be beneficial (e. g. as is found in borderline personality disorder). Doses can be kept low enough that the risk of undesirable side effects like tardive dyskenesia are somewhat reduced. Care must be taken to try agents until one is found the patient tolerates well since mercury toxic individuals tend to have idiosyncratic reactions to a number of drugs. Long term therapy with these agents is highly undesirable. They should be used to control symptoms when necessary, but the underlying problem should be solved and neuroleptics should not be used as a crutch to put that off.

Caution: don't let anything I say inhibit you from using neuroleptics - even in high doses - to control acute psychotic conditions or prevent predictable relapses. But ignore incorrect information from physicians who may tell you that neuroleptics are the cure and detox does nothing. Detox is the cure, neuroleptics are just a comfortable modern straightjacket.

Nefazodone (Rx Serzone®) - an antidepressant that works via serotonin. It inhibits the liver phase 1 3A enzymes.

Nitroglycerin (Rx) - often prescribed for heart pain (angina) which many mercury toxic people get. It releases NO and reduces the heart pain. This also causes a headache and can cause or worsen a migraine for about the next 2 hours. It can also cause tunnel vision so driving may not be safe. Arginine may be a milder way to keep some NO around and reduce angina.

Norpramin® (Rx). See tricyclic antidepressants.

Nortriptyline (Rx). See tricyclic antidepressants.

Nystatin - a yeast killing drug that does not get absorbed. It will kill yeast in the mouth, esophagus, and gut, as well as on the skin. Since it kills yeast directly rather than inhibiting their growth it can result in a worsening of symptoms when the yeast die and release the toxins inside them.

Octacosanol increases muscle oxygen use and muscle glycogen.

Ordinal (US). See alpha agonists.

Oxazepam® (Rx). See benzodiazepines.

Pamelor® (Rx). See tricyclic antidepressants.

Paracetamol. See acetaminophen.

Parnate® (Rx). See monoamine oxidase inhibitors.

Paroxetine (Rx). See selective serotonin reuptake inhibitors.

Passion flower - is a sedative and relieves anxiety. One cup of tea made by steeping a teaspoon of dried leaves for 15 minutes is taken 3 times a day. To induce sleep, stronger tea is taken near bedtime. Passion flower should not be used by pregnant women since it induces uterine contractions.

Descriptions of things you can take

Paxil® (Rx). See selective serotonin reuptake inhibitors.

~~Penicillamine~~ (Rx) - trade name ~~Cuprimine®~~ - is not really a chelating agent in the chemical sense. It is a prescription drug for heavy metal poisoning. It also has other off label uses[1]. All patients who take it experience unpleasant side effects. Penicillamine is contraindicated for mercury poisoning victims in all cases due to its propensity to redistribute mercury rather than cause excretion. Adverse drug reactions are common.

Pertofrane® (Rx). See tricyclic antidepressants.

Phenelzine (Rx). See monoamine oxidase inhibitors.

Phenylalanine and tyrosine are the amino acid precursors to dopamine, epinephrine and norepinephrine. In the body phenylalanine is converted to tyrosine and that in turn makes the neurotransmitters. These amino acids have a similar effect to pseudoephedrine. They can be antidepressive in people who are low in them. You can take one or the other. Two grams of phenylalanine is equivalent to about one gram of tyrosine. They decrease liver phase 1 metabolism. Those who respond well to monoamine oxidase inhibitors may respond well to these.

Phosphatidylcholine (concentrated lecithin) 5 grams - helps the liver move fats around, controls blood cholesterol, is used to make cell membranes which is the part of the body mercury beats up on the most, and is used to make the neurotransmitter acetylcholine in the brain. This is useful for people with things like Alzheimer's disease which do bear some biochemical similarity to mercury poisoning.

---

[1] For example, it often ameliorates rheumatoid arthritis. This might make RA sufferers consider more effective protocols for heavy metal detoxification, such as those in this book, as potential treatments.

Phosphatidylserine 300 mg - helps make better brain cell membranes. It is a good antidepressant and brain tonic - much more effective than phosphatidylcholine and lecithin. Unfortunately phospatidylserine is also much more expensive.

Piracetam (US) is synergistic with phosphatidylcholine and lecithin in enhancing memory and mental capacity for some.

Prednisone and prednisolone - these glucocorticoids may be used in "tapers" to suppress immune effects like allergy or inflammation. If used too often they suppress the body's ability to respond to stress with its own glucocorticoid (cortisol) which can be life threatening under some circumstances. They can also be used routinely by patients with frank adrenal insufficiency, though if the adrenal insufficiency is later cured it takes a couple of years to get the patient weaned of these. They can also be used in doses of 1-3 mg/day to support underactive adrenals as are common in amalgam illness. Indications for this would be excessive immune activation along with hypoglycemia. Glucocorticoids reduce NK cell numbers and should not be used in patients with low NK counts or in patients with impaired ability to fight off viral infections in the absence of an NK cell count. Five day tapers every 2 months are believed to be safe and to enhance energy in chronic fatigue and amalgam illness patients in most cases. Prednisone is inactive and is converted to the active form, prednisolone, by the liver. Prednisolone should be used since it is equally inexpensive and mercury toxic people often have uncharacterized problems with their liver metabolism.

Pregnenolone 100 mg (women) or 300 mg (men) - is the metabolic precursor to DHEA. It can also be converted to progesterone and cortisol, which DHEA can't. Taking pregnenolone makes it easier for your body to make the hormones it needs. Pregnenolone helps the brain work better. Depressed people have lower cerebrospinal fluid pregnenolone than nondepressed people. Taking pregnenolone may improve depression. It may also improve memory and concentration.

Intravenous procaine (not a mainstream thing to do except for certain heart conditions) reset the limbic system and are often quite effective in reducing chronic fatigue and fibromyalgia symptoms for several days to weeks. These can also be self-administered intramuscularly by very daring patients who have doctors who are very daring about what they are willing to prescribe, though very large doses are needed.

Protriptyline (Rx). See tricyclic antidepressants.

Prozac® (Rx). See selective serotonin reuptake inhibitors.

Quercetin is a citrus bioflavinoid which has antiviral and antitumor activity.

SAMe - S-adenosyl methionine - 100-600mg - is the ultimate methyl donor in the sense that it actually is the compound that your body uses to transfer methyl groups. It can be taken orally and a reasonable amount of it makes it into your body and gets where it is needed. For people who are not having any luck with other methyl donors and transfer agents it is worth a try. Methyl donors or transfer agents may well work better for certain people than SAMe depending on where their metabolic problem is and where in the body the methyl groups are needed.

Schizandra enhances cognition and accelerates phase 1 liver metabolism.

Selective Serotonin Reuptake Inhibitors (SSRI's Rx) are fluoxetine (Prozac®), fluvoxamine (Luvox®), paroxetine (Paxil®), sertraline (Zoloft®), and venlafaxine (Effexor®). If you respond to 5-HTP or tryptophan you should respond to these. They are not effective for a lot of mercury toxic people because depression is often due to something other than low serotonin. They also may not be tolerated, so start at a quarter or half the usual dose. These medications also slow down liver phase 1 metabolism. Prozac®, Paxil® and Zoloft® reduce anxiety. Nefazodone and trazodone also affect serotonin though in a different way than the SSRI's do. See Goodman and Gilman for a useful summary table of antidepressants.

Fluoxetine, fluvoxamine, paroxetine and sertraline are both metabolized by and slow down various liver phase 1 enzymes. Care should be taken in using the SSRI's if your liver metabolism is abnormal.

Selegiline (Rx). See MAOI's.

Selenite - a form of selenium that is similar to sulfite. A lot of people respond poorly to this but do well with selenomethionine.

Selenomethionine 50-300 mcg. Aside from being a good all around antioxidant, selenium compounds bind mercury quite tightly and make it inert in the body. Selenomethionine is also an essential part of some enzymes, so having a bunch of mercury running around will reduce the amount available for these essential functions. Some people find it helps with asthma. Selenium can have side-effect like heart arrythmias, insomnia and irritability. Selenium is potentially toxic at doses not far from those used in supplementation. For many people selenium is something they have to experiment with and customize. A few may choose to omit it due to toxicity concerns.

Serax® (Rx). See benzodiazepines.

Sertraline (Rx). See selective serotonin reuptake inhibitors.

Serzone® (Rx). See Nefazodone.

Silymarin. See milk thistle.

Sinequan® (Rx). See tricyclic antidepressants.

Skullcap is sopoforic. It may help with insomnia.

Descriptions of things you can take

St. John's Wort (containing hypericin) - is an Antidepressant which is believed to be a natural MAO inhibitor. It is also known to inactivate retroviruses in vitro. Becoming allergic to it is fairly common. St. John's Wort is discussed in more detail by Murray (1995).

Suma is an immune system stimulant.

Surmontil® (Rx).   See tricyclic antidepressants.

Taurine 500-3000 mg - helps you think clearly by reducing anxiety. Taurine is often used as an anxiolytic. It also suppresses seizure like activity. It helps form bile salts, reducing cholesterol and possibly increasing the rate of toxin elimination in bile. The taurine formed bile salts also make cholesterol more soluble which protects against gallstones.   It assists with kidney function.   It is necessary for brain development during childhood, and possibly for neurohealing later. Zinc helps cells - especially in the brain - absorb taurine. It occasionally helps with depression, and may help with some forms of epilepsy. It also improves pituitary function. Taurine also helps control heart arrythmias and hypertension by holding calcium and potassium in.   Estradiol (a female sex hormone) reduces the liver's ability to produce taurine so women are more likely to need to supplement it.   Stress elevates women's estrogen levels and thus reduces taurine availability. Taurine can stimulate the release of extra stomach acid. It may also help improve compromise immune function. Taurine should only be supplemented if needed - some mercury victims have defective amino acid metabolism that elevates taurine in which case supplementation might be harmful.   Others have defective metabolism that doesn't make taurine and supplementation is essential.   Taurine stimulates insulin production and lowers blood sugar which can be a problem for hypoglycemics.

Tea Tree Oil can be used to kill intestinal parasites. It is "strong medicine" and needs to be used carefully under appropriate supervision (ND, chiropractor, or by yourself if you really know what you are doing). Tea tree oil is discussed in more detail by Murray (1995).

Terbinafine (Rx) - Lamisil® - A systemic yeast fighting prescription drug which keeps yeast from growing. The least toxic of the yeast fighting agents. Has no negative effect on the liver.

Testosterone (Rx) - The major physiological anabolic steroid and androgen. Men who are low may benefit from replacement therapy. Testosterone cyprionate or enanthate given by injection are easier on the liver (a target organ for mercury poisoning) than are oral preparations or the longer acting alkylated preparations. Testosterone controls heart pain (angina) in about half of cases in men when it is restored to young male levels. There are transdermal patches, though most people eventually develop allergies to them. Compounding pharmacies can make creams and gels which are absorbed through the skin and which are less expensive than the patches - and also less likely to cause allergic sensitization. Transdermal delivery may result in excessive levels of dihydrotestosterone - which makes the skin oily, accelerates male pattern baldness, and causes prostate problems. This can be controlled by taking saw palmetto extract.

Testosterone is a schedule 3 controlled substance[1] and are only available by prescription. Attempting to import it without a US doctor's prescription can cause serious legal difficulties.

Thyroid hormone:
~~Thyroxine alone~~ should never be used to treat any thyroid condition. It should always be combined with triiodothyronine in a natural or synthetic product.

Thyroid hormone - is well known that some depressed patients who do not respond to other treatments and who have perfectly normal blood test results for thyroid

---

[1] Subject to strict record keeping and tracing requirements by the DEA.

hormones can have their depression lifted by receiving thyroid supplement, most often in the form of T3[1]. Some of them require rather large doses, especially if T4[2] is used, though some have their depression relieved by doses that leave their blood test results in the normal range.

Thyroxine (T4) 50-200 mcg and triiodothyronine (T3) 15-50 mcg - correct the body and brain symptoms of hypothyroidism. Some T3 is required to really do this - taking all T4 doesn't feel the same and is not as effective. Natural forms of thyroid contain T3 an T4 in a ratio of about 1:4. If the synthetics are used, a timed release version of T3 is often employed. Some patients benefit from having "Wilson's Syndrome" treated by raising and lowering dosages of timed release T3 to encourage the liver to increase its conversion rate for T4 to T3. Some don't.

Dessicated thyroid 1-5 grains per day. This is the natural form of T3 + T4 - desiccated animal thyroid. Most physicians familiar with the use of thyroid hormone in mercury toxic people or environmental illness use desiccated thyroid rather than the synthetics. In their clinical experience patients do better on it.

Tofranil® (Rx). See tricyclic antidepressants.

Tranylcypromine (Rx). See monoamine oxidase inhibitors.

Trazodone (Rx, Desyrel®) is an antidepressant that often reduces anxiety. It also helps with insomnia in low doses. It works through serotonin. See Goodman and Gilman for a useful summary table of antidepressants.

Tricyclic antidepressants (Rx) - these work by inhibiting the reuptake of norepinephrine (noradrenaline). They are likely to be effective for mercury toxic people in general, whether or not they respond to the SSRI's. Tricyclics generally have a broader spectrum of side effects than SSRI's, but less than MAOI's. The tricyclics may be synergistic with selective serotonin reuptake inhibitors.

The tertiary amine tricyclics, amitryptyline (Elavil®), clomipramine (Anafranil®), doxepin (Adapin®, Sinequan®), imipramine (Tofranil®) and trimipramine (Surmontil®) all uniformly are very sedating, very drying to the mucous membranes, reduce blood pressure a lot and have other side effects.

Amitriptyline in low doses helps reduce insomnia. It can produce posturally mediated hypotension as well as reduce potassium levels. Amitriptyline has been known to cause visual hallucinations in mercury toxic individuals, highlighting their propensity to have unexpected adverse drug reactions.

Doxepin is a tricyclic antidepressant which has strong antihistamine action as a side effect. It also has strong anticholinergic actions, which are troubling for many people - particularly for those with attention deficit. It may be helpful for those who don't tolerate other antihistamines because of their depressive side effects. Doxepin is known to be helpful to some sulfite sensitive asthmatics. In low doses it stimulates cellular immunity. It may sometimes reduce the pain associated with fibromyalgia. Mercury toxic people may only be able to tolerate it in low doses (10 mg).

The secondary amine tricyclics, amoxapine (Asendin®), desipramine (Norpramin®, Pertofrane®), maprotiline (Ludiomil®), nortriptyline (Pamelor®) and protriptyline (Vivactil®) have lesser and more diverse side effects.

Desipramine is an antidepressant that may also be helpful for fibromyalgia pain without insomnia.

Nortriptyline is an antidepressant that may be helpful for fibromyalgia pain.

See Goodman and Gilman for a useful summary table of antidepressants.

Many of the tricyclic antidepressants are metabolized by the liver phase 1 2D6 enzyme.

Trimethylglycine (TMG) - 1.5-3 g - is another methyl source that is NOT a

---

[1] the proper chemical name for T3 is triiodothyronine.

[2] the proper chemical name for T4 is thyroxine.

Descriptions of things you can take

precursor to acetylcholine. Effects are similar to choline.

Trimipramine (Rx). See tricyclic antidepressants.

Tryptophan - is the metabolic precursor to serotonin. It is more effective at making serotonin in the brain versus body than 5HTP. It was banned by the FDA in 1989, but it is now available by prescription. Many foods are good sources of tryptophan. Tryptophan helps with some migraines. In addition to being antidepressive, it induces satiety, is analgesic, calms restless legs, aids digestion, and is immunostimulatory - but thus may worsen asthma or autoimmune disease. It is also useful for Parkinson's disease patients who are taking levodopa. The l-tryptophan sold by veterinary sources is not legally permitted to be used by humans under FDA regulations.

Tylenol®. See acetaminophen.

Tyrosine. See phenylalanine.

Una de Gato. See cat's claw.

Valerian - is sopoforic. It may help with insomnia if 300-400 mg of standardized extract are taken at bedtime. It can also be used to control anxiety if 200 mg are taken in the morning. In antianxiety doses valerian does not interfere with alertness. Discussed in more detail by Murray (1995).

Valium® (Rx). See benzodiazepines.

Venlafaxine (Rx). See selective serotonin reuptake inhibitors.

Vinpocetine - an extract of periwinkle - 15 mg/d - is used to improve memory and cognitive function and increase brain function and blood flow. It raises cyclic GMP by inhibiting the enzyme which degrades that. Vinpocetine is known to prevent and reverse neurological damage caused by aging, and to assist in healing some closed skull brain injuries. It makes you more aware, alert, able to concentrate, and brightens you emotionally. It increases turnover of the neurotransmitters serotonin and noradrenaline. It also helps alleviate phenomena like hot flashes that occur during menopause. Migraines are due to excessive blood flow caused by increased blood flow to the front part of the brain caused by extra cGMP so vinpocetine may aggravate them. Typical dosage is 5 mg three times per day. Substantially impaired patients often experience greater relief if started on 10 mg three times per day for 30 days and then switch over to 5 mg three times per day. Vinpocetine can have some heart side effects such as arrythmias. People who have all three of the following symptoms may have too much cGMP and should avoid vinpocetine or take it gingerly: migraines, changes in color perception, easy engorgement of the genital tissues.

Vitamin A - most people make this from beta carotene in their livers. Vitamin A increases nonspecific immunity, increases the number of T helper (CD4+) and natural killer (NK) cells, increases maturation of B cells, increases the rate at which phagocytes eat bacteria cells, and increases secretory IgA. Those with low sIgA may wish to supplement with vitamin A itself rather than or in addition to beta carotene on the assumption that mercury is interfering with liver production of the active vitamin. Vitamin A increases the size of the thymus gland - an important part of the immune system. Vitamin A also helps with skin conditions like psoriasis, hyperkeratosis, or others due to excessive proliferation of skin cells. People with low thyroid also do not adequately convert beta carotene to vitamin A. During pregnancy or when trying to become pregnant, vitamin A supplements should be kept below 10,000 IU per day. Otherwise a reasonable maintenance dose is 20,000 IU per day. 50,000 IU per day can be taken for up to a month during infections. 100,000 IU may be taken for the first 3 days of an infection if a 20,000 IU maintenance dose has been the maximum used over the last month.

Vitamin B1 - 100-500 mg - helps the liver metabolize xenobiotics. It may also be calming and helps stimulate the appetite. Blocks the M1 acetylcholine receptor and allows people with MCS or who are very sensitive to choline precursors like DMAE to use more of them. Necessary with B2 for proper function of insulin and thyroid hormone.

Vitamin B2 (Riboflavin) - 50-100 mg - absorbed better if taken in divided doses. Riboflavin has many functions, including preventing leaky gut and fostering formation of red blood cells. Necessary with B1 for proper function of insulin and thyroid hormone. Riboflavin accelerates phase 1 metabolism.

There are two related forms of vitamin B-3. Niacin and niacinamide. They have many similar and a few different functions. Those functions important for treating mercury poisoning will be described here.
Niacin speeds up phase 1 metabolism.
Niacinamide slows down phase 1 metabolism.
Niacinamide 1-3 grams - may relieve anxiety in people who get it from hydrocarbons like exhaust fumes. It may do this by slowing down fast phase 1 metabolism.
Niacinamide 1-3 grams per day is also antidepressive.
Niacin increases brain circulation. Niacinamide does not.
Niacinamide has been shown to reduce autoimmune diabetes and would be expected to stop other autoimmune problems from developing. It has been shown to help in rheumatoid arthritis. It may also be helpful with allergies.
Timed release niacin is very hard on the liver and should not be used.
Immediate release niacin causes histamine release with consequent flushing and itching. This can be helpful for certain patients with schizophrenia spectrum disorders caused by low histamine. The rate of dissolution and absorption of the niacin can be quite brand specific. The most rapid absorption possible is desired, and can be determined by how quickly you flush in response to it.
Niacin also lowers copper levels.

Vitamin B5 - also called pantothenic acid or pantothenate - 1-3 grams - Helps with the liver, and also helps the brain make acetylcholine. Suppresses rheumatoid arthritis and supports adrenal function.

• Vitamin B6 - 50-100 mg several times per day - mercury appears to cause chronic fatigue by interfering with brain uptake of B6 and B12. B6 may reduce anxiety. B6 also helps the liver do its work. It stimulates antibody response. In women it lowers estrogen and increases progesterone. It often helps with PMS, especially if taken with a lot of magnesium. B-6 works best if taken several times per day in doses of 50-100 mg. A few people get tingling or pain in their hands and feet (peripheral neuropathy) if they take more than 500 mg/day. People who have great difficulty metabolizing aldehydes (such as those who turn beet red from alcohol) may not tolerate B-6 because it is an aldehyde. They flush, feel "drunk," and get sick from it.

Vitamin B 12 - 1-12 mg (not mcg) - lack of adequate B-12 is a big cause of deranged brain metabolism. It is involved in all kinds of methylation reactions. The body has an active transport mechanism in the gut, so if you need to get more into you than that transport mechanism wants to move it has to be done either by taking extremely large quantities (12 mg is 2,000 times the recommended daily allowance) or through a needle. Yeast, parasites, low thyroid levels and adrenal insufficiency all reduce B-12 absorption. In addition a lot of mercury toxic people get allergic to the transport protein so they can't even get normal amounts of B-12 if they don't take high doses of it as a supplement. 1.2% of goes down your throat ends up in your blood. Thus swallowing 83 1 mg tablets is the same as getting a 1 mg injection. Sublingual tablets probably do better than this. People's need for vitamin B-12 is highly individual, but people with fibromyalgia or chronic fatigue need more than most. If B-12 seems to help, try taking more and more until things stop getting better to find out how much you need.

Descriptions of things you can take

• Vitamin C: 4-12 grams - The general purpose do everything antioxidant vitamin. It supports adrenal function, lowers blood histamine[1], and has many other functions. A buffered form is preferred. Taking it in the acid form is more than most people's digestive systems can handle. As the dose is increased absorption becomes less efficient. Taking it several times per day leads to better absorption. Economics may dictate dosages in the lower range.

Vitamin D3. This vitamin helps your body use calcium properly. It can reduce heart arrythmias by helping the heart control calcium levels which are used in the clock whose ticks cause your heart to beat.

• Vitamin E 1000+ IU - is a general purpose lipid soluble antioxidant which is not toxic. It is useful in large amounts to counteract the damage mercury causes by catalyzing oxidation of cell membranes. Vitamin E has been shown to be protective in brain diseases such as Parkinson's that are believed to be caused by oxidative stress[2]. It can also indirectly inhibit arachidonic acid release from cell membranes by interfering with lipid peroxidation, which relieves allergies. It is also an immune system stimulant, and if you aren't getting enough[3] your immune response to infection will be poor. Vitamin E protects LDL cholesterol from being oxidized and forming arterioschlerotic plaques, and it protects all the essential fatty acids in your cell membranes from being destroyed by oxidation too.

Vivactil® (Rx). See tricyclic antidepressants.

Wellbutrin® (Rx). See bupropion.

Whey. See branched chain amino acids.

Yarrow - has a healing effect on mucous membranes. It is useful for ulcerative colitis, irritable bowel, leaky gut, etc. It reduces inflammation, improves blood clotting (and controls excessive menstrual bleeding), and increases sweating.

~~Yohimbe~~ - an alpha 2 antagonist (thus having a similar effect to regular alpha agonists) which raises blood pressure, and is reputed to elevate testosterone and facilitate erections in males - its major OTC use. It apparently does not correct hypoglycemia. Generally advised not to be used in women. ~~Yohimbe~~ is discussed in more detail by Murray (1995) who points out that it has a high rate of adverse reactions and does not usually recommend its use.

• Zinc 50-100 mg - generally competitive with mercury and copper, so taking it keeps mercury from exerting some of its toxic effects. It inhibits copper and manganese absorption from the intestines. It stimulates cellular and humoral immunity. Zinc is a mitogen[4]. It directly inhibits cold viruses. It should be taken at 100 mg per day to start, then reduced to 50 mg per day once you begin using lipoic acid as a chelating agent[5].

Zoloft® (Rx). See selective serotonin reuptake inhibitors.

Zolpidem (Ambion® Rx) is a hypnotic which is a good sleep aid. It is not a benzodiazepine type drug but acts similarly, is taken near bedtime and wears off by the morning, and is sedating, relieves anxiety, relaxes muscles and is anticonvulsant. It is generally used for a week at a time with a break of a few days. It works by stimulating the same receptor that GABA does, the GABAa receptor.

---

[1] people who do not wish to lower their blood histamine, such as those with schizophrenia like symptoms from low histamine, should take no more than 500mg to 1 gram 2-3 times per day.

[2] Mercury poisoning places oxidative stress on the brain.

[3] Megadoses aren't required, but it takes a lot more than the RDA. The exact amount is not known but 400 IU per day is certainly more than enough even for mercury toxic people.

[4] It makes more of the immune system cells called lymphocytes grow.

[5] Don't increase it back up when you are taking breaks from LA.

Appendix

Useful books

Physician's Desk Reference, 53rd edition is 1999. This is a book published every year that contains a couple of pages of information about prescription drugs describing their FDA approved uses (seldom what you want them for), mechanism of action, cautions, etc. It primarily has information on newer, more expensive drugs. The PDR is easy to find. Most libraries and some individuals have it. Some information can be found online at www.pdr.net.

Martindale's Extrapharmacopoeia, Published every 3 years. It contains more abbreviated information than the PDR, but better coverage on what the drugs are actually used for. It covers all drugs used anywhere in the world. Better academic libraries have this.

Drug Facts and Comparisons, updated monthly. Most pharmacies have this and will copy a few pages for a customer. Will usually let you read about a drug or two at the consultation window if they aren't too busy. Some libraries also have it. It contains information on all prescription drugs and related medical materials used in the US. It also lists and discusses 'off label' use[1], which is to say uses doctors often put drugs to other than the ones the FDA approved.

Mosby's 1999 Medical Drug Reference, edited by Allan J. Ellsworth and others. Mosby publishing, St. Louis. Available at many larger or academic libraries. It contains information on many prescription drugs (including older ones), plus how to figure out things like "body surface area," "creatinine clearance," "body mass index," etc. which are referred to in the drug information section and in medical texts. Gives both on and 'off label' uses[1] of the drugs.

Harrison's Principles of Internal Medicine, edited by Anthony S. Fauci and others. Fourteenth edition is 1998. McGraw-Hill, New York. ISBN 0-07-020292-3. This is a thorough, comprehensive textbook of how the body works, what can go wrong with it (the politically correct stuff), and how to diagnose that by ordering tests and examining the patient, plus how to treat it by prescribing medicines. If you can figure out what part of your body is messed up by mercury, you can learn a lot about the conventional handling of things that can go wrong with that body part from Harrison's. It is invaluable in figuring out the standard allopathic approach to helping you by ameliorating symptoms, and at giving you a good idea of what ELSE to look at once you know one thing is not right. Some of the sections have very good, clear descriptions of symptoms from which you can get a good idea of whether you have to worry about something or not.

Tietz Textbook of Clinical Chemistry, edited by Carl A. Burtis and Edward R. Ashwood. Third edition is 1999. W. B. Saunders, Philadelphia. ISBN 0-7216-5610-2. A comprehensive description of clinical laboratory tests and and their uses. The discussion of use is somewhat oversimplified, typically covering the major cause of a given condition and omitting the less frequent causes. It is an excellent guide to the physiology these tests explore. It has a very good appendix containing test normal ranges.

Cecil Textbook of Medicine, edited by J. Claude Bennett and Fred Plum. Twentieth edition 1996. W. B. Saunders, Philadelphia. ISBN 0-7216-3573-3. Similar to Harrison's, though perhaps requiring

---

[1] Off label use is perfectly legal and legitimate. Most drugs prescribed are actually for off label use. However, the drug companies themselves can't advertise these uses or provide much information about them.

Appendix

more background to read. Coverage is not identical to Harrison's, so if you are routinely using one and don't find something, it is worth checking the other.

William's Textbook of Endocrinology, edited by Jean D. Wilson and Daniel W. Foster. Ninth edition 1996. W. B. Saunders, Philadelpha. ISBN 0-7216-6152-1. It is a thorough and reasonably clear discussion of the endocrine aspects of medicine. Endocrinology consists of the effects of various hormones and metabolic factors on the body. Thus, adrenal hormones, thyroid hormones, sex hormones, water regulation, sugar metabolism, etc. are discussed here. Clear, complete descriptions of the effects of hormone excess and deficiency. It also describes the hormone control system flowing from the brain through the hypothalamus and pituitary to the glands that release hormones into the bloodstream. The seventh edition discusses leukotrienes, prostaglandins, and related compounds. This material has been deleted in the eighth edition. The table of contents is a suitable guide to using the book.

Robbins Pathologic Basis of Disease, Cotran, Kumar and Robbins (5th ed.). Sixth edition 1999, fifth edition 1994, fourth edition 1989, third edition 1984, second edition 1979, first edition 1974. W. B. Saunders, Philadelphia. ISBN 0-7216-5032-5 (5th ed.). A clear description of what the different parts of the body are and how they interact in health and disease. This book helps you understand how everything fits together - something you will have a very difficult time doing from the other books unless you know a lot of physiology beforehand. Each edition covers somewhat different material, so if you are trying to understand a particular disease process and don't find it in one edition, check the others. When you need to understand WHY things happen and WHAT you are doing to fix them, go back and forth between *Robbins* and the other books.

Kaplan: *Comprehensive Textbook of Psychiatry,* edited by Harold I. Kaplan and Benjamin J. Sadock. Sixth edition 1995. Williams and Wilkins, Baltimore. ISBN 0-683-04532-6. This is not useful in the same sense as the above books. There are two useful things. One is that in reading through this you will see MUCH discussion of physical abnormalities that go along with conditions asserted to be "psychiatric" and "all in your head." This will convince you that there is indeed some physical cause for these conditions and that psychiatrists are remiss in failing to seek and correct these causes. You will cease to wonder why psychiatrists are unable to cure the conditions they treat - the best they can do is provide partial and inadequate control leading to a lifetime of slightly reduced suffering. The other useful thing is that there is a small amount of guidance for how to deal with someone while he is experiencing these conditions - and what to expect - which is quite relevant to helping him even when the conditions do turn out to be based on some underlying and curable medical problem such as mercury poisoning.

Note: the doctor's textbooks above are VERY EXPENSIVE. Many academic libraries and a few public ones have them. Many libraries which have them let earlier editions circulate. The PDR is not too expensive and older editions are frequently on sale. The books below are more economically priced, though word for word the medical books are no more expensive than popular stuff - they really do cover EVERYTHING and it takes a lot of words to do that!

Teitelbaum: *From Fatigued to Fantastic: a Manual for Moving Beyond Chronic Fatigue and Fibromyalgia,* Jacob Teitelbaum, ISBN 0-89529-737-X. This is a comprehensive description of chronic fatigue and fibromyalgia and what the patient can do about them with an excellent appendix for physicians. This book is about halfway between conventional medicine's lack of any real therapeutic approach and the present work's focus on chronic mercury poisoning as causal for these conditions in that it does have useful therapeutic suggestions and tests to identify elements of the disease process but it does not address a root cause. It also provides information regarding the diagnosis and treatment of yeast problems.

The Life Extension Foundation's Disease Prevention and Treatment Protocols, second edition, c 1998, ISBN 0-9658777-1-X, Life Extension Foundation (954) 761-9199. The contents of this and related works are also available on the web at www.lef.org. It has useful suggestions for alleviating some of the problems consequent to mercury intoxication. It is difficult to understand how everything this book suggests fits together metabolically unless you have a good understanding of human physiology, but it is useful at any level.

Murray (1996): *Encyclopedia of Nutritional Supplements,* Michael Murray, c 1996, ISBN 0-7165-0410-9, Prima Publishing, (916) 632-4400. There are many such books on the market. This one is clear, comprehensible, correct and arranged so people at different levels of knowledge can all find something helpful in it.

Murray (1995): *The Healing Power of Herbs,* Michael Murray, c 1995, ISBN 1-5595-8700-8, Prima Publishing, (916) 632-4400. A good, clear, accurate guide to the actions and uses of selected medicinal herbs and their uses in treatment. Many of the herbal supplements discussed in the present book are discussed in great detail by Dr. Murray.

Other references cited

ADA Council on Scientific Affairs. (1998) Dental amalgam: update on safety concerns. *J. Am. Dent. Assoc.* **129**: 494-503.

Al-Shahristani H. and Shihab K. (1974) Variation in biological half-life of methylmercury in man. *Arch. Environ. Hlth* **28**: 342-344.

Anon. *Federal Register* April 22 1998; 19799-19802.

Aposhian HV, Bruce DC, Alter W, Dart R, Hurlbut KM, and Aposhian MM. (1992) Urinary mercury after administration of 2,3-dimercaptopropane-1-sulfonic acid: correlation with dental amalgam score. *FASEB J.* **6**: 2472-2476.

Barregård L, Sällsten G, and Järvholm B. (1995) People with high mercury uptake from their own dental amalgam fillings. *Occ. Environ. Med.* **52**: 124-8.

Barregård L, Linstedt G, Schültz A and Sällsten G. (1994) Endocrine function in mercury exposed chloralkali workers. *Occ. Environ. Med.* **51**: 536-40.

Begerow J, Zander D, Freier I, and Dunemann L. (1994) Long-term mercury excretion in urine after removal of amalgam fillings. *Int. Arch. Occ. Environ. Hlth.* **66**: 209-212.

Belsky P. (1998) MCS and mercury. *Chemical and Engineering News* **76**: (41) 11-12.

Bjorkman L, Sandborg-Englund G, and Ekstand J. (1997) Mercury in saliva and feces after removal of amalgam fillings. *Toxicol. Appl. Pharmacol.* **144**; 156-62.

Bradley W, Daroff R, Fenichel G and Marsden C. (1996) Neurology in Clinical Practice - the neurological disorders. Two volumes. Butterworth-Heinemann, Boston.

Bunevicius R, Kazanavicius G, Zalinkevicius R, Prange A. (1999) Effects of thyroxine as compared with thyroxine plus triiodothyronine in patients with hypothyroidism. *N Engl J* Med **340** 424-9.

Appendix

Clarkson TW. (1972) The pharmacology of mercury compounds. *Ann. Rev. Pharmacol.* **12:** 375-406.

Cutler E (1998) Winning the war against asthma and allergies. Delmar Publishers. ISBN 0-8273-8622-2.

Echeverria D, Aposhian HV, Woods JS, Heyer NJ, Aposhian MM, Bittner AC Jr., Mahurin RK and Cianciola M. (1998) Neurobehavioral effects from exposure to dental amalgam Hg°: new distinctions between recent exposure and Hg body burden. *FASEB J.* **12:** 971-980.

Echeverria D, Heyer N, Martin M, Naleway, A, Woods J and Bittner A. (1995) Behavioral effects of low-level exposure to Hg° among dentists. *Neurotoxicol. Teratol.* **17:** 161-8.

Ellingsen D, Thomassen Y, Langård S, and Kluus H. (1993) Urinary mercury excretion in chloralkali workers after the cessation of exposure. *Scand. J. Work. Environ. Hlth.* **19:** 334-341.

Eneström S, and Hultman P. (1995) Does amalgam affect the immune system? A controversial issue. *Int. Arch. Allergy Immunol.* **106:** 180-203.

Engel P. (1998) Observations on health before and after amalgam removal (translated from original german) *Schweiz Monatsschefte für Zahnmedizin* **108** nr 8.

Ewers U, and Erbe R. (1980) Effects of Lead, Cadmium and Mercury on Brain Adenylate Cyclase. *Toxicology* **16:** 227-237.

Friberg L, Nordberg GF and Vouk VB. (1986) Handbook on the toxicology of Metals. Volume II. Specific Metals. Elsevier Science, New York.

Gerhard I, Roller E, *et al.* (1997) Reporting a study performed at the University Gynecological Clinic, Heidelberg.

Bundesinstitut für Arznemittel und Medizinproducte.

Gerstner H. and Huff J. (1977) Clinical toxicology of mercury. *J. Toxicol. Environ. Hlth.* **2:** 491-526.

Goodman and Gilman: Hardman J, Goodman-Gilman A and Limbird L (1996) *Goodman and Gilman's The Pharmacological Basis of Therapeutics,* 9th edition, McGraw-Hill, New York, ISBN 0-07-026266-7.

Grandjean P, Guldager B, Larsen I, Jørgensen P and Holmstrup P. (1997) Placebo response in environmental illness. *J. Occ. Environ. Med.* **39:** 707-14.

Haddad, LM, Shannon, MW, Winchester, JF, (1998) Clinical Management of Poisoning and Drug Overdose, third edition, W.B Saunders, Philadelphia. See page 753.

Hanson M, and Pleva J. (1991) The dental amalgam issue. A review. *Experientia* **47:** 9-22.

Harrison's Principles of Internal Medicine - see useful books.

Henningsson C, Hoffmann S, McGonigle L and Winter J. (1993) Acute mercury poisoning (acrodynia) mimicking pheochromocytoma in an adolescent. *J. Pediatrics* **122;** 252-3.

Hodgson E. (1987) A textbook of modern toxicology. See pp 240-243. Elsevier Science, New York.

Huggins H. (1993) It's all in your head, the link between mercury amalgams and illness. Avery publishing group, Garden City Park, NY.

Ingbar J, Borges M, Iflah S, *et al.* (1982) Elevated serum thyroxine concentration in patients receiving "replacement" doses of levothyroxine. *J Endocrinol Invest* **5** 77-85.

Amalgam Illness: Diagnosis and Treatment

Jaffe M (1977) Effect of testosterone cypionate on postexercise ST segment depression. *Br. Heart J* **39**: 1217-22.

Johnson J. (1998) Mercury summit planned. *Chemical and Engineering News* May 11; **76**: 22-3.

Kishi R, Doi R, Fukuchi Y, Satoh H, Satoh R, Ono A, Moriwaka F, Tashiro K, Takahata N, et al. (1993) Subjective Symptoms and Neurobehavioral Performances of Ex-Mercury Miners at an Average of 18 Years after the Cessation of Chronic Exposure to Mercury Vapor, *Environmental Research* **62** 289-302.

Kussmaul A. (1861) Untersuchungen über den constitutionellen Mercurialismus und sein Verhältness zur constitutionellen Syphilis, Würtzburg.

Langworth S. (1997) Experiences from the amalgam unit at Huddinge hospital - somatic and psychosomatic aspects. *Scand. J. Work. Environ. Hlth.* **23**: 65-7.

Larsen P. (1972) Direct immunoassay of triiodothyronine in human serum. *J Clin Invest* **51** 1939-49.

Lazarau J, Pomeranz BH and Corey PN. (1998) Incidence of adverse drug reactions in hospitalized patients. *JAMA* **279**: 1200-5.

Lesser M. (1946) Testosterone propionate therapy in one hundred cases of angina pectoris. *J Clin Endocrinol* **6**: 549-57.

Levy M. (1995) Dental amalgam: toxicological evaluation and health risk assessment. *J. Cdn. Dent. Assoc.* **61**: 667-8, 671-4.

Lichtenberg H (1993) Elimination of symptoms by removal of dental amalgam from mercury poisoned patients, as compared with a control group of average patients. *Journal of Orthomolecular Medicine* **8** 145-148.

Lichtenstein M *et al.* (1987) Sex hormones, insulin, lipids and prevalent ischemic heart disease. *Am J Epidemiol,* **126**: 647-57.

Marlowe M, Errera J, Stellern J and Beck D (1983) Lead and mercury levels in emotionally disturbed children. *Journal of Orthomolecular Psychiatry,* **12**: 260-270.

Marlowe M, Moon C, Errera J, Jacobs J, Brunson M, Stellern J and Schroeder C (1986) Low mercury levels and childhood intelligence. *Journal of Orthomolecular Medicine,* **1**: 43-49.

Merrit (1995) Merritt's Textbook of Neurology, ninth edition, Williams and Wilkins, Baltimore. See page 688.

Nakagawa R (1995) Concentration of mercury in hair of diseased people in Japan. *Chemosphere* **30**: 135-40.

Phillips H (1994) The association of hypotestosteronemia with coronary artery disease in men. *Atherosler Thromb,* **14**: 701-6.

Pleva J (1983) Mercury poisoning from dental amalgam. *Journal of Orthomolecular Psychiatry,* **12**: 184-193.

Pollard KM and Hultman P (1997) Effects of mercury on the immune system. *Metal Ions in Biological Systems,* Sigel and Sigel, eds., Marcel Dekker, New York, **34**: 421-440.

Richardson GM, and Allan M. (1996) A Monte Carlo Assessment of Mercury Exposure and Risks from Dental Amalgam. *Human and Ecological Risk Assessment,* **2**: (4) 709-761.

Roels H, Boeckx M, Ceulemans E and Lauwerys R. (1991) Urinary excretion of mercury after occupational exposure to mercury vapour and influence of the chelating agent meso-2,3-dimercaptosuccinic acid (DMSA). *Brit . J. Ind. Med.* **48**: 247-253.

Sandborg-Englund G, Dahlqvist R, Lindelöf B, Söderman E, Jonzon B,

Appendix

Vesterberg O and Larsson KS. (1994) DMSA administration to patients with alleged mercury poisoning from dental amalgams: a placebo controlled study. *J. Dent. Rsch.* **73**: 620-8.

Silberud RL, Motl J and Kienholtz E (1998) Psychometric evidence that dental amalgam mercury may be an etiologic factor in manic depression. *Journal of Orthomolecular Medicine,* **13**: 31-40.

Skare I and Engqvist A. (1994) Human exposure to mercury and silver released from dental amalgam restorations. *Arch. Environ. Hlth.* **49**; 384-394.

Skog E, and Wahlberg J. (1964) A comparative investigation of the percutaneous absorption of metal compounds in the guinea pig by means of the radioactive isotopes: ^{51}Cr, ^{58}Co, ^{65}Zn, ^{110m}Ag, ^{115m}Cd, ^{203}Hg. *J. Invest. Dermatol.* **43**: 187-92.

Stenman S. and Grans L. (1997) Symptoms and differential diagnosis of patients fearing mercury toxicity from amalgam fillings. *Scand. J. Work. Environ. Hlth.* **23**: 59-63.

Teitelbaum (1996) - see useful books appendix.

ThyagaRajan S, Felten S and Felten D (1998) Selegiline accelerates re-ennervation of rat noradrenergic spleen and lymph nodes and improves cellular immunity, *Journal of Neuroimmunology* **81** 144-57.

Diagnostic tests - when to perform them and what they mean

I am going to cover material not covered adequately in standard medical textbooks. Some of it is just additional detail there isn't room for in these texts, and some of it is "alternative" or controversial material. Do not lose sight of all the STANDARD indications for STANDARD diagnostic tests directed at WELL ACCEPTED conditions. You may have a complication of amalgam illness or have something other than amalgam

Van Benschoten M. (1994) Acupoint energetics of mercury toxicity and amalgam removal with case studies, *American Journal of Acupuncture* **22** 251-262.

Weiner JA, and Nylander M. (1995) An estimation of the uptake of mercury from amalgam fillings based on urinary excretion of mercury in Swedish subjects. *Sci. Total Env.* **168**: 255-265.

Williams Textbook of Endocrinology (1996) - see useful books appendix.

Ziff MF and Ziff S. (1994a) The Missing Link? A Persuasive New Look at Heart Disease as it relates to Mercury. Bio-Probe, Orlando.

Ziff S and Ziff MF. (1994b) Infertility and Birth Defects - Is Mercury from Silver Dental Fillings a Hidden Cause? Bio-Probe, Orlando.

Ziff MF and Ziff S. (1994c) Silver Dental Fillings - The Toxic Time Bomb. Aurora Press.

Zorn N and Smith J (1990) A relationship between vitamin B-12, folic acid, ascorbic acid, and mercury uptake and methylation. *Life Sciences* **47**: 167-173.

Zuichik V, Tsyb A and Vtyurin B (1994) Trace elements and thyroid cancer. *Analyst* **120**: 817-21.

illness, or insurance company or state licensing board officials may assert such if appropriate testing is not documented in your chart.

The interpretation of many of these tests is discussed in greater detail in the medical treatment section.

Most, but not all medical test 'normal ranges' are defined so that they include 95% of a healthy population, with 2.5% expected to be high and 2.5% expected to be low randomly. Most parameters tested for are found to be normally distributed or log-normally distributed. In plain english this means a graph that looks like a bell curve on regular or logarithmic graph paper if you plot how many healthy people show up with each test result.

Test results aren't really "random," in that your have a set point for most of the things tested and will give results close to that number on repeated re-testing.

Most physicians are not familiar with the statistical implications of all this. Someone who tests "abnormal," but relatively close to the normal range, will be giving a result NORMAL FOR THEM in one person out of 20. Conversely, some people whose set point is in the "abnormal" range can give NORMAL results when they in fact are high or low (respectively) for them. Thus the merits of treating the patient rather than the lab report when it comes to things like endocrine problems. Laboratory tests are intended to uncover serious and acute pathological processes that drive the test result well outside the normal range. They are not useful for deciding on the exact level at which a patient becomes "ill" or "well" in a slowly developing disease process like chronic mercury intoxication. They are very useful for guiding therapy if you pay attention to how the numbers change and how symptoms follow that and ignore the "normal ranges."

Some lab test ranges are defined by what is believed to be "good" for us. The upper ranges given for cholesterol, triglycerides and blood pressure are not the limits beyond which only 1 normal person in 40 lies. They are limits determined from epidemiological studies and large fractions of the population have "high" cholesterol, triglycerides and blood pressure. These limits are not useful in determining whether someone is mercury poisoned. Actual "normal ranges" for these tests can be found in the back of some medical textbooks, e. g. *Harrrison's Principles of Internal Medicine*. *Tietz Textbook of Clinical Chemistry* has the most comprehensive tables.

Many test normal ranges depend on age and sex. Few labs list age and sex related norms. Many of these are given in tables in the back of standard medical textbooks or can be found by a thorough literature search if needed. Laboratory standard ranges are often developed for the population the lab thinks is being tested - e. g. most labs that show a single male normal range for testosterone show one appropriate for 85 year olds since these represent the population most likely to have a problem and get tested.

A good example of sex specific cutoffs is alanine transaminase, ALT. Men have higher values than women, but this is seldom shown in lab normal ranges. A good approximation to the proper upper end of the normal range cutoffs (in units per liter) can be given by: proper adult male cutoff = listed cutoff + 4, proper adult female cutoff = listed cutoff - 8[1].

Serum creatinine is also sex specific, and approximate normal ranges are 0.7-1.3 for males and 0.6-1.1 for females. When a laboratory lists a single serum creatinine normal range it is appropriate to consider women within 0.2 of the upper limit to have high creatinine.

Another age specific test is alkaline phosphatase. It is much higher in growing children than in adults because it is used in the process of bone growth.

It is also necessary to bear in mind that most clinical laboratory tests only measure one parameter related to a disease process that has many potential points of pathological derangement. Before the test was invented, diagnosis was based on signs and symptoms and therapy was optimized according to clinical response. This ensured that patients with a derangement of any metabolic process relevant to the disease were properly treated. By relying solely on laboratory test results to direct treatment, patients with less common metabolic causes of the condition are not

---

[1] This was arrived at by considering the table in the back of *Tietz Textbook of Clinical Chemistry*.

treated properly. Case in point: by relying on elevated TSH to diagnose hypothyroidism, pituitary, hypothalamic, and end organ resistance caused disease are missed[1]. While these are presumed to be reasonably uncommon, in aggregate their known incidence accounts for approximately 1,000,000 patients in the United States. Laboratory tests supplement the clinical picture formed by the time consuming and unglamorous process of history taking, examination and getting to know the patient - they do not replace it.

Many laboratory tests are automated, well standardized and use commercially available reagents. These depend on the operator having a reasonable amount of technical skill, keeping the sample from being confused with other samples, etc. Other laboratory tests - particularly those involving a person looking through a microscope - are highly dependent on the skill of the operator, and on the time available to them to perform the analysis. The accuracy rate of such tests (ova and parasite exam, stool analysis, pap smear, mammogram interpretation) are known to be disturbingly low at some HMO's and large chain laboratories. It is best if the physician ensures that this sort of testing is performed at a smaller laboratory specializing in such analyses that is known for quality work. Less routine analyses such as tissue biopsy examination have a higher, but not excellent, accuracy rate. If insurance and financial constraints require that a lab not known to the physician be used, the suspicion of possible

false - normal test results should always be retained.

The accuracy issue is particularly important for tests - like urine mercury tests - that are statutorily mandated for certain workplaces and where the laboratory expects to get normal or low results. Great care may not always be taken to do these tests accurately since the technicians may not expect to find abnormal results and may not believe the results matter in the diagnosis and treatment of disease[2]. Thus for certain tests it is best to identify laboratories which specialize in them for medical - usually alternative medical - purposes and handle each sample with great care because they do believe your health and perhaps life do depend on an accurate analysis. This seems to be particularly problematic when analyzing for toxic elements.

I will give a few "normal ranges" and useful numbers here for tests relevant to amalgam illness. Some of them involve comparing numbers from two different tests - something almost never done on the lab report itself.

Certain metabolic tests may be performed after you have been off of supplements and medications for the past several days or may be performed while you are taking such supplements and medications. The primary consideration is whether it is necessary to understand or document the your untreated metabolic state - which can be very unpleasant - or whether understanding the present state as corrected by supplements so as to identify further defects in need of treatment is the goal. Documentation of the

---

[1] There actually are tests for these, but those tests aren't used to work up patients unless they are considered hypothyroid, and nowadays most physicians ignore the patient and only pay attention to the TSH result. Thus they never diganose hypothyroidism due to any cause but thyroid gland failure. If the physician does not trust his clinical impression that the patient actually is hypothyroid MORE than he trusts the TSH test result which says the patient is NOT hypothyroid, he will never order the existing tests to check for the other less common forms of hypothyroidism and they will always be missed.

[2] Certainly many technicians at major chain laboratories do take each analysis very seriously, and many major chain laboratories do have strict quality control programs in place. However, since federal and state laws prohibit these laboratories from talking to you and giving you enough information to find out if they are among the careful ones you are pretty much forced to use the "alternative" labs that base a large fraction of their business on these kinds of tests if you want any real assurance that your test results are accurate.

untreated state is primarily useful for legalistic and rarely diagnostic reasons. Determination of the present partially compensated state is useful in guiding future therapy and is often adequate for diagnostic purposes. Since you can be very miserable for a long time if you skip your supplements for a few days it is recommended not to do so unless the doctor and lab can give you a better reason than "that's how we always do it."

The most common error when you collect a 24 hour urine sample is to start the collection by urinating into the container rather than into the toilet. This will result in somewhat higher for creatinine and whatever is being measured than would result if the test were performed properly.

Total creatinine is often measured when taking a 24 hour urine collection to ensure that all urine was collected and the sample was handled properly. If the sample was mis-handled as indicated by an incorrect creatinine value, it should be presumed that other handling errors were also made and the test result may be invalid. If in doubt, repeat the test rather than scaling the results. Creatinine is produced by muscle tissue and some also comes from meat in the diet. Mammals are the source of most dietary creatinine. A person taking supplementary creatine will excrete much higher creatinine than expected. The amount of creatinine excreted in urine in 24 hours can be calculated from the following formulae:

Creatinine = $5.7 \times 10^{-6} \times$ (height in inches)^3 for men; and

Creatinine = $4.4 \times 10^{-6} \times$ (height in inches)^3 for women.

The actual amount excreted will be between this amount and this amount + 0.4. Excessively muscular or excessively thin people will excrete more or less. Weight is not a strong determinant - muscle mass, which depends primarily on height and sex, is.

Lab normal ranges are for people of all sizes and many labs give normal ranges for men and women combined. The procedure shown above gives a MUCH more accurate determination of the "normal range" for the person taking the test.

A person doing several 24 hour urine collections under constant dietary conditions will almost always give creatinine results + 0.1 g/d from prior tests.

Expected 24 hour urine creatinine levels for men and women are:

Height	Men	Women
4' 10"	1.11-1.41	0.86-1.09
4' 11"	1.17-1.47	0.90-1.13
5'	1.23-1.58	0.95-1.22
5' 1"	1.29-1.64	1.00-1.27
5' 2"	1.36-1.71	1.05-1.32
5' 3"	1.43-1.79	1.10-1.38
5' 4"	1.49-1.84	1.15-1.42
5' 5"	1.57-1.97	1.21-1.52
5' 6"	1.64-2.04	1.27-1.57
5' 7"	1.71-2.11	1.32-1.63
5' 8"	1.79-2.19	1.38-1.69
5' 9"	1.87-2.27	1.44-1.75
5' 10"	1.96-2.36	1.51-1.82
5' 11"	2.04-2.49	1.57-1.92
6'	2.13-2.58	1.64-1.99
6' 1"	2.22-2.67	1.71-2.06
6' 2"	2.31-2.76	1.78-2.13
6' 3"	2.40-2.90	1.85-2.24
6' 4"	2.50-3.00	1.93-2.32
6' 5"	2.60-3.10	2.01-2.39
6' 6"	2.70-3.20	2.08-2.47
6' 7"	2.81-3.31	2.17-2.56
6' 8"	2.92-3.42	2.25-2.64

It is appropriate to determine creatinine clearance in combination with any convenient 24 hour urine collection to look for unrecognized kidney problems. Mercury is widely reputed to damage the kidneys. While this is rare in chronic poisoning, it can happen. If it occurs in chronic poisoning it is due to autoimmune mechanisms. If there is kidney damage and blood in the urine, determine urine mercury levels as there may have been a recent high exposure and immediate action to stop further exposure is mandatory[1].

Blood is detected in urine by routine urinalysis. Mercury makes blood to appear in the urine during acute poisoning only by causing nephrotic syndrome - a condition where high levels of mercury in the bloodstream actually kill specific kidney cells. If there is not also a relatively high level of mercury in urine and blood at this time then something else is causing blood to be in the urine.

If there is blood in your urine and it is caused by mercury, have your serum creatinine measured. If it is elevated, or significantly higher than your usual level, then significant kidney damage is occurring and you must reduce your mercury exposure promptly.

If you have blood in your urine and elevated serum creatinine it is an urgent matter to reduce your mercury exposure and you need to work with a doctor and a dentist who understand this - whether or not the current ones do. Also note that if you have fillings removed it is key to take precautions to avoid additional exposure at that time.

If medical records are available, erythrocytes seen on routine urinalysis at any time during the period of illness or one year prior to perceived onset suggest mercury. Routine UA is likely to be normal even in serious cases of amalgam illness, so it is not worth getting as a screening test unless there is a history of pink urine within the past year. In this case, if substantial numbers of erythrocytes do not show up, get a fractionated urine porphyrin test[2]. It is of course necessary that women not be having their menstrual period when they give a urine sample for this test.

If routine blood chemistry is to be drawn, it is informative to ensure it includes ALT, AST, Mg, K, Na, Glucose, BUN, creatinine, venous CO_2, HDL cholesterol, total cholesterol, and triglycerides.

Low glucose on any measurement or indications of hypoglycemia suggest adrenal insufficiency. Hemoglobin A1C can be measured to see if you have hypoglycemia a lot. If you do, it will be low.

Treatment with carbamazepine suggests testing for ALT as therapy is initiated, then every few months.

Low essential elements across the board in hair element analysis suggests testing for malabsorption, which will usually be evident as low total cholesterol (<130) and serum triglycerides (<40 for women, <50 for men). Reasons for malabsorption may be found through digestive stool analysis.

Low HDL cholesterol suggests mercury. If records are available it may be possible to see this change with exposures. If not, the test should be ordered only if a standard blood chemistry panel is reasonable to order at that time.

Low magnesium (Mg) in serum (with a standard chem panel) or red blood cells (a special test) indicates deficiency. Deficiency is still possible even if these results are normal since it is the amount inside the other cells in your body that is most important. If you are deficient in magnesium and it is normal in urine[3] then magnesium wasting is occurring and continuous supplementation at

---

[1] Sources of high mercury exposure might be dental work that placed some other metal in direct contact with amalgam thus creating a battery in the mouth and dissolving mercury rapidly, sudden corrosion of an old filling due to decay under it, application of a mercury containing antiseptic to a large area of skin, or exposure to an unrecognized source of mercury like broken fluorescent light tubes.

[2] and ensure that the sample is handled properly per instructions on that test.

[3] during 24 hour urine essential elements determination.

high levels is required. Magnesium wasting suggests evaluating adrenal status, androgens and the body's apparent response to the level of thyroid available.

Signs of adrenal problems or frequent muscle spasms should lead to tests for Potassium (K) and Mg in red blood cells as the cellular content is physiologically important and is not necessarily well reflected by serum. Fibromyalgia should always lead to determining magnesium status. If your body is functioning properly, your K and Mg levels in serum should be about the same place in the normal range as they are in red blood cells. If the level of these in serum is much higher than their level relative to the normal range in red blood cells, then your body is not pumping them into your cells like it is supposed to.

Achiness that can't be diagnosed as fibromyalgia suggests testing sedimentation rate, CPK, and for rheumatoid arthritis and lupus.

Hair element analysis should be considered as a reasonable screening test for people suspected of amalgam illness or other element intoxication, especially if they don't yet take much in the way of supplements. The most suggestive result for mercury intoxication is Hair calcium >1,150 ppm with hair lithium below 0.004 ppm. Mercury intoxication is possible even at very low hair MERCURY levels. Reasonably high silver, tin and nickel confirm that amalgam is the mercury source. It is wise to ensure that the laboratory conducting the analysis does measure silver, tin and nickel as well as mercury. Hair mercury >3.0 ppm is strongly suggestive of intoxication.   Some patients (of both sexes) have long hair and it is not bleached, permed, or dyed. Don't let the nurse snip away and get the roots then discard the rest. Either use the ends of it, or keep the strands and keep them aligned as you might want to reconstruct a history later. If the patient is currently taking supplements and the analysis is ambiguous it may be helpful to analyze the distal ends if they are old enough that supplements were not being taken at the time they grew. Hair element

analysis of this sort also screens for other types of poisoning - copper being one of the more common ones that might be confused with amalgam illness.

Other things that can be seen in hair element analysis: malabsorption shows up as most of the essential elements being low. Mercury intoxication tends to make the essential elements vary widely, while copper intoxication results in greatly elevated copper but most other elements within normal limits and reasonably near the average. Low hair magnesium implies low body magnesium (which can cause fibromyalgia and assorted heart conditions including angina). Low potassium and sodium are suggestive of mineralocorticoid deficiency, which implies that the adrenal glands may be beaten up.

Hair element analysis is controversial among mainstream medical practitioners. Authoritative sources such as Tietz state is is a good screening tests for certain conditions like lead and arsenic intoxication. The virtues of hair element analysis are it is inexpensive and provides a lot of information.   It is appropriate to confirm the results using other tests if diagnostic or treatment decisions will be made based on them and either you or your physician are not completely comfortable with the reliability of the test. No laboratory test is perfectly reliable and I recommend careful thought and further testing if the results of hair element analysis or of any other test lead to a confusing overall picture when combined with all the information available from other tests, symptoms, history and examination results.

Urine mercury is not recommended as a diagnostic test in and of itself. It can be a good tracking test. If urine mercury exceeds 10 mcg/24h in the absence of industrial exposure it is strongly suggestive of mercury intoxication. Low urine mercury levels do not exclude amalgam illness or make it less likely that someone has it. Urine copper will be high in copper poisoning, and if normal means there is not a copper problem.

Copper and iron can be high or low in amalgam illness.   Low copper causes reduction in the sense of taste. Red blood cell copper is a good measure. Standard serum iron, serum ferritin and total iron binding capacity tests are useful.

Elevated uric acid, hair lead, urinary lead or basophilic stippling of blood cells suggests lead. This can be checked by a blood test for ALAD, free erythrocyte protoporphyrin and zinc protoporphyrin, or a urine test for aminolevulinic acid. Lead is synergistic with mercury and other heavy metals, so lead or lead marker levels that would not otherwise be considered quite high enough to be clinically significant should be viewed with great suspicion if there is evidence of significant levels of other heavy metal toxins.

Any reason to suspect cadmium poisoning suggests testing for urine ß-2 microglobulin.

No challenge test is really all that good a diagnostic tool for chronic mercury intoxication. However challenge tests are often accepted as proof of intoxication for a variety of reasons - e. g. determination of insurance coverage.

The mercury section of the 1998 edition of *Harrison's Principles of Internal Medicine* describes a challenge test using a 2 gram oral dose of succimer (DMSA) to check for past exposure to mercury. It is towards the end of the section.

This challenge test described in a widely used medical textbook will be considered legitimate proof of intoxication by people not thoroughly familiar with the subject - especially if they are shown a highlighted copy of the relevant section.

Elevated urine porphyrins or other markers of intoxication without indications of heavy metals on hair, urine and blood testing suggest the toxin is either arsenic or an organic material. You should decide based on your history and symptoms whether to test for arsenic or organics first. Arsenic is tested for by mobilization with lipoic acid as described below. DMSA may be omitted if only arsenic is being tested for, though it will increase the amount of mercury observed

if a significant amount of mercury was deposited in your brain long ago during some unrecognized exposure.

What you do is : first, you do an "unchallenged" 24 hour urine mercury test. I strongly recommend that you actually do a "toxic and essential elements" test just to be sure to catch other stuff that might be odd - like copper. No matter what the doctor says, you MUST use a competent lab, and the ones I KNOW are competent are Doctor's Data, Great Smokies and Metametrix.

Now you will need another test order for a 24 hour urine mercury test. You will also need a prescription for DMSA. If you want to get it from more or less any pharmacy, you have this prescription written for Chemet 100 mg #20. This is about $90-100 worth. If you want to keep the cost down, you use either that prescription or have one written for DMSA 250 mg #8 and fill it at the cheapest compounding pharmacy you can. Call for quotes. Some charge shipping, some don't. This is about $30 worth of compounded DMSA.

Now you do the challenge test. The textbook says take ALL the DMSA at once. You won't do that. It is a lot safer and a lot more comfortable to spread it out. Spreading the DMSA out makes somewhat more mercury come out in the sample. This should not change the interpretation. If the physician or insurance company is concerned they can use the pharmacokinetics given in another appendix to correct the result. If you just say "I took all the DMSA and collected the 24 hour urine sample like I was supposed to" it won't occur to them that exactly how you took it might be important.

To collect a 24 hour urine specimen and do the challenge test, you get up in the morning, pee in the toilet, not the container, and note the time on the collection container. Now you take two of the 100 mg capsules if that is what you have, or one of the 250 mg capsules if that is what you have. From now on, you put your pee in the container. All of it. For the next 24 hours.

Every two hours after you started, you take your 2 x 100 mg caps or your 1 x 250 mg cap, depending. You do that until they are all gone (about bedtime - 14 hours later for the 250's, 18 hours later for the 100's).

Make sure to wake up in time so that EXACTLY 24 hours after you started collecting your urine, you can pee, put it in the container, and stop the collection. You now have a 24 hour urine sample that needs to be mixed, put in a little bottle, and sent to the lab.

The sample kits have instructions about collecting samples, using the preservative that has to go in with the pee when you start to collect it, etc. Your doctor will decide whether you should prepare the sample and ship it or her office staff should. You should measure the volume in the container(s) using the graduations on the side and keep your own record of it. If the report comes back with different volume, talk to the doctor about it. Something is wrong. It is unfortunately very common for the staff at physician's offices to mishandle urine specimens, confuse them with other people's, etc. It is best if you prepare your own specimen (since you will be very concerned and thus very careful to follow instructions) or if you watch the technician prepare it and have them explain what they are doing and why as they do so. Also calculate the amount of creatinine that ought to be in the sample by using the formula or table in the "tests" appendix and make sure the number on the lab report is the number you calculated. If it isn't, something is wrong. Talk to the doctor about it and insist on redoing the test[1].

Women have to make sure not to collect the sample during their menstrual period.

_____

[1] If your doctor argues that an incorrect volume or creatinine are not significant, or that you didn't get them right, or that you shouldn't worry about it because doctor knows best, you have just performed the most important possible test. Can this doctor help you. Result: no. Therapeutic measure: find another doctor.

If you go through all this and the 'challenged' sample still shows low mercury and you are pretty sure you got poisoned by it but don't have current exposure, you can repeat the challenge test and take lipoic acid 50-100 mg with the DMSA. This will mobilize mercury from your brain and internal organs. It will also cause significant side effects. If you are emotionally volatile or have mood disturbances you need to tell everyone these might get a LOT worse when you do this test.

Of course, if you start to do this and are feeling really really bad after a few doses of the chelating agents, STOP TAKING THEM. One of the reasons this is a safer protocol than taking all the chelating agents at once is that you can STOP before you get the whole day's worth into you if you are having an adverse reaction!

If your post challenge - prechallenge number is greater than 20 micrograms, you 'pass' the textbook challenge test and according to Harrison's Textbook of Internal Medicine you have mercury poisoning. Most physicians will interpret a post challenge result of close to 20 mcg/day as indicating mercury poisoning, due to individual variability - some people are more sensitive than others. As a rule, women are more sensitive to toxins than men and women are also usually smaller than the large and muscular male factory workers these "challenge test" results came from.

If you have to pee more than about 8 times per day you should get two collection containers so you don't run out of space. The containers are usually 3 liters and "normal" people supposedly make less than 2.5 liters per day. Most mercury toxic people need 2 containers. Some need 3. By doing the unchallenged measurement first you can determine the number of containers you need without having to take the medicines. If you filled a container most of the way up, get an extra container for use during the challenge test since people usually urinate somewhat more during chelation.

Appendix

There are two DMPS challenge tests. One uses injected DMPS, which should never be used due to the high rate of death and adverse drug reactions. The other is to take 300 mg of DMPS by mouth and is described in the literature by Aposhian and others. It appears to have a higher rate of side effects and adverse reactions than the DMSA test, is not well standardized, and is not discussed as diagnostic in any medical text to the best of my knowledge. Additionally, DMSA is FDA approved in the United States, while DMPS is investigational at this time. You should not use a DMPS challenge test.

Treatment with carbamazepine combined with periodic treatment with DMSA suggests blood counts every few months. Both of these agents very rarely cause bone marrow suppression which can lead to agranulocytosis[1]. CBC's are suggested during treatment with each individually.

High eosinophils in a blood count suggest food allergies.

If there is any question an infectious agent might be involved in your illness, you or your doctor may wish to test for or consider candida, giardia, amoeba, cryptosporidium, clostridia dificile, Lyme disease, mycoplasma, HHV-6, EBV, coxsackie virus, hepatitis, helicobacter pylori, chlamydia and HIV. Do not consider this list exclusive. Reasons to do this include unexplained periodic fever, recurrent viral infections, recurrent unexplained symptoms of any of these diseases, or if your "chronic fatigue" or "amalgam illness" sounds suspiciously close to any of these or had a sudden and well defined onset.

Substantial asthma or allergy problems suggest testing for IgE. Many mercury toxic people do not have a runny nose (rhinitis) even with vastly elevated IgE. However, they do have the fatigue and malaise allergy causes. Fatigue and malaise that is induced by outside air, on windy days, or that varies predictably with the seasons indicates testing IgE regardless of whether rhinitis is present. Note: the 'average' allergy sufferer has an IgE of about 180 IU, but no nonallergic people have IgE numbers above this. Over 292 is a 'pathological' allergy, since less than 2.5% of the nonallergic population exceeds this level.

Immunoglobulin E values are difficult to interpret because the range for allergic and nonallergic people overlaps extensively. Since most labs use a standardized set of lab equipment and reagents for this the numbers are comparable. The upper limit above which only 2.5% of the NONALLERGIC population lies is 292 IU. Above this is the range of "pathological" allergies. About 1/3 of allergy sufferers have "pathological" allergies. Above 806 IU it is more likely the IgE is caused by helminthic parasites than allergies if you don't know which you have (you will experience severe allergies either way since helminth infection causes IgE production and sensitization to go out of control). A value above 2840 IU is "abnormal" even for allergy suffers and is very strongly suggestive of helminth infection or some other pathological process that elevates IgE.

A history of unexplained occasional jaundice, or spines in urine, or rising IgE during mercury detox suggests helminthic parasites. There are blood tests for antibodies to these but the blood tests are not completely reliable. The only reliable test is wedge liver biopsy which is generally not a good idea since it is more hazardous than treatment for the parasites with Biltricide® (praziquantel). Reaction to the medication confirms the diagnosis. Serious reaction to the medication may require prednisone to control immune system activity for the next month or two.

If you have an IgE < 60, you may test positive to antigens and have a history of "allergies," but below this level of IgE the symptoms are seldom significant enough to bother you or interfere with your activities or general energy level.

---

[1] low granulocytes in the blood, plus lesions of the mucus membranes and skin.

Amalgam Illness: Diagnosis and Treatment

Autoimmune markers should be tested if appropriate. It is best to err on the side of overtesting, but symptoms must be a guide to avoid excessive testing. Autoimmunity does not rule out mercury intoxication - this can cause autoimmunity - but it provides a clinical marker to follow and suggests regimens for symptom control.

Difficulty fighting off infections suggests testing the assorted Ig's. Specific difficulty fighting off viral infections suggests testing NK cell number and the IgG subclasses.

Highly elevated IgE, other inappropriate antibody levels, or impaired immune competency suggest testing for T helper, T suppressor, B and NK cell numbers.

Gastrointestinal complaints or suspected malabsorption should lead to digestive stool analysis. It is best to order an ova and parasites exam with this (including giardia antigen and serum antibodies for amebas etc.) rather than depending on history alone to exclude parasites. False negatives on parasite antibody tests are common, and people with low secretory IgA and no other apparent reason for malabsorption should be presumed to have parasites regardless of test results until that is excluded by therapeutic trial or other findings.

Yeast problems can be confirmed by blood tests for anti-candida antibodies. It is useful to test for both IgG and IgM. Elevated IgG indicates candida was getting loose in the bloodstream from your intestines recently, and elevated IgM indicates it is still doing that. If these antibodies are elevated, you may also wish to take a "leaky gut" test.

Food allergies suggest testing for leaky gut and for adequate pancreatic secretion of digestive enzymes. If this is not informative, or diet restriction information suggests it, test for lactose intolerance or for anti-gliadin antibodies, or exclude gliadin (grains) from the diet for a week long trial.

Pancreatic secretion of protease enzymes can be tested for by the chymex test where a synthetic peptide is taken and urine collected for 6 hours. The urine is tested for PABA. Since this is present in many supplements at high enough levels to interfere with the test (and erroneously make it look like your pancreas is fine when it is not) you will need to read your supplement labels thoroughly and leave any suspect supplements out of your regimen for a few days beforehand. If this will make you miserable, it is usually possible to find a similar supplement that does not contain PABA.

Suspicion of mercury or other heavy metal intoxication suggests testing for fractionated porphyrins in urine or feces. Urine is preferred. Elevated coproporphyrin in urine or feces suggests mercury or another toxin or a rare genetic condition. If uroporphyrin is also elevated then the porphyria must be due to intoxication rather than genetics.

In collecting a urine specimen for a 24 hour fractionated urine porphyrin test it is essential that the collection be refrigerated or kept on ice at all times, contain preservative, not be shaken or agitated, and not be exposed to light even briefly. At the end of the 24 hours the collection should be mixed by gently rocking or inverting the container. It must never be shaken. Seemingly trivial errors in sample handling technique - e. g. measuring volume by pouring the collection into graduated cylinders - will lead to a false negative test result.

Most labs that perform the fractionated urine porphyrin test run the standard profile of porphyrins. A few (e. g. Metametrix) also run precoproporphyrin, which is a specific biochemical marker for mercury intoxication. Toxic porphyria without elevation of precoproporphyrin indicates intoxication - but by something other than mercury. Common materials causing toxic porphyria in addition to mercury are: lead, arsenic, other heavy metals, alcohol, chloral hydrate, halogenated organics, particularly aromatic or unsaturated ones, and some drugs such as morphine. Coproporphyrin can be elevated by liver disease, malignancy, and other non-toxic causes as well.

Appendix

It is generally not necessary to test for vitamins, nutrients, essential fatty acids, etc. These are supplemented on the presumption that they are treating symptoms, are being consumed rapidly by the disease process, or their metabolism is defective. If flax oil supplementation is not relieving inflammation after 2-3 months it is appropriate to determine the fatty acid profile to see if the conversion of linolenic acid to EPA and DHA is blocked. It may be appropriate to document that fibromyalgia and chronic fatigue symptoms are indeed due to an elevated ratio of arachidonate to omega 3 fatty acids in patients who have not yet begun supplementation with significant quantities of linolenic acid[1] in patients who do not otherwise have any laboratory abnormalities or distinct signs verifiable on examination.

After months of detox, asthma, allergy or continuing low grade inflammation with malaise, lethargy and fatigue suggest testing for essential fatty acids to determine the balance between pro- and anti-inflammatory mediator precursors. Appropriate supplementation can be chosen based on this test which otherwise might not be apparent since mercury can interfere with the production of fatty acids healthy people are able to make in adequate amounts from dietary precursors.

Plasma amino acid analysis is helpful in suggesting which amino acids to restrict in the diet and which to supplement. This usually improves patient well-being substantially. It often suggests effective treatments for depression, anxiety, and lack of energy or of motivation.

Anxiety should motivate a test for plasma taurine, phenylalanine, tyrosine and tryptophan (amino acids on most aa panels). If taurine is low, supplementing it is anxiolytic. High phenylalanine or tyrosine suggest dietary restriction to reduce epinephrine and norepinephrine. Low tryptophan suggest supplementation or dietary modification to raise serotonin.

Each laboratory's plasma amino acid analysis contains a slightly different set of analytes. It is a good idea to check which ones each lab does beforehand to ensure that the analytes of interest are determined in that test - e. g. carnitine is sometimes a separate test.

Some patients will have reduced histamine levels. This is especially relevant to those patients who have behavioral disturbances similar to the schizophrenia disorders or borderline personality disorder. These can be caused by low systemic histamine. Low histamine also prevents the patient from mounting an appropriate inflammatory response to certain infectious agents.

Reduced histamine levels can be determined by tests such as platelet neurotransmitters or inferred from allergy testing in which there is a strong wheal in response to histamine, very little or no wheal response to known antigens (e. g. candida, to which most people do have antibodies), and RAST results showing positive antibody responses to common allergens which do not raise wheals on skin or subdermal testing. Suspect this condition if the patient experiences a variety of emotional responses and memories during allergy testing.

Elevated histamine can also cause behavioral disturbances similar to schizophrenia in some people.

Liver detoxification capacity tests that measure both phase 1 and the various phase 2 pathways will be helpful in almost any mercury toxic person, and should be performed immediately if there are unusual food sensitivities, chemical sensitivity, or a history of attention deficit, autism or hyperactivity.

Patient imposed food restrictions that do not relate to test determined food allergies suggest metabolic problems which should be explored using the Comprehensive Liver

---

[1] six or more grams per day of flax oil or equivalent.

Amalgam Illness: Diagnosis and Treatment

Detoxification Profile[1]. Chemical sensitivities also suggest immediately performing this test.

High blood pressure or the patient's spontaneous dietary exclusion of some or all 'sulfur foods' should lead to a test for plasma cysteine (not cystine) which is part of the Great Smokies Comprehensive Liver Detoxification Profile but not of most amino acid panels.

The average or expected blood pressure for an adult is a function of age. The systolic number (the first, larger one) is $106 + 0.6*age$. The diastolic number is $74 + 0.15*age$. Some physicians become concerned if your BP is more than 140/85. About 40% of the adult population is over this value. If you are concerned you have amalgam illness, you have much more serious problems to consider and should only worry about BP if it routinely is more than 160/95.

Classic signs of adrenal insufficiency such as weakness, malaise, depression, hypoglycemia, anorexia, weight loss, low blood pressure, or electrolyte disturbances should lead to serum or 24 hour urine cortisol determination or if possible several determinations of salivary cortisol during the day to track the patient's diurnal rhythm. Regardless of results, the response of ACTH to stress (exercise) should also be determined.

Hypoglycemia symptoms are: shaky hands, weakness, nervousness, headaches, lethargy, that improve with caffeine or something to eat, loss of capacity to think clearly that returns after eating something or taking stimulants like caffeine that increase blood sugar. In this case glucose should be determined under a variety of conditions and adrenal function should be investigated if there is no other obvious reason found for hypoglycemia.

A history of performing well during exercise, or travel, or work, followed by long "recovery periods," illness, etc. suggests testing for a decline in cortisol or ACTH in response to stress (e. g. exercise), which should then be directly measured.

In performing the ACTH before and after exercise stress test the doctor must be aware of how you - the patient - perceive blood draws. If you have not had many of them, have not become accustomed to them, and do not like them then the blood draw itself is a source of stress which might make the test difficult to interpret. In this case it is best to perform this test after you have gone through a couple of rounds of testing with an experienced phlebotomist who is able to draw your blood quickly and without undue discomfort and who does not make you feel apprehensive. Ensure that both of the blood draws for the ACTH exercise stress test will be drawn by that phlebotomist. The point of the test is to determine your response to the well defined physical stress of exercise alone.

Low potassium (K) suggests secondary - pituitary - adrenal insufficiency. High potassium levels and salt craving or high salt intake suggest primary adrenal insufficiency, as does easy tanning. Electrolyte balance, mineralocorticoids, adrenaline, DHEA-S and, in women, androgens, are guaranteed to be problems in primary insufficiency. In secondary insufficiency only cortisol, DHEA-S, and in women, androgens, are certain to be low.

Figures giving the approximate relationship between ACTH and cortisol (without stress in the preceding few hours, test done at 8 AM) for normal people, and also showing the relationship between TSH and fT4 in normal people are shown. These figures may be useful in detecting abnormalities that would be missed if each result were interpreted alone.

---

[1] offered by Great Smokies Diagnostic Laboratory. The author is not aware of an equivalent test, but any tests which determine the same values are suitable.

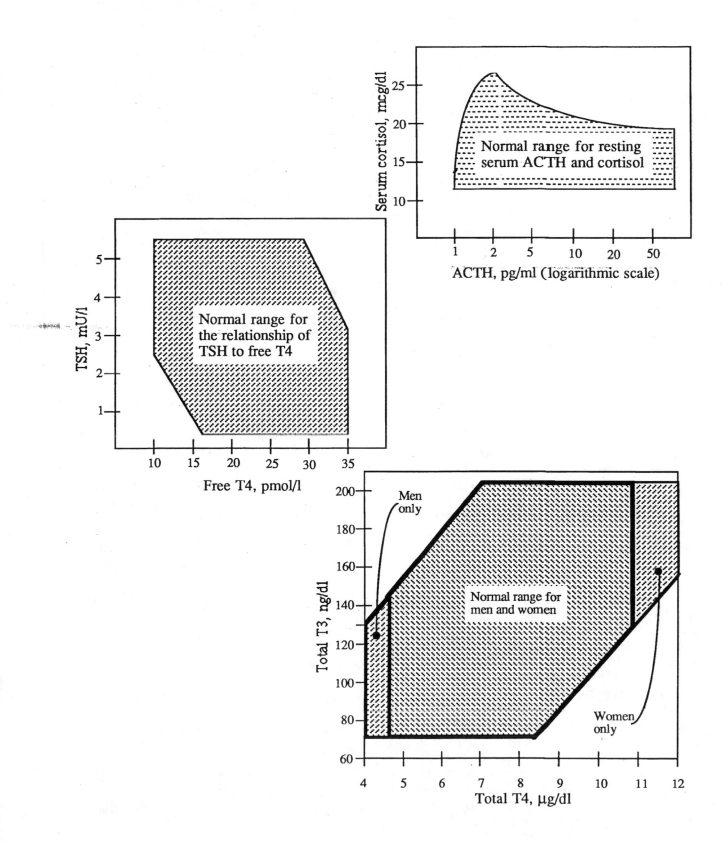

Amalgam Illness: Diagnosis and Treatment

DHEA and DHEA-S are adrenal hormones that should be tested if there are adrenal problems, or autoimmune markers, or if the patient is over 35.

The ratio of DHEA-S to DHEA in serum or plasma is high. Most labs do these tests. DHEA is sulfated in the liver. If there is a reason to suspect liver phase 2 sulfation is deficient and it is impractical to test it directly, testing DHEA-S and DHEA and seeing if DHEA is much higher compared to its normal range than DHEA-S is provides an indirect way of inferring that phase 2 sulfation is slow. This will show up most clearly in a morning specimen.

The lower limit cutoff for DHEA-S for adult males is about 1.7 - 0.02 * age. The lower limit for adult females is about 0.85 - 0.01 * age. Values below this are abnormal for a patient of that age and sex.

People who are sluggish, have dry, coarse skin, reduced body temperature, constipation, proptosis (bug eyes), repetitive thinking patterns, cold intolerance, or other typical thyroid symptoms should have appropriate thyroid tests. T3, T4, T7, and TSH are most commonly run. Free T3 and T4 are more informative. Basal body temperature should also be measured by the patient since this is the most informative indicator of positive response to thyroid supplement. Mercury poisons the hypothalamus, so TSH is not an informative test for thyroid function in a person who might have mercury poisoning.

The appropriate relationship between total T3 and total T4, and what actually happens when supplementary T4 only is given, was shown in a figure on the page before this.

Men should have testosterone, LH and FSH tested if: their arm span to height ratio is >1.00; if their lower body to upper body height ratio is >1.00 (from floor to pubic symphisis - the bone hiding behind the pubic hair, and from there to top of head) if they exercise but have slight musculature; if they have low libido; if they have general feelings of reduced well-being; if the veins on their arms do not stand above the skin and their skin is smooth and thin. If there is any question, determine testosterone levels.

For males between the ages of 30 and 85, the approximate lower limit value of serum testosterone at 8 AM is given by the equation 5.92 - 0.0288 * age in ng/ml. At 10 AM it is 83% of this, 66% at noon, 57% at 2 PM, 48% at 4 PM and 39% at 6 PM. Testosterone also fluctuates quite a bit during the day, so in theory the proper way to obtain an accurate sample is to draw blood three times 15 to 20 minutes apart and pool the serum. Most labs don't do this unless specifically instructed to in writing by the physician. The practical approach sometimes is to order the test more than once if values come in within 20% of the boundary the first time, the average of two within 15%, the average of three within 10%, or the average of four within 5%. The average of five or more measurements should be considered accurate. If the tests are drawn at different times of day they can't be "averaged" directly, but each can be divided by the normal value for that time of day and the results averaged. In this case, use the following interpretive table.

Number of tests	low	normal
1	<0.80	>1.20
2	<0.85	>1.15
3	<0.90	>1.10
4	<0.95	>1.05
5	<1.00	>1.00

A test from pooled samples should count as however many samples were pooled to perform that test.

Women with a history of amenhorrea should have appropriate endocrine evaluations. Women whose hairline is relatively far back on the forehead with indentations at the temples need to have extensive endocrine evaluations of both their adrenal and sex hormones. A hormone profile is usually more informative than a single blood test.

Appendix

A hormone profile is often useful for anyone who has difficulty keeping a "normal" schedule, or the schedule most convenient for their work and social life. Mercury poisoned people often have deranged circadian rhythms for some hormones and feel much better if these rhythms are restored by appropriate supplementation. Such a hormone profile will determine cortisol, DHEA, melatonin, and male or female sex hormones at specific times during the day.

If $2 \times Na$ + glucose/18 + BUN/2.8 is >290 on blood chemistry panels then partial diabetes insipidus is possible. A daily urine volume: > 2.5 liters is abnormal. Another indicator to look at is if you urinate more than 5 times per day (prostate problems should not be assumed in men unless verified by prostate exam and PSA). With this condition you are chronically dehydrated and at risk for serious dehydration if not able to drink water freely. This condition can be due to the kidney or the hypothalamus. Hypothalamic (central) PDI suggests other endocrine abnormalities, and also suggests that the standard tests for them may not be completely informative.

Some physicians may not remember the discussion available in, e. g. *Harrison's Principles of Internal Medicine* regarding partial diabetes insipidus. This is a common condition that results in excretion of more than 2.5 liters of urine per day, but less than the 18-24 characterizing complete diabetes insipidus. The kidney's ability to concentrate urine adequately is impaired - in chronic mercury intoxication due to inadequate release of antidiuretic hormone from the pituitary. To determine whether the test result is "normal" or "abnormal" requires two numbers - serum osmolality and urine osmolality, both measured at the same time after the patient has avoided consuming water for 12-16 hours. If the urine osmolality is > 1,000 mosm/kg, the result is normal. If the urine osmolality is less, the following calculation is performed:

Serum osmolality - 284 - (0.164 * Urine osmolality) ^ 0.5

If the result is a positive number, it is abnormal and you have partial diabetes insipidus. The pituitary versus nephrogenic nature of the disease can be demonstrated by taking DDAVP or vassopressin (any form) and observing further concentration of the next urine sample. An increase in urine concentration of more than 10% indicates that the excessive urine volume is due to a lack of antidiuretic hormone (ADH - also known as arginine vasopressin or AVP) release from the pituitary.

Another test may be used to determine whether excessive urine volume is caused by a lack of antidiuretic hormone. You restrict water for >12 hours and have blood drawn to determine serum osmolality and antidiuretic hormone levels. For serum osmolalities greater than 295 mosm/kg, the lower limit of normal plasma ADH in pg/ml is given by the formula

ADH = 0.6 * (serum osmolality - 293)

If this number is greater than the measured plasma ADH then there is deficient pituitary release of antidiuretic hormone.

It may be helpful in the face of assorted endocrine abnormalities such as low-normal thyroid or testosterone to test for pituitary releasing factors (LH, FSH, TSH, PRL, and ACTH) to decide whether the problem is more one of autoimmune endocrine gland attack, poisoning of certain glands (thyroid + adrenal being most common), or hypothalamic/pituitary poisoning.

Provocative endocrine testing is seldom useful in diagnosing or treating chronic mercury poisoning. There are presently no treatment decisions that depend on knowing whether the pituitary is poisoned or only the hypothalamus is, so there is no reason to perform testing to figure it out.

It may be incorrectly asserted from time to time that an ACTH stimulation test verifies that the entire HPA axis is intact. This is not strictly correct. Mercury poisoned people are an exception. What an ACTH stimulation test verifies in fact is that the adrenals have not atrophied. If the hypothalamus and pituitary never provide any adrenal stimulation, the adrenals will atrophy, otherwise they will not. The ACTH test is a test that the hypothalamus and pituitary provide some sort of adrenal stimulation at least every few days. It is not a test that they provide adequate adrenal stimulation, or that they stimulate adrenal steroid production at appropriate times. An exercise stress test is a direct verification that the hypothalamus and pituitary are activating the adrenals at the appropriate time.

Therapy with Prescription Medications

THERAPEUTIC TRIAL FOR MERCURY POISONING

When a definitive diagnosis cannot be made because of economic or other constraints on testing or in cases of truly ambiguous test results, a therapeutic trial to observe the effects of agents that alter the amount of mercury in circulation is warranted. Such trials will in general be conducted while you still have your amalgams in and are subjected to continuing exposure. Part of the point of such trials is to observe side effects that may be induced. Thus these trials are NOT 100% safe, and the agents are NOT equivalent to aspirin! However, such trials can quickly answer the question of whether mercury is contributing to your problem.

The point of a therapeutic trial is to provide enough information to you that you can decide whether or not to have your amalgam fillings replaced. Therapeutic trials should not be conducted unless they are needed to make a treatment decision.

The best agent for therapeutic trials is DMPS administered orally. DMPS is investigational in the United States. Thus it may not be available or it may not be appropriate for a given physician to prescribe

it. DMPS gives a MUCH sharper suppression of symptoms than DMSA and thus a much more clear cut response or nonresponse to a therapeutic trial.

These agents do not change the body burden of mercury significantly during the trial. They simply change the amount of free mercury in plasma. Thus, they suppress symptoms for a few days during and after administration.

Giving chelating agents while mercury exposure is ongoing will also mobilize additional mercury, so extensive therapy should not be used.

Since these agents induce side effects by redistributing mercury, the presence of side effects confirms the presence of toxic levels of mercury. Since some of these side effects can be severe and they are not predictable, no attempt should be made to induce them for diagnostic purposes! However, if they do occur, or did occur earlier during another physician's chelation therapy performed on an inappropriate administration schedule, they are diagnostic.

The most typical side effects are soreness, particularly of the lower back. This soreness is over the kidneys, but is actually muscular soreness and is not caused by kidney problems. Large single doses of chelating agents such as are used for challenge tests lead to an energized slightly euphoric state followed by achiness, lower back soreness, and mild depression.

Sulfur food exclusion will make most mercury toxic people feel better in a few days. Reintroduction of sulfur foods will make them feel worse. People with high thiols will feel MUCH better and MUCH worse. People with normal or low thiols will feel slightly better for a couple of days. This is because the sulfur foods mobilize mercury. If there is some concern that the person may have slow phase 2 glutathione conjugation or low tissue levels of glutathione this trial can be conducted while administering 600 mg NAC daily. Sulfur food exclusion will make many people feel worse if conducted for a

Appendix

prolonged period. Only people who have elevated plasma cysteine and are sensitive to dietary thiols should exclude sulfur foods indefinitely.

An appropriate DMPS therapeutic trial is 50-100 mg every 8 hours for 5 days. An appropriate DMSA therapeutic trial is 100-250 mg every 4 hours for 5 days. The effects of the DMSA are subtle enough that some care must be taken to evaluate patient mood, energy, symptoms, and behavior several times during the two weeks starting with the trial.

Lipoic acid should not be used for therapeutic trials before amalgam removal. If it was taken as a nutritional supplement without understanding of its nature as a chelating agent, the typical effect will have been to feel better for a few days, then progressively feel worse until it was discontinued.

The largest effects of chelation will be on subjective symptoms. Careful evaluation of these is necessary.

THERAPEUTIC TRIAL FOR YEAST (CANDIDA) OVERGROWTH

Intestinal overgrowth of yeast is common and often goes along with mercury poisoning. It can cause a great amount of discomfort independent of the mercury. There are a variety of laboratory tests for yeast infection.

One very direct test for yeast infection is to administer a medicine - nystatin - that kills yeast and see if you react to it. If yeast is causing a problem, killing it will exacerbate this problem. Whatever symptoms flare up when enough yeast are killed are due to the yeast. If no symptom flareup occurs, then intestinal yeast is present at an appropriate level and no intestinal yeast problem exists.

Since the test is designed to cause symptoms, it is done following a procedure to ensure that it does not cause wildly excessive symptoms by killing far more yeast

at once than your body can handle. The proper way to do this is to administer slowly increasing amounts of nystatin so that a level is reached at which just enough yeast are killed to cause significant symptoms.

The doctor should give you about 5 grams of Nystatin powder in the purest obtainable form.

Each day, you take a glass or plastic jar, a half cup of <u>distilled</u> water, a quarter teaspoonful of baking soda, and that day's nystatin and mix it up in the jar. Keep the jar refrigerated.

The first day, 1/16 tsp of nystatin is used. The next day, 1/8, the next, 1/4, the next, 1/2, the next 1 tsp.

You mix up that day's nystatin, the baking soda, and the water in the jar and refrigerate it. Each two hours or thereabouts, you take a sip from the jar. More or less a half ounce. This is done all day until bedtime. Any liquid left at bedtime is discarded.

Whenever you experience a definite worsening of symptoms that you are sure is due to the nystatin, stop taking it. After waiting a day or two, try again using the same amount of nystatin. If the symptom recurs, the test is over, you have a yeast problem, and there is some information available (from the amount of nystatin required) as to its severity.

Therapy with candidastatic agents is then used to keep you comfortable during mercury detox. A sulfur food exclusion diet is also likely to be helpful, and may resolve the yeast problem. The yeast will not stay in control if you do not also take things to restore your normal intestinal flora, like lactobacillus acidophilus, bifidobacteria, and fructooligosaccharides.

If you worked up to a teaspoon of nystatin in a day using this method and had no worsening of symptoms, you do not have a significant yeast problem at this point and

Amalgam Illness: Diagnosis and Treatment

therapy directed at yeast is not presently required.

MYCOPLASMA THERAPEUTIC TRIAL

Take 100 mg doxicycline (or any tetracycline) twice a day for 3 weeks. Feeling better towards the end of the trial and for a week or two afterwards implies mycoplasma are part of your problem. Note that this therapeutic trial will also affect gut flora and exacerbate yeast problems.

PREDNISOLONE TAPER

A quick therapeutic trial may be conducted with a 5-7 day prednisolone taper with the following number of 5 mg tablets administered at 8 AM and noon (with meals!!!).

Day:	1	2	3	4	5	6	7
8 AM	6	5	4	3	2	1	0.5
Noon	3	2.5	2	1.5	1	0.5	0

Omit days 1 and 2 for a 5 day taper. Have 32 tablets prescribed for 7 days and 16 tablets for 5 days. Count them out into weekly 'pill minder' boxes, or have the pharmacist dispense them that way. People lighter than 100 pounds should consider reducing the rate at which the dosage falls.

Remember, this is not like taking an aspirin or an antihistamine. Do it thoughtfully - it has a lot of profound effects on your body. If you do it properly, and for the right reason, some of them can be quite magical and good. They can also be pretty devastating if you play around.

Tapers like these can dramatically reduce allergy problems for a month or more, suppress inflammation or autoimmune problems, promote healing, and greatly relieve chronic fatigue. They are also mood elevating in the long term and euphoric in the short term for most people.

You can expect to experience some symptoms of temporary adrenal insufficiency - tiredness and achiness in the evenings being the most common, with a reduced heart rate and blood pressure in the evenings on high dose days - when you are tapering down the dose. If these are too uncomfortable, taper the dose off more slowly.

If a longer and higher dose taper is needed, it can be taken from the following tables. The 'short taper' above is just the first 7 days of the 50 kg body weight table. These tables are given for people of varying weights - use the table for your weight OR LESS. Using a lower weight table means the dose is tapering down more slowly for you.

These tables give doses for a taper starting at EXTREMELY HIGH LEVELS, and the total number of tablets that must be prescribed to do the taper. Glucocorticoids can cause psychiatric problems. By far the greatest risk of is on the high dose days[1]. Sometimes the taper feels like a wild roller coaster ride. Other times you wonder if anything is happening. Your subjective response to them is unpredictable.

The taper should be started at whatever is considered the highest reasonable dose and go down from there. It is also perfectly reasonable to start it at a given dose and use that dose for 1-5 days, then taper down as shown. Tapers with an initial hold at relatively low doses (less than 0.5 mg/kg

---

[1] The risk rises exponentially with dose, and reaches 1 chance in a hundred per day at 2 mg/kg. Every conceivable kind of problem occurs. People with a history of psychiatric problems are no more at risk than others. People who have experienced psychiatric problems from glucocorticoids before are no more at risk than others. Even if such problems occur, the taper schedule must be continued, though your physician should be notified immediately and you should work with him to keep things under control. The risk for a significant emotional disturbance to occur during the course of a taper is 4% or 1 in 25 for a taper starting at 2 mg/kg, 2% or 1 in 50 for a taper starting at 1.5 mg/kg, 0.6% or 1 in 167 for a taper starting at 1 mg/kg, and 0.2% or 1 in 500 for a taper starting at 0.5 mg/kg.

Appendix

prednisolone at a constant level for a few days, then tapering off) increase immunoglobulin levels and reduce T suppressor cell numbers. Tapers at high doses (greater than 1 mg/kg prednisolone and immediately tapering off) reduce immunoglobulin levels and reduce B cell number.

For a 50 kg (110#) person,

mg/kg	2.0		1.5			1.0				0.5			
7-8 AM	13	11	10	9	8	7	6	5	4	3	2	1	0.5
12-2 PM	7	6	5	4	4	3	3	2.5	2	1.5	1	0.5	0
Total number of tablets	119	99	82	67	54	42	32	23	16	10	5	2	1

For a 65kg (145#) person,

mg/kg	2.0		1.5			1.0				0.5			
7-8 AM	18	15	13	12	11	9	8	7	5	4	2.5	1	0.5
12-2 PM	9	7	6	6	5	4	4	3	2.5	2	1	0.5	0
Total number of tablets	156	129	107	88	70	54	41	29	19	12	6	2	1

For a 80kg (175#) person,

mg/kg	2.0		1.5			1.0			0.5				
7-8 AM	22	18	16	14	13	11	10	8	6	4	3	2	1
12-2 PM	11	9	8	7	6	5	5	4	3	2	1.5	1	0
Total number of tablets	191	158	131	107	86	67	51	36	24	15	9	4	1

For a 95kg (210#) person,

mg/kg	2.0		1.5			1.0			0.5				
7-8 AM	26	23	19	17	15	13	11	9	7	5	3.5	2	1
12-2 PM	13	11	10	8	7	6	5	4.5	3.5	2.5	1.5	1	0
Total number of tablets	225	186	152	123	98	76	57	41	27	17	9	4	1

On the days where dosage is 0.5 mg/kg or above, 1 mg prednisolone or 5 mg hydrocortisone with dinner may make the evening more comfortable.

2 mg/kg is an EXTREMELY LARGE dose with DRAMATIC side effects. 1 mg/kg is a VERY LARGE dose with SUBSTANTIAL side effects. 0.5 mg/kg is a BIG dose with SIGNIFICANT side effects.

Overweight people should calculate a dose based on their ideal body weight unless they have done this before and have a clear idea of how it affects them.

You and your doctor can design your own taper too. If the doctor has experience with a particular way of doing it, by all means use that! The basic rule of thumb when coming up with your own is that you should not have the dose fall by more than 33% from one day to the next (which is much more rapidly than in the tapers above) or you are sure to get adrenal insufficiency problems for a few days. If you do get the achey, spaced out, low blood pressure, slow heart rate adrenal insufficiency symptoms they mean you are tapering your dose down too fast and need to change your dosage schedule to a longer, gentler taper.

IMPORTANT PRECAUTIONS: Once you start a taper, you can't just stop it cold turkey - you have follow it down to the end. It can be very dangerous to stop cold turkey and you MUST have medical supervision if you need to do that, or to change how you are tapering.

The prednisolone will cause your stomach to make a LOT of extra stomach acid. You are likely to get gastric acid reflux. Taking H2 blockers for a few days and lots of antacids helps[1]. ALWAYS take the medicine with food! ALWAYS!! If you wake up at night with a LOT of pain in your chest, all the way from your stomach to your throat, it is probably reflux. Sip baking soda dissolved in water, stay upright, and be patient - the pain will get better in about an hour. Try to sleep sitting up after reflux if you can. If you are able to sleep with the head of your bed elevated, or in a reclining chair, you are less likely to have reflux. Also, do not eat less than 2 hours before you go to bed. Try not to eat a high carbohydrate meal or other acid producing meal (e. g. not spicey) after noontime. Do not do tapers more closely spaced than ever 2-3 months without talking to your physician about "HPA suppression" and wearing a medical alert bracelet if s/he thinks it is appropriate. The 2 month interval is most appropriate for relatively short 5-7 day tapers.

MAGNESIUM AND VITAMIN C INJECTIONS

Many mercury toxic or otherwise fibromyalgic people are low on magnesium because they do not absorb or retain it well. Magnesium may be administered by injection to correct this and alleviate a number of symptoms until the body is able to absorb and retain it naturally. In addition, intravenous vitamin C, or vitamin and mineral drips, are often used for symptom control. This appendix presents recipes and protocols on how to administer magnesium, and vitamin C, taken from a variety of sources including *Harrison's, Teitelbaum*, correspondence with a number of patients, and protocols provided by assorted physicians and compounding pharmacies. Many compounding and other pharmacies can provide more extensive or specialized protocols. Some compounding pharmacies can also provide preservative free vitamin solutions for sensitive people.

If magnesium deficiency cannot be corrected through oral therapy, it can be corrected by injections. It takes a lot of them, though, and they have to be continued until your body absorbs magnesium well. If potassium is low as well, 10 meq (750 mg) standard potassium chloride supplement pills can be given just before and 4 hours after the magnesium injections. It is not generally a good idea to include potassium in solutions for injection. If you need to also get potassium at the same time you get magnesium, you can take 10 mmol (750 mg - a standard prescription potassium tablet) by

---

[1] This is the one exception to the general rule that H2 blockers should be avoided.

Appendix

mouth just before the injection, and then another 4 hours afterwards.

The amount of magnesium in 4-5 ml of 50% $MgSO_4$ for intramuscular injection is about the same as is in 10 ml of $MgCl_2$ for intravenous injection. Intramuscular injections are quick and many people find they can do it themselves instead of having a doctor or nurse do it for them. Intravenous injections must be given by a doctor and take a while. The reason for intravenous administration of magnesium is so that additional helpful things may be included at the same time.

According to *Teitelbaum*, 50% magnesium sulfate can be injected intramuscularly, 2 ml into each buttock. 0.1 to 0.2 ml of lidocaine should be mixed in with this as it is VERY PAINFUL otherwise. Harrison's does not mention the lidocaine, suggests 5 ml in one injection, and euphemistically notes that patients "do not tolerate this well." Many patients are able to give themselves intramuscular injections of 4-5 ml of 50% magnesium sulfate + 0.5-1.0 ml of lidocaine in the hip or thigh using a 1.5" 23 to 25 gauge needle after their doctor has taught them how to do it properly. People who do this do not report it being painful when they use the lidocaine.

Regardless of whether you get injected with magnesium intravenously or intramuscularly, you may experience greatly reduced blood pressure (hypotension), dizziness, and even fainting for up to a half hour afterwards. You will also feel warm and sweat. You should stay around the doctor's office for half an hour to let this run its course. If you do it yourself at home, make sure you have experienced it a few times before, sit or lie down, and don't plan on doing anything for half an hour after the injection.

Harrison's notes that to replenish the body stores of magnesium in someone deficient in it, such injections should be given 3 times a day for 5 days. This is in the context of hospitalized patients with cardiac problems.

Some physicians administer magnesium injections 3-4 times a week for the first month, then once or twice a week thereafter. Others simply start on a weekly schedule.

Your magnesium levels will not stay up in the normal range when you stop getting periodic injections until you have corrected or healed whatever is causing your body to not absorb enough magnesium or not hold on to it properly. It is not uncommon to get magnesium injections for several months to a year or two before this happens.

Most physicians are familiar with injecting vitamin B-12 to correct deficiency. Some physicians also inject other B vitamins for other uses. The amount of vitamin C that can be administered intramuscularly is not large enough to be significant if you are able to take vitamin C orally.

Harrison's describes the intravenous administration of 10 mmol (10 ml $MgCl_2$ solution) over 15 minutes with great attention to hypotension and other side effects. These side effects are greatly reduced by including calcium in the solution for injection. A typical magnesium containing solution for intravenous administration would contain:

Magnesium chloride	10 cc
Calcium chloride or gluconate	10 cc
Sodium ascorbate (250 mg/ml)	15-30 cc
Lidocaine 1%	2 cc
Sterile water for injection, if needed	25 cc

All this is drawn up into one syringe. The solution is hypertonic, and will cause pain if it infiltrates an area outside the vein. The solution is infused slowly over 10-30 minutes through a 25 gauge butterfly needle. It is best for the doctor to inject the first 0.5-1.0 ml and wait one minute to see how you respond.

Your veins are very likely spasm due to low magnesium and the doctor may need to stick several different veins to get the whole injection done. If you take your magnesium iv's on a schedule and start your program with several closely spaced intramuscular magnesium injections the vein spasm problem will be reduced since it is partly due to low magnesium.

Sodium ascorbate for injection should be used, not ascorbic acid. The pH of the solution should be approximately 7.2-7.4.

If you have low plasma sulfate or slow liver phase 2 sulfation the 10 ml magnesium chloride may be replaced with 5 ml magnesium sulfate + 5 ml sterile water for injection to provide sulfate.

The beneficial effects of the vitamin C in the intravenous injection may last longer than the magnesium. Thus a schedule such as one intramuscular magnesium sulfate injection per week and one intravenous magnesium injection per week may be appropriate.

Intravenous vitamin C as typically discussed in the context of amalgam illness or alternative medicine typically consists of administering 20-50 grams of vitamin C and possibly other materials. This is most commonly done by intravenous drip into a peripheral vein over a period of about 2 hours. Three to seven vials of sodium ascorbate (19.98 to 46.62 grams vitamin C equivalent) are added to a 500 ml standard iv bag containing sterile water for injection or 0.45% saline or ringer's solution. These solutions are hypertonic, ranging from 378 mOsm/kg for 3 vials of sodium ascorbate in sterile water to 836 mOsm/kg for 7 vials in 0.45% saline. It is not uncommon to add other materials, e. g. 1-5 standard vials of multivitamin concentrate for injection (similar to that made by Fujusawa USA or Lyphomed), individual vitamins, trace minerals, a mixture of magnesium and calcium as above in the magnesium iv, or specific preservative free vitamins.

The purpose of intravenous administration of vitamin C and other materials is to obtain blood levels well above those possible with oral administration. Normal individuals can absorb approximately 500 mg of vitamin C per hour regardless of how much is given orally[1]. Many people also have trouble with limited magnesium absorption.

Further information, protocols, and more specialized supplies may be obtained from:

Apothe'cure   (800) 969-6601 US
Dallas, TX   (800) 203-2158 Canada

Key Pharmacy   (800) 878-1322
Kent, WA   (206) 878-3900

Central Avenue Pharmacy
                  (800) 501-9715
Pacific Grove, CA (408) 373-1225

Food

Lists of foods with certain basic chemical components in them follow. These lists are NOT complete! You don't need to exclude ALL of these things from your diet! If something is giving you trouble, you need to figure out what is and limit or exclude the relevant foods. You can be allergic to more or less anything. If you have trouble with foods in the following classes it is not an allergy problem - it is because your liver is not metabolizing one of the basic components in the food.

None of this material is relevant to a rotation diet.

TYRAMINE

Things that contain tyramine are: all cheeses except cottage cheese and farmer's cheese, plus sour cream and yogurt; liver (beef, chicken, or any other), meat

---

[1] Most mammals make vitamin C metabolically and produce it in large quantities during illness and other stress. Humans do not make their own vitamin C. The average human taking oral saturation doses (which induce diarrhoea) has 5-10 grams of vitamin C in their body. Administering significantly more than this parenterally increases the ability to respond to physiological stress.

Appendix

prepared with tenderizer, fermented sausages, unrefrigerated or fermented meat or fish, game meat, dried fish, pickled fish, shrimp paste, beer or ale, nonalcoholic beer, red wine and chianti, sherry, avocados, yeast extracts such as marmite, bananas, honeydew melons, canned or overripe figs, raisins, soy sauce, miso soup, bean curd, fermented beans, and fermented seasonings.

OTHER MAO PROBLEM FOODS

Other things that can cause elevated blood pressure and other interesting symptoms in someone whose MAO isn't doing its job: overripe fava beans (dopamine); things with caffeine in them such as coffee, tea, and many sodas like colas, Dr. Pepper®, Mountain Dew®, and similar products; chocolate, and ginseng.

SULFITES

Things that contain sulfites are: (>100 ppm) sauerkraut, wine, grape juice, processed lemon and lime juice other than frozen, dried fruits, molasses, (10-100 ppm) pectin, gravies and sauces, fruit toppings, maraschino cherries, pickled peppers and other brightly colored things, pickled onions, pickles and relishes, wine vinegar, fresh shrimp, dried potatoes, (<10 ppm) cornstarch, hominy, frozen potatoes, canned potatoes, fresh fruit salad, fresh mushrooms, grapes, beer, malt vinegar, dried cod, dry soup mix, instant tea, soft drinks, syrup, sugar, jams and jellies, gelatin, coconut, cookies, frozen pizza dough, pie dough, crackers, canned items that are brightly colored, such as garbanzo beans.

Many pharmaceuticals also contain sulfites.

MELATONIN

Foods high in melatonin: oats, sweet corn, rice, japanese radish, ginger, tomatoes, bananas, and barley.

Melatonin is partially metabolized by MAO.

TRYPTOPHAN

Foods high in tryptophan: spriulina seaweed, soybean, cottage cheese, chicken liver, pumpkin seeds, grapefruit, turkey, chicken, watermelon seeds, almonds, peanuts, brewer's yeast, malted milk, milk, ice cream, and yogurt.

ASPARTAME

A very concentrated dietary source of phenylalanine is the artificial sweetener aspartame, trade name Nutrasweet®. Some people seem to react poorly to aspartame. There are many hypotheses as to why, such as that it degrades to methyl (wood) alcohol on storage.

Meat is the main dietary source of phenylalanine and tyrosine.

SALYCILATES

Foods high in salycilates and other things that require sulfation are excluded from the Feingold diet which is described in various sources. The Feingold association maintains up to date lists of foods which do not contain synthetic colors, synthetic flavors, the preservatives BHA, BHT or TBHQ, and which have certain levels of naturally occurring salycilates. They can be reached via www.feingold.org or at (516) 369-9340.

SULFUR FOODS (THIOL FOODS)

"Sulfur foods" are foods that contain free thiol groups, not literally foods that contain sulfur in any form. Things like sulfate as in epsom salts are perfectly safe for people who have trouble with "sulfur foods." If an alternative health practitioner suggests a diet that contains more "sulfur," they are actually referring to thiols.

The <u>sulfur foods</u> are: eggs, dairy products, bakery products containing whey, cysteine, eggs, or "enzymes," cabbage, bok choy, cauliflower, broccoli, broccoflower, brussels sprouts, kale, turnips, rutabagas, asparagus, onions, shallots, leeks, garlic, and coffee. If you think it is related to one of these, don't eat it. If you are very sensitive it also helps a lot to restrict your total protein intake. If you are really desperate, you can cut it as low as about a pound of meat, poultry or fish per week. If you have to do this, supplement the essential amino acids your body seems to need. This is the minimum required for to prevent protein malnutrition presuming you absorb it adequately. Take branched chain amino acids and glutamine if you have to restrict your protein intake.

If you need to avoid sulfur foods the following discussion will be helpful.

Menus based on celery carrots eggplant peppers lettuce tomato dumplings biscuits pasta rice corn cornbread (that you make) tomato sauce, canned tomatoes (Read the labels carefully, most of them have added ingredients), beans, peas, squash, etc. are good. Most fruit is fine and is pretty convenient. Apples peaches pears plums berries and melons are sulfur free, though DRIED fruit almost always has sulfites ("preserved with SO$_2$" is chemically the same as sulfites).

Bananas, avocados and honeydew melons don't have sulfur but they do have other things some people have trouble with.

If you go to a reasonably high class grocery store and look around at the upscale bread you will often find a brand that is made traditionally and has no cysteine or related sulfury things in it. Such breads have flour (or assorted kinds of flour) with all the usual enriching additives in it, plus water salt and yeast as their ingredients.

Things you need to exclude from the vitamin stack if you are "sulfur food" sensitive are cysteine, glutathione, msm (methylsulfonylmethane), DMSO, extracts of the vegetables mentioned above, chlorella, dairy source acidophilus, and you need to be aware that other stuff - particularly herbal extracts - might also be contributing to the problem by having thiol groups in them. Don't freak out and stop the vitamins - just read the labels and pull or replace any specific ones you see a clear problem with.

COPPER

Copper containing foods: organ meats such as beef liver or kidney, chicken liver. Bone meal; shellfish, salmon, seafood; nuts, almonds, pecans, walnuts, pistachios; wheat germ, wheat bran, barley, oats; avocados, mushrooms, radishes, beets, green leafy vegetables; corn oil and margarine; yeast, brewer's yeast, garlic, blackstrap molasses, oranges and raisins, many kinds of dried fruit.

Beans and lentils, especially dried ones, are particularly high in copper. Soybeans and soy products like tofu contain much copper. Many fast food products such as hamburgers are "extended" with soy protein. "meatless" sausages, burgers, bacon, etc. is usually soy based.

Vegetarian diets are often high in copper.

Other copper sources:

Copper sulfate is also used in swimming pools to prevent algae growth, and is often sprayed on fruits and vegetables as a fungicide. If you cook in copper pans a large amount of copper can dissolve into your food. Some houses with copper plumbing have significant amounts of copper in the water.

How to get your medical records

Different states have different laws on whether you have a right to your records. Regardless, if you want a complete copy of your records, most physicians will charge you for them. If you request copies of test results as they come in these will usually be given to you for free.

If your physician doesn't want to give you your records and you don't live in a state where you have a right to them or you don't want to make a fuss insisting on it, most physicians will send your records to ANOTHER physician if you sign a release authorizing them to do so. They can charge you for this if they wish, but many do not. It is of course best to have your records sent to a physician you already know is willing to give you a copy.

Once you start collecting records, it is best to routinely get copies of test results at each appointment. You should also keep your own notes of what happens during the appointment.

When you get copies of records you should go over what the physician wrote down - they will often make interesting notes of things they observed that they didn't mention to you.

Many large practices and HMO's don't do a very good job of record keeping and much material may be missing from your chart. If it is really important to you, sometimes laboratories can generate another report from old test reports on microfilm or their computer. Laboratories can only send these to a physician - some will send it to any physician you request, others only to the physician who ordered it. They usually will tell you over the phone whether they can find anything. You of course have to figure out which laboratory was used.

Sources

Clinical laboratories:

Accuchem
(a division of FHS inc.)
990 Bowser, Suite 800
Richardson, TX
(972) 234-5412

(800) 451-0016

Accuchem offers blood tests for organic solvents and pesticides that are suitable for diagnosing and treating environmental illness and toxicities due to environmental exposure.

Diagnos-techs
POB 58948
Seattle, WA 98130-1948
(425) 251-0596

Diagnos-techs offers various tests, including an adrenal stress index that includes diurnal cortisol rhythm, and a saliva test for sIgA and anti-gliadin antibodies.

Doctor's Data Inc.
PO Box 111
West Chicago, IL 60186-0111

(800)323-2784
(630)231-3649 voice
(630)231-9190 fax
inquiries@doctorsdata.com

Doctor's Data offers urine, hair and blood elements, plasma and urine amino acids, and a variety of other tests relevant to liver metabolism.

Great Smokies Diagnostic
Laboratory, Inc.
63 Zillicoa Street
Asheville, NC 28801

(800)522-4762
cs@gsdl.com
www.greatsmokies-lab.com

Great Smokies offers a wide variety of tests relevant to amalgam illness and other conditions, and also has a readable and informative laborabory manual explaining the tests in detail that they will send to any licensed health care practitioner of any sort. Their web site is also quite informative.

Metametrix, Inc.
5000 Peachtree Industrial Blvd.
Norcross, GA 30071
(800)221-4640
(770)446-5483 voice
(770)441-2237 fax
meta@atlanta.com
www.metametrix.com

Metametrix offers a wide variety of tests relevant to amalgam illness and other conditions. They have a useful packet of information they will distribute to anyone interested. Their web site is quite informative.

Specialty Laboratories
2211 Michigan Avenue
Santa Monica, CA 90404-3900
(310)828-6543
(800)421-4449

Specialty Laboratories offers a wide variety of tests to evaluate the immune system, endocrine system, nervous system, autoimmune processes, and gain the type of precise information needed to figure out what is happening and what to do about it when run of the mill health plan lab panels aren't adequate.

This list is not intended as an endorsement of any particular laboratory and is certainly far from complete. These laboratories offer specialized tests that are not widely available from other laboratories, and are not yet well known among physicians.

Nutritional supplements are widely available through health food stores, stores specializing in supplements, and also via mail order and on the web. In addition many common supplements are available at grocery and drug stores.

Mail order has great advantages for seriously ill mercury poisoned people, and a few good sources are:

The Vitamin Shoppe
4700 Westside Avenue
North Bergen, NJ 07047

(800)223-1216
www.vitaminshoppe.com

The Vitamin Shoppe has an extensive catalogue that includes the product lines of many other manufacturers as well.

HealthSmart
1921 Miller Drive
Longmont, CO 80501

(800)492-3003
www.HSvitamins.com

Bronson
1945 Craig Road
PO Box 46903
St. Louis, MO 63146-6903

(800)235-3200

Vitamin Research Products, inc.
3579 Highway 50 East
Carson City, NV 89701

(800)877-2447
www.vrp.com

Life Extension Foundation
PO Box 229120
Hollywood, FL 33022-9120

(800)544-4440
www.lef.org

The LEF has a very informative web page explaining what to do with the vitamins and herbal supplements, as well as what they are.

Appendix

Allergy Research Group
30806 Santana Street
Hayward CA 94544
(800)782-4274
(510)487-8526
(800)688-7426 fax
(510)487-7427fax
www.nutricology.com
order@nutricology.com

ARG has particularly useful products for highly allergic and reactive individuals. The products are fairly pure and are often derived from other than the usual source so that they are tolerated by people who react to the small amount of source material that comes through in the purified products (e. g. beet derived vitamin C rather than corn derived vitamin C).

Chelation Considerations

My basic approach in determining an appropriate chelation schedule is to minimize the redistribution of mercury which occurs following a substantial decline in chelator blood concentration. This redistribution appears to be less when the decline happens after a period of chelation - and the number of redistribution events can be minimized for a given amount of chelation by using relatively long chelation campaigns.

Side effects can never be eliminated. You will always have some. The more poisoned you are, the worse they will be. But these protocols will give you the least side effects you can get. A proper protocol will also vastly reduce the risk of adverse reactions - those times when really nasty things happen and you get a lot worse for a long time. There is no reason to take a chance on these.

First, here is the basic chemistry of chelating agents and what they do. The body is full of thiol groups. Chemically, these are -SH groups attached to body tissues that grab onto things like mercury ions and hold them.

Thus a medicine or nutrient with ONE thiol group will make the mercury in a person's body bounce around faster. This will cause a lot more damage, but it makes the mercury come out a little faster. A chelating agent is something with TWO OR MORE thiol groups in the same molecule which holds onto the mercury more tightly than a lone thiol group. Thus a chelating agent is more likely to pick up a mercury and move it a long ways - perhaps out of the body - before redepositing it and allowing it to do more damage. Mercury does its damage when it first settles down on the thiol groups that are a natural part of the human body. This is why chelating agents are much safer for mercury removal than penicillamine, glutathione, cysteine, high sulfur foods, chlorella, MSM, etc. Such things are not really chelating agents. Things that have two thiols and actually are chelating agents are DMPS, DMSA, BAL, and lipoic acid. The way chelators and monothiol agents work is shown schematically in the figure on page 200.

For DMSA, literature kinetics in healthy volunteers show that blood concentrations of active, unmetabolized chelator remain within a factor of 2 of the peak for a period of about 4 hours following oral administration. Thus I suggest administration every 4 hours or more frequently during a chelation campaign. For DMPS the appropriate figure seems to be 8 hours. For lipoic acid the literature indicates that it and its metabolite bisnorlipoic acid should be present in reasonable concentrations for 3-4 hours.

Exacerbated symptoms occur about 6 hours after taking a single dose of DMSA and about 10-12 hours after taking a single dose of DMPS. These exacerbations do not occur during a series of doses spaced more closely together. Taking DMSA every 4 hours and DMPS every 8 hours greatly reduce side effects and practically eliminate adverse reactions. The figure on page 201 shows how taking closely spaced doses of a chelating agent maintains a steady blood level, while taking it at too widely separated of intervals leads to spikes or bumps in chelator concentration.

Amalgam Illness: Diagnosis and Treatment

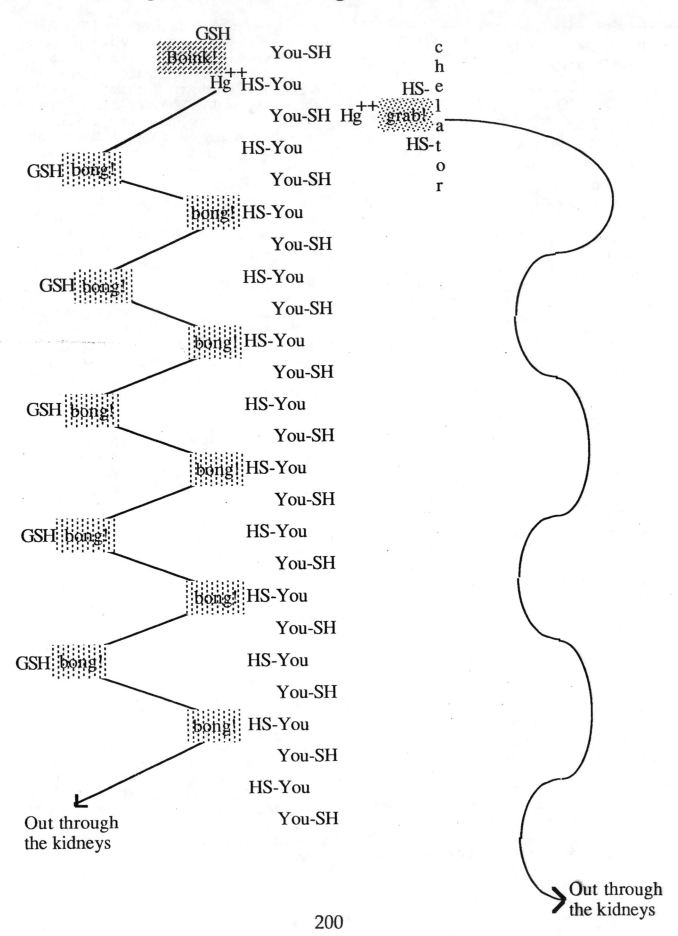

Appendix

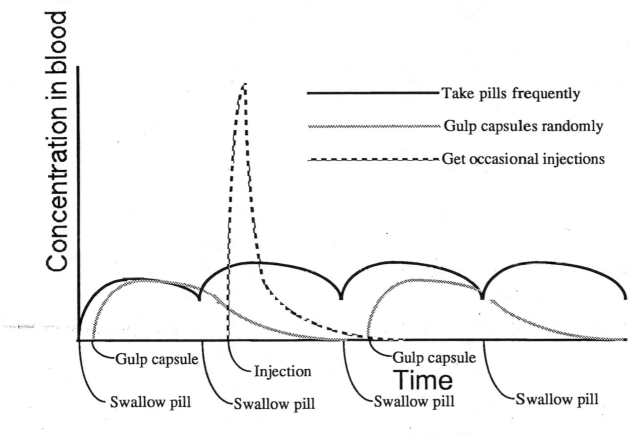

The sharp spike in drug concentration caused by an injection, or the bumps caused by occasional oral dosing, are compared to the relatively steady level of drug maintained in the bloodstream by giving periodic doses by mouth.

Literature reports show that DMPS and DMSA may redistribute mercury to motor neurons in mice if given in well separated periodic high doses. Examples of adverse reactions seen when using DMSA every other day include: marked weakness and ataxia (e. g. going from being an avid dancer to needing a cane and a handicapped parking permit within 3 weeks of commencing therapy), psychosis, dementia, and severe insomnia. This is consistent with redistribution of mercury to selected neurons. My personal experience of reproducible symptoms on single oral doses, or single daily doses of both DMPS and DMSA also indicates redistribution. The "DMPS backfires" discussed so frequently among patients are also believed to be caused by redistribution. The most frequent DMPS reaction is anxious, agitated depression with suicidal ideation leading to suicide attempts, which occurs frequently in individuals with no history of such and no other reason for them.

Thus the protocol is to administer whatever dose of DMSA every 4 hours for several days, and to stop and wait for several days if a dose is missed.

As for starting dosage I have heard of few serious adverse effects at 100 mg, so I suggest starting at 50 mg for the first dose or two, moving up to 100 mg, and going up in steps to whatever target dosage is desired.

When used later, lipoic acid should be administered every 3 to 4 hours and started at 25-50 mg and increased as tolerated. DMSA or DMPS should be used with it if possible.

201

Amalgam Illness: Diagnosis and Treatment

People who experience significant side effects on these dosage schedules may be fast metabolizers and should try more frequent administration. Prompt reactions are probably reactions to the drug. Reactions that grow over a series of doses are probably reactions to mercury redistribution, which would suggest more frequent administration.

Thus the ramping up is an increase in dosage, but the administration schedule should remain fixed at every 4 hours or more frequent. A good initial test is 50 mg every 4 hours for a day (5 doses), followed by a break of a few days.

A note for physicians: Mercury toxic individuals seem not to complain about side effects unless they are serious, and even to tolerate adverse reactions[1]. Thus it seems appropriate to offer them the therapeutic option with the least side effects for a given level of effectiveness rather than simply finding one that is tolerable enough they will continue to follow it.

Since the administration schedule above is based on a combination of theoretical argument and limited practical experience it should not be carved in stone. Anything that suits your particular needs is fine. The art of medicine consists of the clinician selecting a therapeutic regimen that fits each patient's needs without the undue experimentation an entirely theoretical or entirely empirical approach would require.

The basic factor to consider in designing chelation regimes is that DMPS and DMSA in the dosages discussed here do not dramatically accelerate mercury excretion. 100 mg DMSA every 4 hours accelerates mercury clearance by about 30%. The reason to take it is to control the symptoms of mercury intoxication during the prolonged period when mercury is naturally being cleared out of the body. It doesn't make sense to tolerate side effects worse than the original condition to accomplish this.

DMPS and DMSA do not remove mercury from the nervous system and can redistribute mercury to it. It is necessary to use a protocol specifically designed to minimize this - thus DMSA every 4 hours or DMPS every 8 hours. NEVER use DMSA every other day or DMPS injections monthly.

PDR instructions for DMSA are every 8 hours. DMSA was approved for lead poisoning for which the equilibrium between free and bound metal in blood is lower than for mercury - thus redistribution is less of a problem. I think that DMSA should be used more frequently than manufacturer's guidelines because those are for lead treatment. I suggest following following manufacturer's guidelines for DMPS because these were developed for mercury. There are no manufacturer's guidelines for lipoic acid. However the known kinetics of it and its first metabolic product, which should be an equally good chelator, indicate that it should be taken ever 3-4 hours - a little more frequently than DMSA by itself needs to be taken.

Lipoic acid DOES remove mercury from the nervous system, and DOES substantially accelerate mercury clearance. Using DMPS or DMSA with it reduces its side effects, and I speculate[2] that it synergistically accelerates mercury clearance much more than using the agents separately.

Thus from a cost/benefit perspective it seems pointless to tolerate much in the way of side effects from anything other than lipoic acid.

NB: since lipoic acid allows mercury to move through nerve cell membranes, using it when there is a high blood level of mercury, such as while amalgams are in or shortly after amalgam removal can lead to the

---

[1] the ataxia case mentioned above did not consider this to be a good enough reason to ask her physician to consider a different administration schedule.

[2] on entirely theoretical grounds which seem to be borne out by my personal experience - an uncontrolled study with N = 1.

202

Appendix

redistribution of large amounts of mercury into the nervous system with consequent exacerbation of symptoms. I suggest not using lipoic acid until urine or blood mercury is observed to have fallen 80% from its peak value for cases where the onset of poisoning was within the last 2 years, or 50% for cases where the onset of poisoning was much earlier and where it is believed current levels of mercury excretion are lower than those at the onset of poisoning. In any case, there should be a marked rise in urine or blood mercury level at the beginning of lipoic acid administration as mercury moves from the intracellular to the extracellular space. If such an increase is not observed after a week lipoic acid therapy should be deferred until blood or urine mercury fall further. Similar considerations apply to the use of cilantro[1] to chelate brain mercury.

The clinical use of DMPS and DMSA is usually described as involving 'campaigns' with breaks in between. This is necessary with lead since time must pass for it to be redistributed from the skeleton into the circulation where it can be chelated. It is less clear if this is necessary with mercury, but a series of campaigns with breaks is quite effective in suppressing symptoms.

It is important to use LA in campaigns because it reduces the liver's excretion of copper, zinc and methylmercury. Continuous administration would significantly elevate the body inventory of these materials.

Recommendations: DMPS: every 8 hours, start with 50 mg and increase succeeding doses by X1.5 or 2 until target dose is reached. Continue 4-14 days until symptoms are suppressed, then take a break of 4-14 days and repeat.

DMSA: every 4 hours, start with 50 mg and increase succeeding doses by X1.5 or 2 until target dose is reached. Continue 4-14

---

[1] I do not advocate the use of cilantro by anyone who can tolerate lipoic acid, since LA is adequately well characterized to know how to use it properly and cilantro is not.

days until symptoms are suppressed, then take a break of 4-14 days and repeat.

LA: every 4 hours, start with 25 mg and increase succeeding doses by X1.5 or 2 until target dose is reached. Take DMSA 50-100 mg with each dose or DMPS 50-100 mg with alternate doses. If side effects of emotional disturbance become marked, try taking it ever 3 hours. Continue 3-14 days (until emotional side effects become too annoying), then take a break of 4-7 days and repeat.

The specific symptoms lipoic acid exacerbates are:

LA increases urine volume

LA causes more obsessive thinking patterns

LA causes more emotional volatility (however, nothing like "sulfur foods" cause in susceptible individuals)

LA causes difficulty relating to other people and understanding their feelings and intentions

LA causes apathy and lack of motivation

LA causes mild photophobia

LA is euphoria producing so all of this is somewhat pleasant, although distracting.

LA gives the urine a very distinctive "sulfury" smell.

The liver excretes a lot more inorganic mercury when lipoic acid is taken, but excretes a lot LESS methylmercury, copper, zinc and cadmium.

These come out in feces.

LA would not be helpful for methylmercury poisoned patients.

Patients who took LA continuously would build up copper, zinc, and methylmercury (the body does make a small amount from regular mercury). So it should be taken intermittently.

Patients with low liver glutathione should take NAC all the time, especially because LA removes more glutathione from the liver than normal.

Problem: lipoic acid isn't a one way street. It just makes it easier for mercury to go back and forth between the blood and the brain. If you have a LOT in the brain, then taking LA right away will help. However, if you have more in the bloodstream than in the brain and you take LA it will move it INTO the brain.

It takes a long time for the brain to fill up with mercury so most people are expected to have more mercury in their blood. And there is no real test to tell how brain and blood mercury levels relate to each other. So it is best to get the blood (and urine) levels down a lot. If the blood level is way down from where it started, then LA is a good thing to try. Urine level is just as good a measure of mercury as a blood level. The thing to do is have ONE course of LA (with or without another chelating agent like DMPS or DMSA) and then do another measurement a few days after you have stopped taking the chelating agents. If blood or urine level of mercury is HIGHER afterwards than beforehand, that means mercury is coming out of the brain, which is good. If it doesn't go up then use regular chelating agents more and try again later when the blood or urine mercury level is a lot lower.

Suggested target doses: DMPS and DMSA: maximum tolerated dose (up to limiting dose) under ideal circumstances. Often circumstances are less than ideal, and doses as low as 50-100 mg are usually adequate in these cases. LA: half of maximum tolerated dose, with 50-100 mg DMPS/DMSA or prior dosage used (half of it if it was the maximum tolerated dose rather than the dose limit).

Appendix

DMPS, DMSA, LA, BAL, PA AND CYSTEINE STRUCTURAL FORMULAE

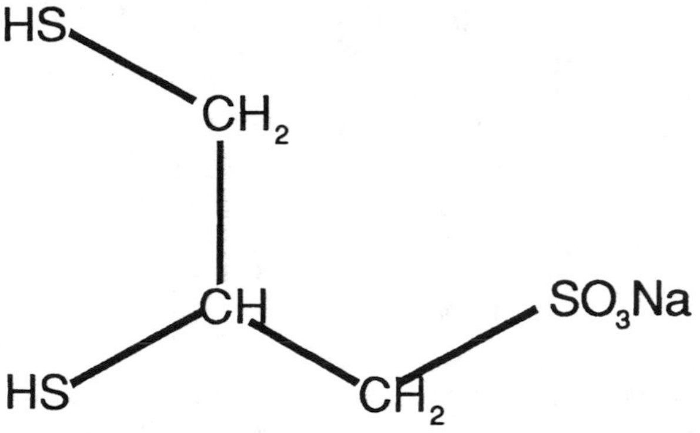

HS—CH$_2$
HS—CH—CH$_2$—SO$_3$Na

DMPS
2,3 dimercaptopropane sulfonate sodium

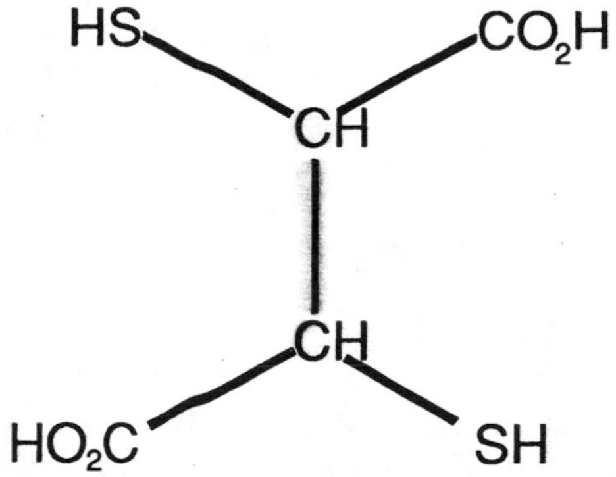

HS—CH—CO$_2$H
HO$_2$C—CH—SH

DMSA
meso-2,3 dimercaptosuccinic acid

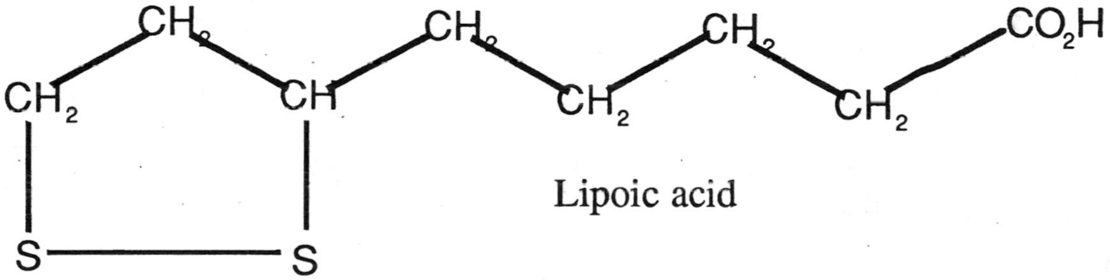

CH$_2$—CH—CH$_2$—CH$_2$—CH$_2$—CH$_2$—CO$_2$H
CH$_2$
S——S

Lipoic acid

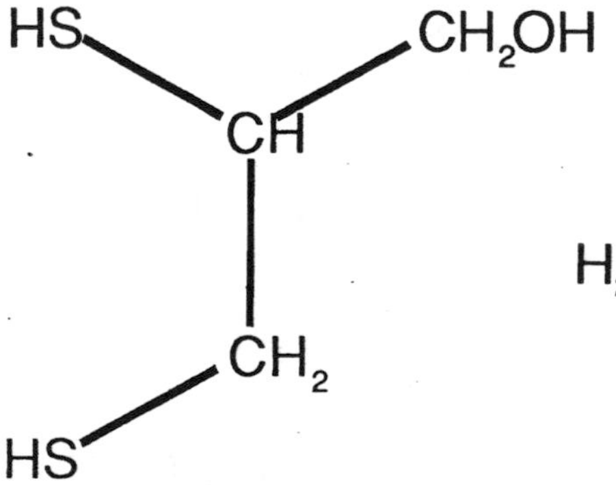

HS—CH—CH$_2$OH
HS—CH$_2$

BAL - Dimercaprol

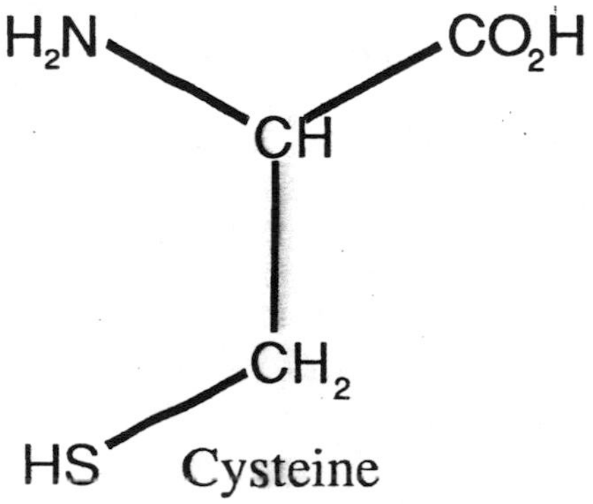

H$_2$N—CH—CO$_2$H
HS—C—CH$_3$
CH$_3$

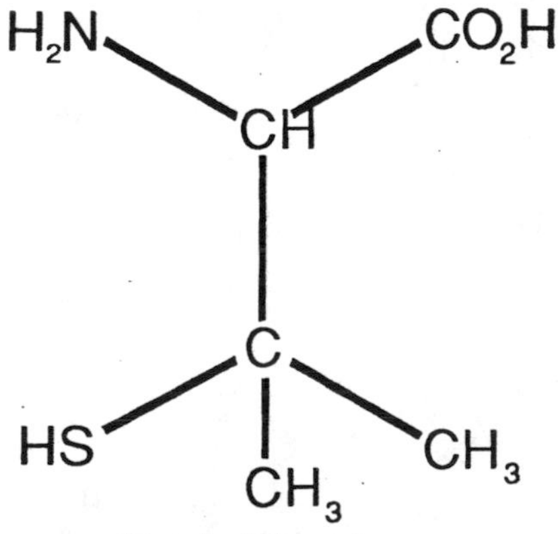

Penicillamine

H$_2$N—CH—CO$_2$H
HS—CH$_2$

Cysteine

Amalgam Illness: Diagnosis and Treatment

Chelating agent pharmacokinetics

The chelating agents DMPS and DMSA increase urinary excretion of mercury. For every 2 units of mercury that come out in urine under ordinary conditions, 5 come out in feces. Thus taking enough DMPS to increase the day's urine level of mercury (250 mg iv) actually only doubles the total excretion that day.

Thus, taking DMPS iv once a month would appear to increase overall mercury excretion about 3%. DMPS IV's have side effects and can also have dangerous adverse reactions. In addition, they are costly. It hardly seems worthwhile.

The side effects seem to be from grabbing a bunch of mercury, stirring it up, and dropping it as the DMPS level goes down. Anecdotally it appears that people who take DMPS by mouth only experience side effects when they STOP taking it. They have to take it every 8-12 hours to have no side effects during therapy. The side effects experienced after oral therapy are quite mild compared to those experienced after parenteral therapy. Intramuscular administration is associated with somewhat greater side effects than is intravenous administration.

As anecdotally reported by amalgam illness victims, 100 mg capsule of DMPS (any brand) increases that day's mercury in the urine by about 50%. So, three capsules a day increases TOTAL excretion by 42%. This is quite different than literature reports relating to the DMPS challenge in mercury exposed individuals, e. g. by Molin or Aposhian, would lead one to believe. Apparently there is a vastly different body distribution or metabolism of mercury in amalgam illness victims versus healthy people that is overlooked in the mainstream medical literature.

Again anecdotally, 100 mg of DMSA every 4 hours approximately doubles the day's urine mercury, increasing total excretion about 28%.

The above figures are consistent with literature reports on DMSA and DMPS. While rate laws for mercury excretion caused by DMPS and DMSA are not reported they are reasonably apparent from the literature. One can compare the effects of different dosages very roughly by taking the ratio of the proposed dose to the dose known and raising it to the 0.63 power. E.g. if an organism ingests 300 mg DMPS and urinary excretion doubles, then taking 100 mg every 12 hours will also double daily urinary excretion, or 100 mg every 8 hours will increase it 2.5 times. DMPS remains in the body long enough that doses closer together than every 8 hours will affect each other (in humans) and the pharmacokinetics becomes much more complex. The corresponding time for DMSA is about 4 hours.

The necessary administration frequency to keep blood concentrations of chelating agent constant within a factor of two can be determined by graphical interpolation from literature reports discussing the pharmacokinetics and metabolism of DMPS, DMSA and lipoic acid. DMPS must be given every 8 hours, DMSA every 4 hours, and lipoic acid every 4 hours. Anecdotally, the exacerbation of side effects by a less frequent administration schedule is less for the lipoic acid than for DMPS or DMSA, but is not negligible.

My current best estimate of the pharmacokinetics of these materials is:

DMSA by mouth: $F_u = 1 + (d/24)^{0.409}$

DMPS by mouth: $F_u = 1 + (d/3.53)^{0.409}$

DMPS by injection: $F_u = 1 + (d/0.20)^{0.409}$

Lipoic acid by mouth: $F_f = 1 + (d/24)^{0.53}$

Lipoic acid also increases urinary excretion, but the exact formula has not yet been developed.

where d is the dose in mg/kg/day, Fu is the factor to multiply unchelated urinary excretion by and Ff is the factor to multiply unchelated fecal excretion by. Splitting the dose into 2 or 3 parts per day does increase excretion for a given amount of chelating agent. These formulae are based on a single daily dose.

Some mercury is apparently excreted in sweat. The amount is not known, and it is also not known whether chelating agents increase this amount significantly.

Since these formulae are less than order one in the chelating agent, there is an economic optimization involved in selecting dosage - increasing the dose increases costs linearly but decreases illness time less than linearly. Thus for a given value of a patient's time there is an appropriate dosage to use. In practical circumstances the numbers work out that this is relevant for DMPS and DMSA since they are so expensive. At US OTC prices lipoic acid is inexpensive enough the amount taken is more likely to be limited by your tolerance for side effects. As DMPS is anecdotally reported to control lipoic acid side effects it is possible a more sophisticated economic analysis would be appropriate for combined therapy - especially since the effectiveness of DMPS for this use, and the level of side effects it causes, are brand dependent. DMSA also controls lipoic acid side effects, though less effectively. DMSA is available by prescription in the US as a regular FDA approved drug and is more economical per unit mercury removed than DMPS - especially if bought from a compounding pharmacy.

Approximate back-of-the-envelope style calculations indicate that in the range of 2-3 DMPS capsules per day or 4-6 DMSA capsules per day the added cost of taking enough more chelating agent to bring the cure forward one day is roughly $50-$100.

Using the above formulae to work examples,

	daily excretion	
urine	//	no
chelating agent		
feces	/////	
total	7	
urine	/////	100 mg
DMPS by mouth every 8 hours		
feces	/////	
total	10	
urine	///// /////	300 mg
DMPS by mouth every 8 hours		
feces	/////	
total	15	
urine	////	100 mg
DMSA by mouth every 4 hours		
feces	/////	
total	9	
urine	//	100 mg
LA by mouth every 4 hours		
feces	///// ///	
total	10	

Alpha lipoic acid is interesting. A related compound, lipoamide, was used in laboratory experiments on chronically mercury poisoned rats in the former Soviet Union. It was also used to treat some mercury poisoned Polish people. It is supposed to work well. It makes the extra mercury come out in the feces. It crosses the blood brain barrier unlike DMPS or DMSA and thus gets mercury out of the brain.

IMPLICATIONS OF KINETICS FOR AMALGAM ILLNESS

Being a chemical engineer and simply viewing the body as a complicated pile of pipes and tanks and pumps instead of the wondrously complex biological system it really is I can use the known kinetics in the literature to say a few things.

The problem in amalgam illness is caused by mercury in the BRAIN, or the IMMUNE SYSTEM, not elsewhere. This is because the mercury builds up to levels that are very toxic to these over a long period of exposure, but can't damage these organs rapidly during short exposures. This is different than what happens during brief large exposures where the kidney is damaged and the other organs are not hurt as much.

It takes a long time to get mercury into the brain, which is why nobody dies or goes crazy the week after going to the dentist.

The poisoning is all brain poisoning and unless it happens in the few months right after a bunch of new dental work, the kidneys aren't going to be involved.

It takes a long time to get mercury OUT of the brain so a person with very low current mercury excretion can be severely mercury poisoned with a high brain burden and a low body burden.

While there is much literature discussion that mercury moves in and out of the human brain quite slowly (and is apparent in the brain at very high levels at autopsy following decades of nonexposure) I am not aware of any literature reports that are detailed enough to allow any estimates to be made of either these rates or simply of the equilibrium amount of mercury in the brain in relation to blood levels.

The therapeutic approach of monthly DMPS injections is ineffective. Since it also has serious risks as well as mundane side effects[1] as well as being expensive, this therapeutic approach is contraindicated in all cases.

Dosage schedules that proved to minimize side effects were what one would expect from the reported literature pharmacokinetics

---

[1] Researchers in the area apparently do not keep statistics. Estimates from anecdotal reports are: risk of death may be as high as 1%, risk of death by suicide consequent to DMPS produced depression is significant, risk of long term or permanent disability is 2-5%. Risks are per patient, not per injection. Adverse events do not always follow the first injection of DMPS. They may occur at any point during therapy.

of these substances in healthy volunteers: DMPS by mouth every 8 hours for 1 week, DMSA by mouth every 4 hours for 1-2 weeks, or LA by mouth every 3-4 hours for 1-3 weeks, with breaks in between. DMPS and DMSA dosages will usually be driven by economics. 50-100 mg of DMPS or DMSA. Up to 1.8 grams per day of LA have been used, with substantial behavioral side effects. Combined therapy with 50-100 mg DMSA + 25-200 mg LA for 3-4 days, both taken at the same time every 3-4 hours has also been used and seems to be especially effective at removing mercury from the brain. The emotional and behavioral side effects from this are very different than from LA alone.

COMPARING ASSORTED URINE MERCURY TESTS TO EACH OTHER:

Using the standard formulae above, I calculate that the relationship between the amount of mercury in a 6 hour plain urine sample and a 6 hour urine sample following 500 mg DMSA po is:

unchallenged value = 0.31 X challenged value

There is of course some variation in the multiplying factor from individual to individual and from time to time, but this will give a reasonable estimate (almost certainly better than $\pm$ 30%) of one result if the other is known.

The amount of mercury expected in a 24 hour iv DMPS challenge test is about 5 X the 6 hour, 500 mg DMSA po challenge amount, permitting comparison.

The amount of mercury expected in a 24 hour 2 gram DMSA po (all at once - not a protocol I recommend) challenge is 2.45 X the 500 mg DMSA po 6 hour value. This is numerically also the same as the amount of mercury expected with a 24 hour 300 mg DMPS po challenge.

An approximate conversion factor table is given below which can be used to convert from or to various chelated or challenge results and unchelated 24 hour urine mercury results. Remember that there is day to day variation if one person repeats the same test many times, and that nobody has exactly the "theoretical" kinetics as given by the equations used to generate this. However, if the numbers are several times different than what this table predicts it is likely there was an error in sample collection, analysis, or challenge agent administration.

Test protocol	to24h	from 24h
300 mg DMPS po[1]	0.51	1.96
2 gm DMSA po 24h	0.48	2.08
2 gm DMSA 200 mg at a time	0.28	3.59
2 gm DMSA 250 mg at a time	0.28	3.61
DMPS 3 mg/kg iv	0.25	4.00
500 mg DMSA po 6h	1.22	0.82
200 mg DMSA po 6h	1.56	0.64
unchelated 24h	1.00	1.00

For example, my personal results before amalgam removal and chelation came out as follows (in micrograms of mercury in a 24 hour urine sample):

Sampling condition	Measured	Calc.
300 mg DMPS po 24h	17, 18	16.4
2 g DMSA po 24h	16	17.5
DMPS 3 mg/kg iv 24h	not meas.	33.9
500 mg DMSA po 6h	not meas.	6.9
Plain 24h mercury	8.4	8.5

Mathematical background for diagnosis

There are many laboratory test abnormalities alleged to go along with amalgam illness. There is no one salient abnormality that is always present.

One may use standard bayesian statistical formulae to address this problem.

$$C = \frac{i * P1 * P2 * P3 * \ldots}{i * P1 * P2 * \ldots + (1 - i) * P'1 * P'2 * \ldots}$$

where C is the chance (probability, $0 < C < 1$) that a patient with certain test results has amalgam illness, P1 is the probability that test 1 comes out the way it did, P2 the probability for test 2, etc, when the patient has amalgam illness. P'1 etc are the probabilities these tests come out the way they do for that patient if that patient is a member of the non-amalgam illness population. i is the incidence of amalgam illness in the general population.

Laboratory test "normal ranges" are defined so that 97.5% of the population lies below the upper cutoff (or above the lower cutoff) and 2.5% on each side of the "normal range." Thus the P' s are 0.975 or 0.025 as appropriate.

The Ps are a bit more problematic, since we don't have good survey data. However, it is a well known approach in this kind of case to use 0.5 as it gives the least sensitivity of the result to variation in the actual value. In a technical sense it is also the rigorous approach. Later estimates of P can be used to improve the procedure.

One may note there is no need to depend on any measurement of mercury, and thus no need to resolve arguments about mercury metabolism and whether some individuals become intoxicated because they fail to excrete it or are unusually sensitive to it.

More sophisticated formulae may be developed using the fact that clinical laboratory test results are assumed to be normally distributed, but it is unlikely practitioners will apply anything more complicated than counting the number of abnormal results on a test panel. The proper statistical problem is to determine the right test panel to run.

One may rewrite this for n abnormal results and m normal results as:

---

[1] po means by mouth.

$$C = \frac{i * P+{}^{\wedge}n * P-{}^{\wedge}m}{i * P+{}^{\wedge}n * P-{}^{\wedge}m + (1-i) * P'+{}^{\wedge}n * P'-{}^{\wedge}m}$$

and take the limit as n+m goes to infinity, for n << m (positives << normals).

$$Clim = \left(\frac{i}{1-i}\right) * \left(\frac{P+}{P'+}\right)^{\wedge}n * \left(\frac{P-}{P'-}\right)^{\wedge}m$$

term a	term b	term c

Now of course we know this limit expression will not be perfectly accurate at n+m < infinity, but we can still deduce some useful things from it. After all, term a is at least 1/1000. Term b is about $20^{\wedge}n$. Term c is about $0.5^{\wedge}m$.

So, to start with, we need about 2 or 3 positives in term b to multiply with term a and get somewhere near one. In addition, we need about one positive in term b for every 4 negatives in term c to 'cancel' them out and keep the result somewhere near one.

What does this mean? If we have a long string of tests that might be affected by mercury, then the number of tests for which actual measurements exist for a given patient is n+m. The probability that the patient in question has mercury poisoning is high if n is appropriately high. The probability is low if n is appropriately low. Further testing or appropriate clinical judgement is required if n is in the middle. The numerical assumptions above suggest the following if we assume about 0.1% of the population has amalgam illness:

total tests (n+m)	n which confirms mercury poisoning	n which excludes mercury poisoning
5	4 or more	0
10	5 or more	0
15	6 or more	1
20	7 or more	2
25	8 or more	3
30	9 or more	4
35	10 or more	5
40	11 or more	6
45	12 or more	7

In this context I have interpreted "excluded" and "included" in the same way laboratory test "abnormal" results are defined: the diagnosis is confirmed if the probability is greater than 97.5 percent, and it is excluded if the probability is less than 2.5 percent.

If one wishes to assume a population incidence of 1 in 50, the table becomes:

total tests (n+m)	n which confirms mercury poisoning	n which excludes mercury poisoning
5	3 or more	0
10	4 or more	1
15	5 or more	2
20	6 or more	3

The use of 'check lists' for diagnosis is not new to physicians. Conditions such as schizophrenia or rheumatoid arthritis are diagnosed when an adequate number of items on a defined checklist are observed. See, for example, *Harrison's Principles of Internal Medicine.*

Symptomatic diagnosis - accurate numeric procedure derived

The diagnostic symptom checklists were derived from data presented by Lichtenberg. The accurate probability factors thus calculated were approximated to create checklists for ease of use. For those who would like to calculate more accurate probabilities than can be done by using the symptom checklist, it may be done as follows:

Check off the symptoms below and multiply together all the factors f by the checked off symptoms. Ignore the unchecked symptoms. This yields one combined factor F.

Appendix

Probability of having amalgam illness
$$= 1 / (1 + ((1-i)/i) * 973.5 * F)$$

where i is the incidence of amalgam illness in the general population ($0<i<1$). Use whichever factor you think is appropriate for that. Personally I estimate it as 1-5% (i = 0.01 to 0.05) and usually use 0.1% (i = 0.001) in statistical calculations like this in order to be conservative.

This probability is based only on the symptoms, and one could then combine it with the probability of having amalgam illness calculated from history, physical examination and laboratory tests, or one could use it alone.

Symptom	factor
allergy	0.473
bleeding gums	0.095
tender teeth	0.103
bad breath	0.412
metallic taste	0.108
blisters and sores in mouth	0.161
sore or irritated throat	0.192
diverticulosis	0.331
Loss of appetite	0.184
diarrhea and constipation	0.362
intestinal cramps and pains	0.483
headache	0.216
fatigue	0.387
lack of concentration	0.217
fear	0.741
irritability	0.464
depression	0.778
dizziness	0.333
muscles tire easily	0.677
muscle tremor	0.267
schiatic pains	0.412
chest pains	0.203
leg cramps	0.426
joint pains	0.555
cold hands and feet	0.577
tachycardia	0.582

The toxic threshold for mercury

Public policy to date has been based on experience with industrial workers. Figure 1 shows that exposed industrial workers are biochemically distinct from the general population in their metabolism of mercury. Exposure guidelines must thus be derived by analysis of more basic research results.

Mercury compounds exert their toxic effects after metabolism to mercuric ion. In acute intoxication differences in prompt tissue distribution patterns lead to different suites of symptoms from different compounds. In chronic intoxication all sources of mercury lead to similar symptoms from equilibrated tissue distribution. Thus the appropriate exposure level to consider is the systemic intake of mercury from all sources.

Inappropriate comparison of intake rates instead of body burden between different species has led to confusion in the literature. Comparison of effects between different species depends on the amount of mercury present in the organism rather than the intake rate (Clarkson, 1972), and proper account of differences in species kinetics must be taken to compare, e. g. the rat or mouse to man. Mercury follows first order elimination kinetics in the situations pertinent to chronic exposure (Clarkson, 1972). The body burden of an organism in equilibrium with a given exposure level is

$$B = [I * t_{\frac{1}{2}} / \ln(2)] = 1.443 * t_{\frac{1}{2}} * I$$

where B is the body burden, I is the constant exposure rate, and the elimination half life of the organism is $t_{\frac{1}{2}}$. B may be calculated in amount / unit weight of organism if I is given in amount / unit weight of organism / unit time. B in units of moles / kg has the same numerical value as B in moles per liter, facilitating comparison between in vitro and in vivo work.

This formula is most familiar to medical professionals in the pharmacokinetic form:

$$B = (V_D / C_L) * I$$

and thus

$$(V_D / C_L) = (t_{\frac{1}{2}} / \ln(2))$$

where V_D is the volume of distribution and C_L the clearance rate. The half life of mercury is about 7 days in the mouse and 16 days in the rat (Clarkson, 1972). The half life of mercury in man is complex. Population exposure guidelines must be based on the longest expected mercury excretion half life in the general population - about 240 days - coupled with the highest expected sensitivity to mercury's toxic effects.

Mercury affects T cell populations and immune function in vitro at 10^{-5} to 10^{-6} $\underline{M}$, [$\underline{M}$ is moles per liter - 10^{-6} $\underline{M}$ (or 1 $\mu\underline{M}$ in customary medical units which will be used throughout this paper) mercury is 200 mcg/l or 200 mcg/kg]. Mercury also affects T cell populations and immune function in genetically susceptible strains of rodents (Eneström and Hultman 1995; Pollard and Hultman 1996) at daily intakes which result in such concentrations according to the above kinetics equations. Measurable immune system effects are also seen in mercury exposed industrial workers. Presumably workers have 'self selected' for those without genetic susceptibility to immune dysfunctions incompatible with continuing employment just as Figure 1 shows they have self selected for rapid elimination kinetics. Population exposure guidelines should prevent anyone from experiencing immune system effects so as to protect those with a genetic predisposition for conditions involving significant morbidity or mortality.

Mercuric ion directly inhibits the activity of the enzyme adenylate cyclase by 50% in brain tissue at concentrations of 0.4-0.9 $\mu\underline{M}$ (Ewers and Erbe, 1980). Behavioral effects and biochemical changes have been observed in dentists (Echeverria, Heyer, Martin, Naleway, Woods and Bittner, 1995) with mercury excretions corresponding to about 1 $\mu\underline{M}$ body burden of mercury (assuming they are all fast eliminators). Dentists, like industrial workers, may be self selected for insensitivity to mercury.

An exposure guideline incorporating no safety factor is to hold mercury below 1 $\mu\underline{M}$, or 200 mcg/kg body burden since physiological changes are observed in occupationally exposed groups at this level which are consistent with in vivo and in vitro research results. The population distribution of sensitivity to toxins is empirically observed to usually be log-normal (that is it falls on a Probit plot. See Hodgson, 1987). While the standard deviation for mercury sensitivity is unknown, the similar toxins lead and cadmium have a factor of two sensitivity deviation (Friberg, Nordberg and Vouk, 1986). Assuming 1 $\mu\underline{M}$ is the average intoxication threshold, and using a factor of 2 deviation, a safety factor of 5 protects 99% of the population, a factor of 8.5 protects 99.9%, and a factor of 13.5 protects 99.99%. The US EPA proposes a safety factor of 10 below the level at which detrimental effects are observed, which corresponds to a body burden below 0.1 $\mu\underline{M}$, or 20 mcg/kg.

It is reasonable to believe that some very sensitive people may have toxic body burdens of mercury when their urinary excretion exceeds 1 mcg/liter, or their daily exposure exceeds 3.5 mcg.

Dental amalgam - major source of mercury exposure

The population distribution for urinary mercury excretion is known (Barregård, Sällsten and Järvholm, 1995). Total excretion is 3.53 times urinary excretion (Bjorkman, Sandborg-Englund and Ekstand, 1997). Assuming equilibrium, intake is thus 3.53 * urinary excretion. Most of this mercury is believed to come from dental amalgam (Barregård, Sällsten and Järvholm, 1995; Skare and Engkvist, 1994). Illustrated mass flow calculations (Skare and Engkvist, 1994) show that the 'average person' absorbs $8.5 * 10^{-10}$ moles of amalgam derived mercury / kg / day. Thus a person with a 240 day elimination half life will achieve an equilibrium body concentration of mercury of 0.3 $\mu\underline{M}$ on the average. Given a log-normal distribution for the population's intake of mercury from their fillings with a mean of $5.4 * 10^{-10}$ moles / kg / day and a standard deviation of $6.5 * 10^-$

10 moles / kg / day[27] one can estimate that 4% of that fraction of the general population with an elimination half life of 240 days will exceed 1 μM. About 0.03% of individuals with 'short' excretion half lives of 72 days will also exceed this level due to their dental amalgams. Combining the Iraqui data on mercury excretion kinetics with the log-normal distribution of population mercury exposure allows one to estimate that at least 0.5% of the population has $\geq$ 1 μM systemic mercury concentration from their amalgams. These people are composed of roughly equal numbers of individuals with short, medium and long excretion half lives. This appears to be so for the 'environmental illness' cases shown in Figure 1 in the main text.

Exemplary numbers have been used for the sake of argument. While accurate modeling of average response to amalgam has shown that the adult population as a rule has more amalgam restorations than can be presumed safe (Richardson and Allan, 1996), and the statistical distribution of mercury uptake from amalgam has been reviewed (Weiner and Nylander, 1995), inadequate information is available in the literature to make accurate estimates of the population distribution of excretion half lives, of the actual concentration of mercury that causes adverse effects, or of interindividual variation in sensitivity to mercury. Despite these uncertainties, one must conclude that some fraction of the population greater than 1 in 200 is definitely experiencing adverse health effects from their dental amalgam. This is a large number from a public health perspective, but is dwarfed by the 30% who exceed the "safe limit" of 20 mcg/kg.

Cutaneous absorption of mercury

Solutions of mercury salts are readily absorbed through intact skin in the guinea pig (Skog and Wahlberg, 1964). Absorption was most rapid at about 1% mercury content and did not depend strongly on the other chemical constituents of the salt. Typical absorption rates were 0.15 to 0.25 μmoles/cm^2/h. Continuous exposure of 0.05

cm^2/kg of intact skin to topical solutions containing 1% mercury, e. g. merbromin or merthiolate, will result in a systemic concentration of 1 μM in a fast excreter. In practical terms this means using a bottle of mercury containing antiseptic on a 30 kg child over a period of 15 months certainly maintains systemic mercury $\geq$ 1 μM. These materials are not usually applied to intact skin - thus absorption may be greater. Mercurial preservatives are also used in assorted eye care products, vaginal contraceptives and hemorrhoid remedies. It is reasonable to assume that absorption via the eye and associated mucus membranes, vaginal mucosa, or irritated rectal mucosa is at least as high as through intact skin.

Iatrogenic exposure to mercury

Vaccines and certain other injectables are variously reported to contain thimerosal at between 1:1,000 and 1:10,000. Vaccines are typically administered in 0.5 ml doses, containing 0.124-1.24 micromoles of mercury. The recommended pediatric administration schedule brings a typical child up to between 0.04 and 0.7 μM by 4 months of age. This leaves very little safety factor for additional sources of exposure, further vaccinations, administration of several vaccinations at once or of additional thimerosal preserved injectables, or individual susceptibility. Diaper rash remedies are also preserved with thimerosal. An infant's T cells are iatrogenically exposed to a LARGE amount of mercury at a time when the immune system is maturing and, for example, deciding whether it will respond to innocuous antigens with vast amounts of immunoglobulin E for the rest of the individual's life.

Iatrogenic self exposure to mercury

It is generally recognized that dentists are at risk for mercury intoxication and must use appropriate hygiene. Other health care professionals (e. g. optometrists), may have received very large unrecognized mercury exposures from skin contact with thimerosal preserved solutions, etc., which are no longer widely used and which have indeed recently been banned in the United States (Anon., 1988). An optometrist exposing 400 cm^2 of skin (fingers and palms) to 1:10,000 thimerosal preserved contact lens cleaning solution 1 hour per working day would be expected to achieve a body concentration of 1 μM mercury before a year passed. Since the half life of mercury in the brain is variously estimated as 16-25 years and neurological impairment is observed decades after exposure ends [Kishi *et al.*, 1993], these people would reasonably be expected to experience lifelong neurobehavioral impairments while exhibiting normal levels of mercury excretion.

Index

Index

Index

Index

Index

Index

Amalgam illness: diagnosis and treatment

Tear this page out and send it in!

To order another copy of Amalgam Illness: Diagnosis and Treatment, or any of the other books on this page, you can mail this sheet in, fax it to (425) 557-2104 or phone your order in to (425) 557-8299. You can also order online at www.noamalgam.com/buythebooks.html.

Mail this form to:
Andrew Cutler
3006 230th lane SE #X103
Sammamish, WA 98075

Or fax it to (425) 557-2104
Or phone it to (425) 557-8299
Or order online
www.noamalgam.com/buythebooks.html

Circle the books you want

	Price	Tax if sent to WA state
Hair Test Interpretation: Finding Hidden Toxicities	$35.00	$3.08
Amalgam Illness: Diagnosis and Treatment	$35.00	$3.08
Biological Treatments for Autism and PDD	$25.00	$2.20
Natural Healing for Schizophrenia and other common mental disorders	$26.95	$2.37
What your Doctor might NOT Tell You about Children's Vaccinations	$5.99	53¢
What your Doctor might NOT Tell You about MENOPAUSE	$6.99	62¢
What your Doctor might NOT Tell You about PREMENOPAUSE	$5.99	53¢
Dr. John Lee's Hormone Balance Made Simple	$14.99	$1.32

Shipping and handling charges of $5 for US orders and $10 for foreign orders must be added. For free (glacially slow, media mail) shipping on US orders ONLY mail in a check for the price of the books only and allow one month for delivery.

Amount $_____ Credit card number _____ Exp date _____

Signature _____ date _____
I agree to pay the amount authorized above

Address I want the books shipped to _____

._____.

._____.

My phone number or e-mail in case there are questions _____

Hair Test Interpretation: Finding Hidden Toxicities

By Andrew Hall Cutler, PhD, PE

A surprising number of people diagnosed with incurable health conditions turn out to have a heavy metal problem. Heavy metal problems are easy to correct. Hair testing allows the underlying problem to be identified and treated,

Hair Test Interpretation: Finding Hidden Toxicities is a practical book. It provides a step by step discussion of this with figures and examples using actual hair tests.

Mercury interferes with how the hair element results come out – mercury is often low and other minerals take unusual values. It is crucial for proper hair test interpretation to know how to recognize mercury's characteristic signature.

Mercury often causes retention of arsenic, antimony, tin, titanium, zirconium and aluminum which may show up in the hair test even when mercury does not.

There are 79 example hair tests with background information, interpretation, and how they responded to different treatments. The example hair tests are from people with a wide variety of conditions, ranging from childhood developmental disorders, chronic fatigue and chemical sensitivity to those with schizophrenia, cancer and Lou Gherig's disease. Several families are presented with hair tests and health histories for all members, one including identical twins. Several of the cases have before and after hair tests showing the effects of different treatment regimens on test results.

A detailed discussion is included of the effects of toxicity (and deficiency for nutritional elements) of all the different elements determined on a hair test

Hair Test Interpretation: Finding Hidden Toxicities also explains what to do based on the test results, e. g. how to chelate heavy metalsThis book explains how to identify the derangement of mineral transport that mercury often causes so as to know when someone with low mercury in their hair (and urine, and blood) has toxic levels of it stored in their body. It also explains how to tell what other toxic metals may be present, how to identify the signs of adrenal and thyroid problems as well as signs suggesting osteoporosis.

The book does not stop at interpretation, detailed protocols are presented for chelating or clearing all of the toxic metals that might show up on a hair test.

Biological Treatments for Autism and PDD

By William Shaw, PhD

This book is a uniquely valuable tool for any parent or health care practitioner who wants to help developmentally impaired children improve. Dr. Shaw does not accept the "mainstream" view that autism is incurable and there is no need for medical treatment. How could he? He has seen too many children improve dramatically when their doctor or parent finally provided the proper treatment for their individual biochemistry.

This book provides a detailed discussion of the various biochemical defects that may be present in autism, covers how to identify which ones a given child has, and provides clinically validated information on how to treat those problems.

Natural Healing for Schizophrenia and other common mental disorders

By Eva Edelman

This book is relevant to a wide variety of disorders such as childhood developmental disorders, depression, chronic fatigue, etc. as well as schizophrenia. It covers the role of histamine, copper/zinc balance, allergies, physical illness, mercury and pyrroles in these disorders. It explains what the people with these different problems are like and what to do to help. It updates and extends much of the information in Carl Pfeiffer's work on nutrition and mental illness, as well as incorporating other views and approaches in orthomolecular psychiatry. There is a forward by Abram Hoffer, and Bill Walsh of the Pfeiffer Treatment Center is quoted extensively.

Dr. John Lee's Hormone Balance Made Simple

By John R. Lee, MD and Virginia Hopkins

This book tells you how to use natural hormones to control the symptoms of menopause and premenopause, and to figure out how much of each you need on your own. Most women will find they do not need the help of a doctor to arrive at a program that leaves them feeling better, happier, being healthier and looking younger. Women using this book will usually get better results than simply relying on their doctor's advice since the doctor doesn't live inside their body, feel what they feel, and know what they know. It clearly identifies how to use your symptoms to decide on dosage, timing and selection of hormones, when you DO need to talk to a doctor, and how to tell if you are having some OTHER kind of medical problem that is affecting your hormones. This book is the ideal companion to *What your Doctor might NOT Tell You about MENOPAUSE* and *What your Doctor might NOT Tell You about PREMENOPAUSE*.

What your Doctor might NOT Tell You about Children's Vaccinations

By Stephanie Cave, MD

This book is a uniquely valuable source of information for any parent or health care practitioner who wants to make an informed decision about how to best protect a child from both infectious diseases AND the risks of adverse vaccine reactions. Dr. Cave has gone through the medical literature thoroughly to identify the actual risks associated with specific vaccinations. She has also explained what the risks of the diseases are that we are vaccinating against, and how people are exposed to them. This critical information, never before available in one place, allows parents to make rational decisions about which vaccinations their children need, when they should be administered, and when to say "no, thanks!"

What your Doctor might NOT Tell You about MENOPAUSE

By John R. Lee, MD and Virginia Hopkins

The revolutionary book about bioidentical hormone replacement therapy now fully revised and updated.

Over a decade ago, Dr. John Lee published his controversial conclusions about hormone replacement therapy (HRT): synthetic hormones don't work and they may pose a health threat to women. Years later, research has proven him right. Hundreds of thousands of women have followed Dr. Lee's natural hormone program – experiencing amazing results. Newly revised and updated, this revolutionary book features Dr. Lee's effective plan for restoring balance using bioidentical hormones, including natural progesterone.

Discover the benefits of his breakthrough program:

- Reduce or eliminate premenopausal and menopausal symptoms
- Help eliminate hormone–related problems such as osteoporosis, hot flashes, night sweats,   and vaginal dryness
- Reduce "middle age" weight gain
- Help stop and reverse osteoporosis
- Protect against breast cancer
- Help restore sex drive and energy... slow the signs of aging

What your Doctor might NOT Tell You about PREMENOPAUSE

By John R. Lee, MD, Jesse Hanley, MD and Virginia Hopkins

Do you think you are too young for menopause, but wonder why you feel so bad?

You could be experiencing unexplained weight gain... fatigue... mood swings... loss of libido... fibroids... tender or lumpy breasts.... endometriosis... PMS... infertility... memory loss... migraines... very heavy or light periods... cold hands and feet... or a combination of these symptoms. You may have been told they're "nothing," or stress, or even menopause – and offered surgery, antidepressants or prescription hormones.

But the startling truth is that you may be suffering from premenopause syndrome – and there are simple, safe solutions. When John Lee wrote the groundbreaking What Your Doctor May NOT Tell You About MENOPAUSE, younger women started asking if natural progesterone could help them, too. In this book, Dr. Lee, with women's health expert Jesse Hanley, MD, brings you a revolutionary nonprescription "Balance Program" to restore your gynecological health, energy, and sex drive – and even slow the aging process before menopause, and beyond.